LONGITUDINAL RESEARCH ON DRUG USE

LONGITUDINAL RESEARCH ON DRUG USE

Empirical Findings and Methodological Issues

EDITED BY

Denise B. Kandel
NEW YORK STATE PSYCHIATRIC INSTITUTE
AND
COLUMBIA UNIVERSITY

HEMISPHERE PUBLISHING CORPORATION
Washington   London

A HALSTED PRESS BOOK
JOHN WILEY & SONS
New York   London   Sydney   Toronto

This work was published under grant 5-PO1-DA-01097 to the
Center for Socio-Cultural Research on Drug Use of Columbia University.
The United States Government has a royalty-free, nonexclusive, and
irrevocable license to reproduce, translate, publish, use, and dispose
of, and to authorize others to do so, all or any portion of this work.

Hemisphere Publishing Corporation
1025 Vermont Ave., N.W., Washington, D.C. 20005

Distributed solely by Halsted Press, a Division of John Wiley & Sons, Inc.,
New York.

1 2 3 4 5 6 7 8 9 0   D O D O   7 8 3 2 1 0 9 8

Library of Congress Cataloging in Publication Data

Main entry under title:

Longitudinal research on drug use.

  Includes indexes.
  1. Drug abuse—Longitudinal studies. I. Kandel,
Denise Bystryn.
RC566.L58   362.2'92   78-6093
ISBN 0-470-26287-7

Printed in the United States of America

Contents

v

Preface

Longitudinal studies are among the most powerful available to social scientists because they provide an optimal set of data for the testing of causal assumptions. Analyses of longitudinal data are complex, however, and the methods available for dealing with such data obtained from large-scale surveys are in their infancy. Recently, as social science has moved in the direction of complex mathematical techniques, such as path and regression analyses or the analysis of mean and covariance structure, interest has developed in the application of these techniques to panel data and the study of change. A variety of techniques has been proposed, but few have been applied empirically because longitudinal data are not readily available.

In the last several years, different groups in the United States have initiated longitudinal investigations of drug behavior. These are prospective studies in which respondents are followed over time. The substantive focus has been on the antecedents and consequences of the use of a variety of drugs, including legal and illegal ones. These studies are based on general populations, sampled at approximately the same historical period, with similarly structured instruments. Such convergence in the social sciences is unusual.

To take advantage of this parallelism of research, the Conference on Strategies of Longitudinal Research on Drug Use was organized and held April 7 through 9, 1976 in San Juan, Puerto Rico, under the sponsorship of the Center for Socio-Cultural Research on Drug Use of Columbia University and under support of the National Institute on Drug Abuse. The conference had two interrelated objectives. One was to bring together the drug researchers involved in major longitudinal studies to integrate substantive findings on antecedents and consequences of drug use in various populations and to move toward a theoretical synthesis of these findings. A second objective was to provide an opportunity for detailed methodological critiques of these longitudinal drug studies, in the hope of contributing to the development and codification of methods in longitudinal research, using drug research as a test case.

The chapters in this volume, with the exception of the introductory chapter by Kandel and the concluding chapter by Bentler, are revisions of specially commissioned papers presented at the conference. The studies selected for inclusion in this volume represent, in my opinion, the most significant of their period. The judgment was made on the basis of sample size, the richness of the information

collected, the nature of the theoretical scheme underpinning a study, the sophistication of an analysis, and the strength of the results. Eight empirical studies are
represented, covering populations at various points in the life cycle, from junior
high school to adulthood.

The book is divided into four parts. In a general introductory chapter, Kandel
emphasizes the commonalities among the studies and derives a series of substantive
propositions based on convergent research findings. The empirical papers are
grouped into two major sections covering the high school years in Part II and the
subsequent years in Part III. In a last section devoted to commentaries, the chapters
by Clausen and by Riley and Waring discuss theoretical issues raised by these
studies. The last two chapters focus on methodological issues. Lazarsfeld provides
an historical overview of the various approaches to the study of change. This is the
last manuscript that Lazarsfeld completed before his death in August 1976, and he
did not have a chance to revise it himself. In a summary chapter, Bentler distills,
from the detailed methodological critiques and the discussions that took place at
the conference, the most important methodological points and indicates their
relevance for longitudinal research in general.

In juxtaposition, the eight different studies illuminate and complement each
other. They illustrate the role of social context in the initiation of a particular
behavior (Robins); they document the fact that many of the factors that have been
found to be related to drug use at one point in time, such as low academic performance, crime, depression, or rebelliousness, precede the use of drugs (Johnston;
Jessor; Mellinger; Smith; Kandel); they deal with cohort, maturational, and historical effects on drug behavior (Jessor); they develop the usefulness of the notion
of stages as a strategy to pinpoint the role of specific factors in developmental
transitions (Kandel).

This undertaking would not have been possible without the help of many individuals. Eric Josephson, Director of the Center for Socio-Cultural Research on
Drug Use, provided support for this project from its inception. Seymour Spilerman
was generous with his time and advice. Neil Henry agreed to the delicate task of
reviewing and editing the late Professor Lazarsfeld's unfinished manuscript, and
Donald Pelz reviewed the reference to his own work. Mildred Katz contributed her
unmatched administrative skills and good humor. I am also indebted to Mark
Davies, Theresa Hawthorne, Natalie Gross, and Marta Burns for their help. The
volume greatly benefited from the skillful editorial contributions of Oscar Ochs. I
want to thank especially Dorothy Jessop, who assisted me throughout with utmost
dedication, care, and imagination. The National Institute on Drug Abuse financed
the conference, under grant 5-PO1-DA-01097, to the Center for Socio-Cultural
Research on Drug Use of Columbia University.

My husband, Eric R. Kandel, provided emotional and intellectual support and
was unswerving in his enthusiasm even when my commitments threatened to
interfere with his own scientific activities. To him, as always, I am most grateful.

Special thanks also are due to the many conference discussants and participants.
Unfortunately, it was not possible to include in this volume all their statements and
contributions. Several of the papers were revised to take into account suggestions
that were made during the meetings.

It is my hope that, while the studies included in this volume deal with drug
behavior, they also contribute more generally to our understanding of development
in adolescence and in adulthood.

Denise B. Kandel

I

AN OVERVIEW

Convergences in Prospective Longitudinal Surveys of Drug Use in Normal Populations

Denise B. Kandel
New York State Psychiatric Institute,
and School of Public Health
and Department of Psychiatry, Columbia University

Until recently, most longitudinal data relevant to drug use were obtained in follow-ups of clinical populations of heroin addicts. Subjects were drawn from facilities specifically designed for addicts, or from institutions such as courts or social service agencies set up to deal with deviant or maladjusted individuals. These subjects represented the most extreme segment of the drug-using population (see Ball & Chambers, 1970; McGlothlin, Anglin & Wilson, 1976; O'Donnell, 1972; Stephens & Cottrell, 1972; Vaillant, 1966; Weppner & Agar, 1971). Research based on already addicted individuals precludes the investigation of many issues relevant to our understanding of drug behavior, which takes many forms other than addiction. Furthermore, although longitudinal in character, studies of this nature do not permit a clear assessment of the precursors and the consequences of drug use. Such an assessment requires contact with a population at risk for drug use and follow-up over time in order to identify and to compare the characteristics of individuals who initiate the use of drugs and of individuals who do not. Continued follow-up of such populations also makes it possible to identify both consequences of use and further changes over time of the variables related to use.

Several prospective longitudinal investigations of drug behavior based on general populations were initiated in the United States in the late 1960s and early 1970s. These are epidemiological studies of adolescents or young adults, sampled at approximately the same historical period, and studied with similarly structured instruments. Such convergence is unusual in the behavioral sciences. These investigations collected information on future drug users in their natural settings, before

This chapter is a revised version of a paper presented at the meetings of the Society for Life History Research in Psychopathology, in Fort Worth, Texas, October 1976. Work on this review was partially supported by research grant DA-00064 from the National Institute on Drug Abuse and by the Center for Socio-Cultural Research on Drug Use, Columbia University. The assistance of Dorothy Jessop and Stephanie Paton is gratefully acknowledged.

they had ever used drugs, and therefore included built-in comparison groups of nonusers through which to evaluate and to contrast the users. In juxtaposition, these studies provide data for the development of a comprehensive, although still tentative, understanding of drug behavior. This volume includes reports from the most important of these studies.

Drug behavior, in the context of this volume, refers to the use of illicit drugs. Indeed, the studies were initiated with a specific focus on illegal substances, especially marihuana. The distinction between legal and illegal drugs, however, is arbitrary. To emphasize the point, this review includes a longitudinal study of problem drinking carried out in the same period. In fact, several investigators have felt it imperative to examine involvement in legal drugs in order to better understand involvement in illegal drugs.

My aim in this opening chapter is to synthesize the results of this research so that the reader can place the studies included in this volume within the wider context of existing longitudinal drug studies. The chapter is an overview divided into three major parts. The first is a brief description of the eight studies represented in the volume and specifies their location in time, samples, and methodology. The second includes a series of propositions, derived from summarizing and integrating the research, that pertain to patterns of involvement in illicit drugs, antecedents, and consequences of drug use. The third, a discussion of the implications of the studies for our understanding of drug behavior, points to lacunae and further work needed.

CHARACTERISTICS OF PROSPECTIVE LONGITUDINAL STUDIES OF DRUG USE IN NORMAL POPULATIONS

A total of 21 longitudinal studies have been identified. Of these, 16 had already been completed or were in the last stages of completion as of this writing. There were 5 ongoing or recently initiated projects on which no findings were available, data collection not having yet started in some. One of the studies, that by Cahalan, is exclusively concerned with alcohol and was selected because of its implications for illicit drugs. I have attempted to be as comprehensive as possible, but I may inadvertently have omitted some relevant work.

Selected characteristics of the studies are summarized in Table 1-1, part 1 listing the 16 studies with published data, part 2 listing those for which no results are yet available. Included are the year of the first wave of data collection; the nature of the sample; the number and intervals of the over-time contacts; and the kinds of drugs inquired about. Almost two-thirds of these studies were carried out on samples of college students or young adults; the others on high school students.

This chapter is restricted to the 16 studies that have already published results. Not all these 16 studies are of equal scientific importance. Several are based on very few cases and contain methodological weaknesses that raise serious doubts about the meaning of the results. In the extreme, some of these longitudinal projects only report results based on cross-sectional analyses (Brill & Christie, 1974; Garfield & Garfield, 1973; Goldstein, Gleason, & Korn, 1975). The 8 studies I consider to be the most significant are included in this volume. This is a judgment I have made on the basis of the sample size, the richness of the information collected, the nature of the theoretical scheme underpinning the study, the sophistication of the analyses, and the strength of the results.

The Eight Studies Represented in This Volume

The most important longitudinal high school studies, all represented in this volume, include: Jessor and Jessor's yearly follow-ups over a 4-year period of junior and senior high school students in a small western city (chap. 2); Elinson and Josephson's 2-year follow-up of students from 23 junior and senior high schools representing different kinds of schools throughout the United States (chap. 5); Smith's 5-year follow-up of cohorts of 4th through 12th graders in six schools in the greater Boston area, with an assessment of the youths' personalities as rated by their classmates (chap. 4); and Kandel's follow-up of a representative sample of students from 18 public secondary schools in New York State, with a subsample of graduated seniors contacted a third time after graduation from high school (chap. 3). A distinctive feature of the Kandel study is the collection of data from adolescents' parents and peers so as to assess the impact of a youth's social context on his or her behavior and attitudes. Johnston's (chap. 6) study, which bridges the high school and post-high school years, is a follow-up through 5 years after high school graduation of the Youth in Transition cohort, a representative sample of 10th-grade boys initially selected for a study of school dropouts (Bachman, Kahn, Mednick, Davidson, & Johnston, 1967).

The most important studies of college students and young adults include Jessor and Jessor's 4-year follow-up of selected freshmen in a western university (chap. 2), Mellinger and Manheimer's 2-year follow-up of one freshman and one senior class at the University of California at Berkeley (chap. 7), and Robins's study of Vietnam veterans followed over a 3-year period with a control group of nonveterans interviewed in the last wave (chap. 8). Cahalan and Roizen's work on alcohol use is in this group (chap. 9).

Location in Time

The concentration of the longitudinal studies listed in Table 1-1 within the same historical period is striking, most having been initiated in the 3-year period between 1969 and 1971, but the concentration is even greater than is revealed by the table. In 1970, both Johnston and Smith added a drug component to existing studies that had no earlier concern with illegal drug use. The initiation of these longitudinal studies coincided with a period of spectacular increases in the use of illegal drugs by young people. After a hiatus of several years, a new group of studies was started. Whereas the first group included mainly white respondents or minority individuals in proportion to their representation in the general population, several of the new studies focused specifically on black ghetto youths (Brunswick, 1976; Kellam, Ensminger, & Turner, 1977) or adults (Brook, Lukoff, & Whiteman, 1977).

Samples

Although the samples included in the various studies listed in part 1 of Table 1-1 represent normal noninstitutionalized populations, they are not without bias. Indeed, with the exceptions of Robins's study of Vietnam veterans and Roizen and Cahalan's studies of adult males, the subjects were all sampled from schools. Thus, whereas clinical follow-up studies sample from institutions comprising the most extremely involved segment of the drug-abusing population, the longitudinal

TABLE 1-1 Characteristics of Longitudinal Studies of Drug Use in Normal Populations (Listed by Completion Status and Age of Respondents)

Principal investigators	Population characteristics	Grade or age at Time 1 of sample eligible for panel	Year of first contact	Year of last contact	Total number of contacts	Interval between contacts	Size of sample at Time 1 eligible for panel	Size of matched panel	Methods of data collection[a]	Drugs inquired about
					Part 1. Completed or nearly completed studies					
Smith	Students from grades 4-12 in 6 school systems in greater Boston area, predominantly white and middle-class	Grades 4-11	1969	1973	2-5	1 year	12,000 (approx.)	Variable	Self-administered questionnaires in classrooms; school records; peers' ratings of student's personality	Cigarettes, liquor, marihuana, ups, downs, psychedelics, opiates, inhalants, nonprescription drug store products
Kaplan	Seventh grade students from 18 of 36 junior high schools of the Houston Independent School District	Grade 7	1971	1973	3	1 year	7,620	3,148	Self-administered questionnaires in classrooms	Beer or wine, liquor, marihuana, narcotics
Jessor and Jessor	High school study: random sample of students from grades 7-12 of 3 junior and 3 senior high schools in a small city in the Rocky Mountains, almost all of Anglo-American, middle-class background	Grades 7-9	1969	1972	4	1 year	589	483	Self-administered questionnaires outside of class; school records	Beer or wine, hard liquor, marihuana, amphetamines, LSD, other psychedelics, cocaine, heroin
		Grades 10-11	1969	1972	2-3	1 year	262	Variable		
Elinson and Josephson	Students from 5 junior and 18 senior high schools purposively selected to represent varied regions, community sizes, socioeconomic levels, and racial compositions but not to represent the United States	Grades 7-10	1971	1973	2	2 years	18,363	8,136	Self-administered questionnaires in classrooms	Cigarettes, beer or wine, hard liquor, marihuana or hashish, amphetamines, methedrine, barbiturates, LSD, other psychedelics, cocaine, heroin, inhalants

(See footnote on p. 11)

Author	Sample	Level	Year	Year	N	Interval	N	N	Method	Drugs
Kandel	(1) Multiphasic random sample of New York State public secondary school students from 18 schools and data from mothers or fathers; best schoolfriend in subsample of 5 schools	Grades 9–12	1971	1972	2	6 months	8,206	5,423	Self-administered questionnaires in classrooms (adolescents) mailed questionnaires (parents)	Cigarettes, beer or wine, hard liquor, marihuana, hashish, amphetamines; methedrine, barbiturates, tranquilizers, LSD, other psychedelics, cocaine, heroin, other narcotics, inhalants, cough syrup
	(2) Subsample of 1972 senior class	Grade 12	1971	1973	3	7–12 months	2,386	1,635	Self-administered questionnaires (T1, T2); mailed questionnaires (T3)	Same
Johnston	Youth in Transition cohort—A national random sample of boys in 87 public high schools in continental United States in 1966; drug components added in 1970 and 1974	Grade 10	1966	1974	5	2 years 1 year 1 year 4 years	2,213	1,608	Interviews (T1, T2, T4); self-administered questionnaires (T1–T4); mailed questionnaires (T5); ability tests (T1)	Cigarettes, beer, wine, hard liquor, marihuana, amphetamines, barbiturates, hallucinogens, methaqualone, cocaine, heroin
Jessor and Jessor	College study—random sample of arts and science university students in a small Rocky Mountain city	College freshmen	1970	1973	4	1 year	276	226	Self-administered questionnaires; school records	Beer or wine, hard liquor, marihuana, amphetamines, LSD, other psychedelics, cocaine, heroin
Gulas and King	Seniors at Dartmouth College matched retrospectively to their freshmen-year records	College freshmen	Not given	Not given	2	4 years	90	90	Mailed questionnaires	Marihuana, amphetamines, barbiturates, hallucinogens
Haagen	College juniors at Wesleyan University matched retrospectively to their freshmen- and sophomore-year records	College freshmen	1965	1968	2	3 years	70	70	Self-administered questionnaires; test data on file at Office of Psychological Services	Tobacco, alcohol, marihuana, hallucinogens
Sadava	College freshmen in an English-language Roman Catholic college in province of Quebec	College freshmen	Not given	Not given	2	6 months	358	319	Self-administered questionnaires in classrooms	Cannabis, psychedelics, amphetamines, alcohol

TABLE 1-1 Characteristics of Longitudinal Studies of Drug Use in Normal Populations (Listed by Completion Status and Age of Respondents) (*Continued*)

Principal investigators	Population characteristics	Grade or age at Time 1 of sample eligible for panel	Year of first contact	Year of last contact	Total number of contacts	Interval between contacts	Size of sample at Time 1 eligible for panel	Size of matched panel	Methods of data collection[a]	Drugs inquired about
					Part 1. Completed or nearly completed studies (*Continued*)					
Groves	Full-time students at predominantly white nonspecialized colleges with projected enrollment of over 1,000 in 1970	College freshmen and juniors	1970	1971	2	1 year	7,948	3,961	Mailed questionnaires	Caffeine, alcohol, marihuana, hashish, methedrine, other amphetamines, barbiturates, sedatives, tranquilizers, LSD, other psycedelics, cocaine, opium, heroin, other narcotics, cough syrups
Mellinger	(1) Probability sample of male freshmen of University of California at Berkeley in Fall 1970	College freshmen	1970	1973	2	$2\frac{1}{2}$ years	960	834	Personal interviews and self-administered forms; school records; mailed questionnaires	Tobacco, alcohol, marihuana or hashish, amphetamines, barbiturates, sedatives, psychedelics, cocaine, heroin, opium, other opiates, inhalants
	(2) Probability sample of senior men in class of 1971	College seniors	1971	1973	2	$2\frac{1}{2}$ years	986	821	Same	Same
Garfield and Garfield	Random sample at large private suburban residential western university	College students	1966–1967	1970–1971	4	1 year	300	T2–100 T3–201 T4–100	Personally administered questionnaires	Alcohol, marihuana, hashish, LSD, mescaline
Grupp	Random sample of 1% of students at Illinois State University not reporting marihuana use	College undergraduates and graduate students	1969	1973	3	2 years	127	T2–120 T3–103	Personal interviews at T1, T2; mailed questionnaires for those out of area at T2, and for everyone at T3	Marihuana

Author	Sample	Age	Year	Year	No.	Interval	N	N	Method	Variables
Robins	(1) Vietnam veterans—random sample of army enlisted males who returned from Vietnam to the United States in September 1971, and a supplementary random sample from all men returning that month whose urine had been detected as positive for morphine prior to leaving Vietnam. T2 sampled from reduced T1 target population restricted to men inducted since 1969 and from the 25 more populous states	20 years (mean)	1972	1974–1975	2	2 years	605	571	Interviews; urine samples; military and Veterans' Administration records	Cigarettes, alcohol, marijuana, amphetamines, barbiturates, tranquilizers, hallucinogens, cocaine, narcotics
	(2) Control group at T2—sample of nonveterans matched on Selective Service Board, draft eligibility, age, and education	Matched to veterans	1974–1975	—	1	—	302	284	Interviews; urine samples; Selective Service records	Same
Cahalan et al.	(1) National probability sample of United States adult population; T2 sampled from reduced T1 target population N = 1,810, with abstainers and very infrequent drinkers subsampled at a lesser rate	21 and over	1964–1965	1957	2	2 years	1,810	1,359	Household interviews (T1); mail questionnaires (T2)	Drinking patterns, practices, and problems
	(2) National probability sample of white males aged 21–59, with over-sampling of urban areas	21–59 years old	1969	1973	2	4 years	978	725	Same	Same
	(3) Probability sample of white males, aged 21–59, in San Francisco	21–59 years old	1967–1968	1972	2	4 years	786	615	Same	Same

TABLE 1-1 Characteristics of Longitudinal Studies of Drug Use in Normal Populations (Listed by Completion Status and Age of Respondents) *(Continued)*

Principal investigators	Population characteristics	Grade or age at Time 1 of sample eligible for panel	Year of first contact	Year of last contact	Total number of contacts	Interval between contacts	Size of sample at Time 1 eligible for panel	Size of matched panel	Methods of data collection[a]	Drugs inquired about
					Part 2. Ongoing studies; no findings yet reported					
Kellam	All entering public and parochial school first-grade children in a black community in Chicago with low income and high unemployment	Grade 1	1966	1974–1975	5	3 times during first grade; 2 years; 6 years;	2,000	Grade 3–50% Grade 9–85% (estimated)	Home interviews; school tests (IQ, achievement) and grades; ratings by teacher, clinician, mother (T1–T5); police records, questionnaires (T5)	Marihuana
Bentler	Students in the greater Los Angeles area with oversampling of lower socioeconomic schools	Grades 7–9	1976	Ongoing	5	1 year	1,300 (approx.)	Not yet completed	Self-administered questionnaires from the students, their parents, and peers	Cigarettes, beer, wine, liquor, marihuana, hashish, ups, downs, tripping stuff, cocaine, heroin, drug store medicine, sniffing stuff
Dunnette	All students in selected grades in Minneapolis, Minnesota, and Portland, Oregon, public schools	Grades 7–12	1976–1977	Ongoing	To be determined	Variable	20,000 (10,000 in each city)	Variable	Questionnaires (T1); follow-up strategies to be determined	Alcohol, cigarettes, marihuana, amphetamines, barbiturates, LSD, other psychedelics, inhalants, heroin, tranquilizers, cocaine
Johnston and Bachman	Monitoring the Future—five successive nationally representative cohorts of high school seniors from 115 public and 15 private high schools; repeated annually; entire senior classes in schools with <300 seniors, and subsamples (N = 300) in larger schools	Grade 12	1975–ongoing	Ongoing	6 for each cohort	1 year	17,000 (approx. for each cohort)	7,000 (target for each cohort)	Questionnaires (T1); mailed questionnaires at follow-ups	Alcohol, cigarettes, marihuana, amphetamines, barbiturates, LSD, other psychedelics, heroin, other narcotics, tranquilizers, quaaludes, cocaine, inhalants

Investigator	Sample	Age			Waves	Duration	N		Method	Drugs studied
Brunswick	Representative community sample of Harlem youth	16–17 years old	1969–1970	1975–1976	2	6 years	664	500+ (estimated)	Household interviews	Alcohol, marihuana, amphetamines, barbiturates, acid, cocaine, heroin, glue
Schuckit	Random samples of incoming freshmen at:								Semistructured interviews; mailed questionnaires to non-residents	Tobacco, alcohol, marihuana, hashish, amphetamines, speed, LSD, mescaline, psilocybin, STP, MDA, opiates, medicinal drugs
	(1) Washington University in St. Louis	College freshmen	1970	1974	4	1 year	158	Not given		
	(2) University of California at San Diego	College freshmen	1971	1975	4	1 year	222	188		
Lukoff	Samples of ghetto community stratified for ethnicity, social class, and contiguity with deviance:								Household interviews	Marihuana, ups, downs, psychedelics, heroin
	(1) Children	13–17 yrs	1973	1975–1976	2	$2\frac{1}{2}$–3 yrs	404	Not yet completed		
	(2) Mothers	30–45 yrs					284			

[a]The same methods were used in all waves of data collection of a study, unless specific times are indicated per abbreviations T1–T5.

epidemiological surveys sample from institutions in which membership generally represents fairly good social adjustment. Yet, by restricting themselves to school populations, especially during the high school years, these studies exclude those youths most likely to be involved in drugs. The high school studies do not include absentees or school dropouts, except on those multiwave longitudinal studies in which students missed on one wave might have been included in subsequent testings (see Johnston, 1973, or Smith, 1973). Furthermore, self-reported rates of use vary directly with school absences (Haberman, Josephson, Zanes, & Elinson, 1972; Josephson, 1974; Kandel, 1975c; Kandel, Treiman, Faust, & Single, 1976; Smith & Fogg, 1976) and dropping out of school (Johnston, 1973, 1974). Subsequent interviews with students absent from school on the days the surveys were conducted indicate that chronic absentees are much heavier drug users than regular school students (Kandel, 1975b; Smith & Fogg, 1976).

Ideally, prospective longitudinal studies ought to start with a representative sample of the total population at risk. Adolescents not in school and young adults who have already entered the labor force, as well as those neither in school nor in the labor force, ought to be included. It is to be hoped that several of the recently initiated studies will start filling in these lacunae, for they are studying community samples of youth including those most vulnerable—minority youths in urban ghettos. It must be emphasized that the data available to date and discussed in this chapter do not include the total population at risk for involvement in drugs.

The studies cover the period in the life cycle that is of greatest risk for initiation into drug use, the years between 14 and 22. Although one researcher started with 9-year-old children (Smith), most investigators started with adolescents in junior and senior high school, or in college. The oldest cohort at initial interview consisted of adults 21–59 years old in studies of drinking problems (Cahalan).

The very large samples in the studies provide many methodological advantages. Samples can be partitioned according to different criteria, and sophisticated multivariate analytical techniques can be applied to the data. As a result, findings can be stated and elaborated with an increased degree of precision.

Contacts with Respondents

The modal number of contacts with respondents is two. Several studies made three contacts (Cahalan, Kandel, Kaplan, Robins) but rarely more, although Jessor conducted four waves of data collection, and Smith and Johnston five waves each. The most frequent time interval between waves of data collection is 1 year, but it can be as short as 5–6 months (Kandel, Sadava) or as long as $2\frac{1}{2}$ years (Mellinger, Robins), 3 years (Haagen), or 4 years (Cahalan, Johnston). Respondents are generally followed over a relatively short span of time, ranging from 6 months to a maximum of 8 years (Johnston, Cahalan). The period over which these subjects were monitored is much shorter than the mainly retrospective life histories covered in follow-ups of clinical populations. For example, Vaillant (1966) obtained data over a 12-year period, and O'Donnell (1969) followed former admissions to the Lexington Hospital for approximately 23 years after the onset of addiction. As compared to follow-up studies of clinical populations, prospective longitudinal studies of normal populations start with a younger population and cover a much shorter span of time.

Instruments and Data Collection

In all cases, the data are collected through structured instruments, either personal interviews or questionnaires administered in classroom situations or by mail. In addition to patterns of drug use, information is generally obtained about the respondents' social and psychological characteristics, most often their psychological and personal functioning, and more rarely, the characteristics of their interpersonal and social context. Several studies obtained supplementary information from school records (Brill, Jessor & Jessor, Mellinger, Smith), or school personnel (Johnston, 1973). Rarely were respondents other than the potential drug user contacted. In a most innovative design, Smith obtained classmates' assessments of a young person's psychological functioning. Kandel obtained data from one parent, alternately the mother or the father, of each student in the study as well as the best schoolfriend of each in a subsample of five schools. The group of 16 completed studies made no assessments of respondents' medical histories or physical symptomatology, precluding any investigation of physiological determinants or consequences of drug use. A most important component of Brunswick's (1976) ongoing study is that comprehensive medical examinations of her cohort of Harlem youths are available as of the initial interview at ages 12–17.

SELECTED FINDINGS

The findings from these various studies follow in the form of 19 propositions organized around three aspects of drug use: (1) patterns of involvement in drug use, (2) antecedents of drug use, and (3) consequences of drug use.

Patterns of Involvement in Illicit Drugs

1. *The period for risk of initiation into illicit drug use is over by the mid-20s.*

Cross-sectional studies of representative national samples or of more restricted populations have found that the use of illicit drugs begins in the early teens, peaks in the 18–22 age group, and declines to very low levels by the late twenties (National Commission on Marihuana and Drug Abuse, 1972, 1973). Because these data have been collected at one time point, the findings are confounded by cohort and historical effects. The cohorts, 20 years old in 1972, have not had the same histories or the same opportunities for drug use as more recent cohorts. What will be the patterns of use of later cohorts as they enter their mid and late twenties? Will they experience much higher rates of use than the cross-sectional cohorts studied to date, or will they decrease their use relative to their own level of use at an earlier age? Robins's data on Vietnam veterans and their matched controls suggest that both use among users and the rates of initiation into drugs among nonusers peak at ages 22–23 and decline sharply thereafter (see chap. 8).

2. *A high proportion of youths who have tried marihuana will eventually go on to experiment with other illicit drugs.*

The National Commission on Marihuana and Drug Abuse concluded that most American youth would restrict themselves to the use of marihuana. This may not be the case, however, inasmuch as many young people who have experimented with marihuana appear to go on to try other illicit drugs. Among adolescents in New

York State, 25% of those who were using marihuana exclusively at the beginning of a school year had started to experiment with one of the harder illicit drugs 6 months later (Kandel, 1975d; Kandel & Faust, 1975). Similarly, Mellinger and his collaborators (Davidson, Mellinger, & Manheimer, 1977) reported that 28% of freshmen at Berkeley had used other illicit drugs at time of entry; within $2\frac{1}{2}$ years after entering, an additional 15% had initiated use of these drugs. The probability of becoming a multiple user increases in direct proportion to the recency and extent of initial marihuana use (Davidson et al., 1977; Kandel & Faust, 1975). It is important to stress that these findings do not establish that youths who experiment with these drugs will necessarily become habitual users.

3. *Later age of onset is associated with lesser involvement and greater probability of stopping.*

Brill and Christie (1974) found that those college students who stopped using marihuana within a 2-year period tended to have started using marihuana later (at 21.4 years of age on the average) than those who continued or only reduced their use (18.6 years). Similarly, Davidson, Mellinger, and Manheimer (1977) found that the proportion of college men who began using drugs more than 1 year prior to entering college was highest (61%) among those who were continuous users of multiple illicit drugs over the first $2\frac{1}{2}$ years of college, and lowest (8%) among those who used marihuana exclusively and intermittently between the freshman and junior years.

4. *There are clear-cut developmental steps and sequences in drug behavior, so that use of one of the legal drugs almost always precedes use of illegal drugs.*

A follow-up of two cohorts of random samples of adolescents in New York State, a high school sample and a sample of graduated seniors, indicates four stages in the sequence of involvement with drugs: beer or wine; cigarettes or hard liquor; marihuana; and other illicit drugs (Kandel, 1975d; Kandel & Faust, 1975). The legal drugs are necessary intermediates between complete nonuse and marihuana. Whereas 27% of high school students who smoked and drank progressed to marihuana within a 5-6 month follow-up period, only 2% of those who had not used any legal substance did so. Marihuana, in turn, was a crucial step on the way to other illicit drugs. Whereas 25% of marihuana users progressed to LSD, amphetamines, or heroin, only 1% of nondrug users and 4% of legal drug users did so. This sequence was found in each of the 4 years in high school and in the year after graduation. The reverse sequence held for regression in drug use.

The specific order in which the various illicit drugs other than marihuana are tried is more difficult to determine. In the total New York State high school sample, this sequence followed marihuana: pills (ups, downs, tranquilizers), psychedelics (LSD, other psychedelics), cocaine, and heroin (Kandel, 1975d). Probably, these stages are culturally and historically determined. Subsequent analyses on a sample of young black ghetto adults (Lukoff & Brook, 1974) indicate that although marihuana still precedes the use of other illicit drugs, the order in this black sample is quite different: cocaine, heroin, barbiturates, amphetamines, and psychedelics (Jessop, Kandel, & Lukoff, 1976).

As stressed by Kandel, Kessler, and Margulies (see chap. 3), the identification of stages in drug behavior has important implications for studying the factors that predict, differentiate, or result from drug use. Whereas most studies compare youths within a total population on the basis of their use or nonuse of a particular substance, the results cited above suggest a different strategy, namely the decomposition of the panel sample into appropriate subsamples of individuals at a particular stage who are at risk for initiation into the next stage. Because each stage represents a cumulative pattern of use and contains fewer adolescents than the preceding stage in the sequence, comparisons of users and nonusers must be made among members of the restricted group that has already used the drugs at the preceding stage. Unless this is done, the attributes identified as apparent characteristics of a particular class of drug users may actually reflect characteristics important for involvement in drugs at the preceding level. The usefulness of decomposing samples for isolating special populations at risk has also been stressed by Robins, who identified stages pertaining to narcotic addiction among veterans: use of narcotics in Vietnam, continuation after return, and addiction if use continued (Robins, Davis, & Wish, 1977). Although these developmental stages describe increased involvement with one drug and are specific to a particular cohort of Vietnam veterans, they illustrate the basic principle involved. As Robins states (Robins et al., 1977), "There is nothing new about defining the 'population at risk' in which one is to search for predictors of an outcome. What is less common is sequentially defining successively diminishing populations at risk" (p. 380).

5. *Addiction to heroin is not necessarily a permanent state.*

Most of our knowlege about heroin addiction derives from populations of addicts in treatment or from populations who have come to the attention of the criminal justice system. This is true, not only of the earlier follow-up studies of treated addicts, but also of more recent anthropological community studies (Gould, Walker, Crane, & Lidz, 1974; Nurco, Bonito, Lerner, & Balter, 1975; Waldorf, 1973). The life histories of these individuals have suggested that the cycle of heroin addiction is very difficult to break and that most addicts tend to relapse (O'Donnell, 1972). Most of the individuals released from Fort Worth or Lexington had relapsed into addiction 1 year after discharge. Over time, however (O'Donnell, 1972), "the percentage abstinent increases at a fairly steady rate" (p. 247).

Robins's data on Vietnam veterans provide the first systematic longitudinal data on a population of addicts located within a sample representative of almost the total population of young males in the United States, namely those draft eligible at a time when conscription was universal. These data are striking in documenting that narcotics addition is not necessarily a permanent process and that heroin can be given up more easily than had previously been thought possible. Of the soldiers addicted in Vietnam, only 2% in the general sample, and 7% among those detected as drug positive before discharge, became readdicted in the 8–12 months after returning to the United States. The curves of remission rates for veterans in that period are exact mirror images of the curve for a sample of Lexington-treated addicts 6 months after release to aftercare (Robins, Davis, & Nurco, 1974). Robins (1975) observes that "remission rates of 95% for those who had been addicted in Vietnam . . . [are] unheard of among narcotic addicts treated in the U.S." (p. 6). Furthermore, only 29% of the men addicted in the first interview after discharge reported such addiction in the second interview $2\frac{1}{2}$ years later (Robins, 1974).

The findings on heroin addiction thus confirm those obtained in other areas of psychopathology, such as delinquency (Roff, 1972), character disorders (Robins, 1970b), or alcoholism (Cahalan & Roizen, 1974; Clark & Cahalan, 1976; Roizen, Cahalan, & Shanks, chap. 9). Individuals with certain behavioral disorders who are followed in natural populations have better prognoses than those followed in treatment institutions. Cahalan and his collaborators (chap. 9) stress that the traditional clinical conception of alcoholism as a progressive and irreversible condition does not hold in general populations. Drinking problems are episodic and transitory, with a substantial amount of spontaneous remission.

6. *Occasional use of heroin does not necessarily lead to addiction.*

The Robins data also showed that occasional users of narcotics did not necessarily become addicted, nor were narcotics users more likely to develop tolerance to, or more problems with, their drugs than users of amphetamines or barbiturates. Robins (1973) emphasizes that the findings from her study are striking in two ways: "They showed a surprisingly high remission rate for heroin addiction, and they showed that many men who reported addiction in Vietnam had used narcotics occasionally thereafter without having become readdicted" (p. vii).

In interpreting the results of Robins's study, however, one must keep in mind that this reduction in heroin use took place among men who made a striking geographical transfer from one location to another. It remains to be seen whether the same processes take place in situations in which users remain in the same geographical and social environment.

Antecedents of Drug Use

Although cross-sectional studies have identified a variety of factors correlated with drug use, it is unclear whether they precede or derive from the use of drugs. (For reviews of cross-sectional studies, see Gorsuch & Butler, 1976; Kandel, 1975c; National Commission on Marihuana and Drug Abuse, 1972, 1973.) A most important contribution of longitudinal studies is to suggest a causal order between various factors and drug behavior, although only experimental manipulation of variables can definitely establish a causal sequence (Ricks, 1970; Robins, 1970b). The variables that have been investigated fall into three broad classes: (1) sociodemographic characteristics; (2) intrapersonal attributes, which include (a) personality characteristics and (b) life-style variables; and (3) interpersonal influences of either (a) peer or (b) family. I discuss the substantive results here with respect to antecedents of drug use, and in the next section with respect to consequences.

To date, much more effort has gone into examining the determinants of drug use than the consequences. Most interest in predictors has focused on personality variables, involvement in delinquency, attitudes and values favorable to drug use, and interpersonal influences of family and peers. Two consequences of drug use have been analyzed: criminal behavior and the amotivational syndrome.

The integration of substantive findings originating from these studies is somewhat hampered by the fact that different investigators have focused on different drugs and kinds of use, defined drug behavior differently, and analyzed the data through different techniques. Some examined the predictors of the use of a single drug in a total population, most often marihuana (Elinson, Jessor & Jessor, Sadava, Smith). Others examined the predictors of use of a particular drug in the restricted group that has already participated in use at the stage lower in the sequence. For instance, Kandel examined in turn the predictors of initiation into hard liquor, into marihuana, and into other illicit drugs (see chap. 3). Robins examined the predictors of three developmental stages of Vietnam addiction: narcotic use in Vietnam, continuation after return, and addiction if use continued in the United States (Robins et al., 1977). Robins examined separately marihuana, barbiturates, amphetamines, and narcotics, but many investigators do not distinguish among illicit drugs, except for marihuana. Most frequently, the drugs are grouped together as part of a classification based upon implicit Guttman-scale criteria, with respondents classified in a particular category having experienced the patterns lower on the scale. The most common index has three categories: never used any illicit drugs; used only marihuana; also used other illicit drugs (Johnston, Mellinger). Another three-category index is described by Gulas and King (1976): nonusers of any illicit drugs; light marihuana-only users (defined as having used marihuana no more than 20 times, smoked less than once a week in the 3 months prior to the survey, and not used any hallucinogens); heavy marihuana users (defined as having used marihuana more than 50 times and experimented with hallucinogens and other substances). Johnston also developed two five-category indexes that combine the seriousness of the drugs used and the degree of involvement with each. One index consisted of: no use of illicit drugs; use of marihuana only; experimental use (one to two times) of one, two, or three pills (amphetamines, barbiturates, hallucinogens, cocaine, or methaqualone); more than experimental use of one or two pills; more than experimental use of three pills or any use of heroin (Johnston, O'Malley, & Eveland, chap. 6). A different version included: no use of any illicit drugs; experimental use of marihuana only (one to two times); use of marihuana only, more than twice, and no other illicit drugs; use of hallucinogens; use of one or a combination of heroin, amphetamines, and barbiturates, but no hallucinogens (O'Malley, 1975). Sadava (1973b; Sadava & Forsyth, 1976) described an elaborate four-category classification based on frequency of use and experienced effects of marihuana and other illicit drugs. Smith (1973) developed a four-category classification of degree of drug involvement: no use; infrequent (1–10 times) exclusive use of marihuana; frequent (11 or more times) exclusive use of marihuana; use of hard drugs (heroin, hallucinogens, stimulants, or depressants).

In examining drug use over time, different investigators emphasized different aspects of drug behavior. Most focused on the initiation into drugs, most often marihuana. (Jessor and Kandel also examined onset of drinking, chaps. 2, 3. See also Jessor, R., Collins, & Jessor, S. L., 1972; Jessor, R., & Jessor, S. L., 1973, 1977; Margulies, Kessler, & Kandel, 1977.) Some took into account the time of onset and distinguished early marihuana users (those who started in grade 9 or earlier) from late users (those who started in grade 10, 11, or 12) (Smith & Fogg, chap. 4). Others specified changes in behavior over time. Mellinger examined continuous versus noncontinuous users of marihuana, and of other illicit drugs (Mellinger, Somers, Davidson, & Manheimer, 1976; Mellinger, Somers, Bazell, & Manheimer, chap. 7). Kandel defined status-change groups as well as raw-change scores in the frequency of recent marihuana use (chap. 3, and Kessler, Kandel, & Margulies, 1976).

There were also differences in the definition of drug users. A user was most often defined as an individual who had ever used a particular substance *once* (see also Kandel, 1975a). To be counted as a marihuana user by Jessor and his collaborators, however, a young person had to have used marihuana more than once in the past year (Jessor, R., & Jessor, S. L., 1977; Jessor, R., Jessor, S. L., & Finney, 1973); and Brill and Christie (1974) set a minimum of 10 experiences unless used recently.

Finally, in their analyses, some investigators relied solely upon bivariate relationships between predictors (or consequences) and drug use, whereas others used multivariate techniques of data analysis that controlled for spurious and overlapping effects. Thus, the variations in definitions of drug patterns under investigation and in analytic strategies complicated the task of integrating the substantive findings. Most of the propositions that have been derived pertain to marihuana use. They are obviously tentative and in need of further testing and documentation.

At a most general level, the overall conclusion to be drawn from these longitudinal studies is that dysfunctional attributes of drug users appear to precede drug use. Furthermore, few unfavorable outcomes of drug use have been identified in these noninstitutionalized populations.

7. *Different factors are involved in the transitions into different stages of drug use.*

When the notion of stages has been used, it has pinpointed the importance of different factors at different stages of drug behavior. As noted earlier, two of the studies under review developed the notion of stages, albeit in different ways. Kandel isolated sequences in adolescent involvement from legal to illegal drugs and investigated variables predictive of initiation to hard liquor, marihuana, and other illicit drugs, respectively. Robins defined phases in the process of addiction in a specific cohort of soldiers with Vietnam experience, distinguishing between the use of narcotics while in Vietnam, continuation of use after return to the United States, and addiction to narcotics among those who continued to use in the United States. Similar conclusions, however, are reached by both authors: The specification of developmental phases and the partitioning of the sample into these phases maximize the identification of predictors of specific outcomes of interest.

Sociodemographic variables were of little importance overall in the sample of New York State high school students (Kandel, Kessler, & Margulies, chap. 3), but they were important in explaining first exposure of the Vietnam veterans to narcotics and continuation of use after return, though not to probability of addiction among users (Robins et al., 1977). Prior involvement in a series of precipitating activities such as minor delinquency and use of cigarettes, beer, and wine were the most important predictors of adolescent hard-liquor use. Adolescents' beliefs and values favorable to the use of marihuana and association with marihuana-using peers were the strongest predictors of initiation into marihuana. Poor relations with parents, feelings of depression, and exposure to drug-using peers were most important for initiation into illicit drugs other than marihuana (Kandel et al., chap. 3). Parents' behavior was the only predictor of the last stage (liability to addiction among users of narcotics after Vietnam) of narcotic involvement among the veterans, although it was the weakest predictor of the two earlier stages of addiction. By contrast, preservice drug experience was important only for predicting narcotic experience while in Vietnam (Robins et al., 1977). As stressed by Robins (Robins et al., 1977), unless the sample had been decomposed, several of the findings would not have come to light "because no single variable is a strongly positive predictor at all stages of the development of addiction" (p. 397).

8. *Personality factors, indicative of maladjustment, precede the use of marihuana and of other illicit drugs.*

Most of our knowledge about personality predictors of drug use comes from six studies to date, concerned almost exclusively with the initiation into the earliest phases of marihuana use.

A most extensive set of data was provided by Smith (Smith & Fogg, chap. 4), who administered a 400-item inventory designed to measure attitudes, beliefs, expectations and behavioral predispositions "viewed from the perspective of desires and expectations of parents who hold traditional middle-class values" in each of five waves of data collection (Smith & Fogg, chap. 4, p. 102). In the first wave, parallel assessments were also obtained based on peers' ratings of the junior and senior high school students on each of 20 personality traits. The self-administered battery was reduced first to 7 scales defined a priori, then subsequently, to 8 factor-analytically derived scales: obedient, law abiding; works hard and efficiently; feels capable; confident academically; self-sufficient; likes school and intellectual activities; ambitious; feels valued and accepted. These detailed personality measurements were used to predict time of onset of marihuana use in one of six schools (Smith & Fogg, chap. 4). In earlier analyses, rebelliousness was also examined as a predictor of type and frequency of use among five groups of users (Smith, 1973; Smith & Fogg, 1974a, 1974b).

As in Smith's instrument, the concepts encompassed in Jessor and Jessor's (chap. 2, p. 43) personality system variables emphasize the cognitive aspects of personality, "values, expectations, beliefs, attitudes, orientations toward self and others . . . and reflect social meanings and social experience." The measures cover three structures: (1) motivational instigation, which includes subscales of values and expectations for academic achievement, independence, and affection; (2) personal beliefs: social criticism, alienation, self-esteem, and internal–external locus of control; and (3) personal control: attitudinal tolerance of deviance, religiosity, and importance attached to positive, relative to negative, functions of problem behavior. These measures were used to predict initiation and time of onset to marihuana.

Extensive personality measures were available as of 10th grade on Johnston's Youth in Transition cohort (chap. 6). The personality dimensions covered (1) motives—in particular, attitudes toward school; also needs for achievement, affiliation, social approval, and independence; (2) affective states—including self-esteem, independence, impulse to aggression, depression, anomie, general anxiety; (3) values—such as honesty, social responsibility, academic achievement, religiousness; (4) attitudes—job-relatedness, internal–external control, opposition to the Vietnam war, political alienation; and (5) aspirations—educational and occupational (Bachman et al., 1967; O'Malley, 1975).

The personality measures included in Kandel's study included self-esteem, alienation, normlessness, and a six-item index of depressive mood (chap. 3; see also Paton & Kandel, in press).

I have described the scales in detail to illustrate that the studies include few measures of affective states. Such measures may be particularly difficult to obtain within the context of large-scale surveys. Access to detailed psychological assessments makes the retrospective study by Haagen (1970) so important, despite the small size of its sample ($N = 70$) and the limited assessment of drug use. The marihuana use of selected college juniors was ascertained and then related to scores on extensive batteries of psychological tests taken by those same juniors during orientation week in their freshman year, prior to any drug involvement. These tests included the California Psychological Inventory, the Strong Vocational Interest Blank, the S.A.T. verbal and math tests, Gough's Adjective Checklist, the Myers-Briggs type indicator, and several other attitude and questionnaire forms. In addition, Haagen examined separately the predictors of infrequent, as contrasted with frequent, marihuana use. Gulas and King's (1976) retrospective study of college seniors had access to freshman scores on the Gordon Personal Profile, which measures ascendency, responsibility, emotional stability, and sociability.

It is necessary to note important limitations of these data for understanding the predictive role of personality factors in drug involvement. As noted, the personality variables are mainly cognitive and, by and large, do not deal with affective states. Several of the concepts considered as aspects of personality by the researchers have a strong social-psychological component. For example, concepts such as religiosity or level of educational aspiration would be more appropriately classified as values or attitudes. In addition, though Smith and Jessor presented detailed analyses in which they distinguished early from late drug onset, most studies have dealt exclusively with initiation into drugs rather than with extent of use or changes in degrees of use over time, where psychological factors can be expected to play their most important role. Thus, Haagen (1970) found that, whereas some personality factors had a linear relationship to subsequent extensiveness of marihuana involvement, other measures showed nonusers and future infrequent users to be initially alike but different from future frequent users.

Several themes emerge from the data, suggesting that adolescents who will eventually experiment with marihuana, either at the high school or the college level, are characterized by certain personality patterns that are not socially approved. Furthermore, the higher the scores on attributes predictive of initiation, the earlier the onset of use (Jessor & Jessor, chap. 2; Smith & Fogg, chap. 4). On the basis of data from the Youth in Transition cohort, O'Malley (1975) is the only investigator to conclude, from regression analyses predicting use of any illicit drug, and from discriminant-function analyses classifying students into one of five patterns of illicit drug use, that: "variables which tap into psychological problems, e.g. negative affective states—showed . . . little relationship with later drug use. The notion that drug use is an attempt to deal with problems is deeply ingrained, but there is little support for that notion in the results of this study" (O'Malley, 1975, p. 269). Results of one-way analyses of variance relating these same personality measures at Time 1 to the five-category index of drug use at Time 4 revealed no significant relationships. Jessor found that the same set of personality factors were much poorer predictors of subsequent marihuana involvement at college level than at high school level (Jessor, R., & Jessor, S. L., 1977; Jessor, R., et al., 1973; Jessor & Jessor, chap. 2). According to Jessor (Jessor, R. et al., 1973), this is so because, by the time of college, marihuana use has become the norm: "Under such circumstances of widespread use and availability, the prediction of onset may depend more on factors such as the crowd one happens to find oneself in or the vicissitudes of a particular relationship than on the systematic pattern of variables specified in the problem behavior theory" (p. 14).

The personality variables predictive of subsequent involvement in marihuana are related to the following themes:

- *Rebelliousness.* Smith found that rebelliousness, measured both by self-reports and by peer rating, was monotonically related to subsequent type and frequency of illicit drug use: Nonusing adolescents who subsequently became users of "hard" drugs scored higher than those who subsequently became frequent, but exclusive, marihuana users. The frequent, exclusive marihuana users scored higher than the infrequent, exclusive marihuana users, and in turn, the infrequent, exclusive marihuana users scored higher than those students who remained nonusers of any drug. Self-reported rebelliousness was the best discriminator among five predictors (Smith, 1973). Similarly, both on the basis of self-reports and peer ratings, a low score on the related scale—obedient, law abiding—was the single most important predictor of adolescent involvement in marihuana (Smith & Fogg, chap. 4). Lack of tenderness as assessed by peers was the second-most important personality predictor. O'Malley (1975) found that all drug users scored higher than nonusers on impulse to aggression, and that nonusers scored higher on self-control at Time 1. Furthermore, impulse to aggression was the only affective measure that was a significant predictor of subsequent experimentation with any kind of drug, although it was an extremely weak predictor, explaining .3% of the drug-use variance.

- *Stress on Independence.* Differences on this factor between prospective users and nonusers are among the most consistent findings across studies. Future marihuana users had higher expectations for independence (Jessor & Jessor, chap. 2; Sadava, 1973a) and placed a higher value on independence relative to achievement than did nonusers (Jessor & Jessor, chap. 2). Gulas and King (1976) found that future heavy users scored higher than nonusers or infrequent marihuana users on Gordon's ascendancy scale in their freshman year. O'Malley (1975) also reported that, in the 10th grade, future drug users, particularly those who experimented with hallucinogens, had high scores on all scales measuring various aspects of independence.

- *Low Sense of Psychological Well-being.* Jessor and Jessor (chap. 2) found that prospective marihuana users scored high on personal alienation. The future marihuana users among the high school students studied by Smith and Fogg (chap. 4) were apathetic and pessimistic. Depressive mood predicted onset of marihuana use among high school students who were previous nonusers as well as onset of other illicit drugs among prior marihuana users (Paton, Kessler, & Kandel, 1977). College students in Haagen's (1970) sample who became *frequent* marihuana users in the freshman year had described themselves as dissatisfied, anxious, apprehensive, pessimistic, restless, volatile, and in conflict with people. Positive assessments, however, characterized those who became *infrequent* users. Prior to experimenting with marihuana, they had described themselves as having satisfying social relationships; as having their emotions under control; as being self-confident, spontaneous, and insightful; and as seeking opportunities for change and new experience. O'Malley (1975) found no significant relationship between drug use and prior scores on measures of depression, anomie, anxiety and irritability, or feelings of unhappiness.

- *Low Self-esteem.* In Haagen's (1970) sample, low self-esteem characterized the college students who became frequent marihuana users. Smith and Fogg (chap. 4) reported that adolescents who started marihuana use did not feel capable, valued, and accepted. In an elegant analysis based on three waves of data collection on 3,148 junior high school students, Kaplan (1975a) documented that a lowering of one's self-image between Time 1 and Time 2 increased the probability of subsequent involvement in drug-related activities, such as smoking marihuana or taking narcotic drugs by Time 3. Change in attitude between Times 1 and 2 was examined among students who had not engaged in deviant behaviors before Time 3. The author could clearly establish that a change in self-esteem between Time 1 and Time 2 preceded the initiation of the behaviors between Time 2 and Time 3. Level of self-esteem did not, however, predict subsequent marihuana experimentation among Jessor and Jessor's high school students (chap. 2), nor among the Youth in Transition cohort (O'Malley, 1975), nor among New York State adolescents (Kandel et al., chap. 3).

• *Lower Academic Aspirations and Motivation.* This, too, is one of the most consistent findings across studies. In Smith & Fogg's (chap. 4) high school sample, the following scales were good discriminators of subsequent marihuana use: does not work hard and effectively; is not ambitious; exhibits low intellectual maturity; does not strive for achievement. Similarly, Jessor and Jessor (chap. 2) found that future marihuana involvement was strongly predicted by low value on academic achievement, low value on expectation for academic achievement, and as noted above, high independence-achievement value discrepancy. Finally, Gulas and King (1976) found that future marihuana users among college students had lower scores on the Gordon responsibility scale than those who remained nonusers.

Most of the results presented to date pertain to marihuana. Although the assessment of psychological functioning in Kandel's study was limited, her results illustrate the obvious but important point that different psychological factors antecede involvement in different kinds of drug use. Depression had a low relationship to initiation into marihuana but was an important predictor of subsequent involvement in other illicit drugs (Kandel et al., chap. 3).

The traits that discriminate future users from nonusers are not, for the most part, socially valued ones. Rarely are positive attributes mentioned. Social presence and sociability seem to be the most prominent positive traits of future marihuana users. The early marihuana users in Smith and Fogg's high school sample scored highest of any group, including nonusers, on the peer rating scale "sociable, talkative, outgoing" (see chap. 4). This is consonant with the well-established finding that peer influences are among the strongest predictors of subsequent drug involvement. O'Malley (1975) found that future drug users scored highest on flexibility. As noted above, Haagen (1970) reported that college students who became experimental users described themselves as sociable and well adjusted. Gulas and King (1976), however, found no difference in sociability and emotional stability among future nonusers, experimental users, and heavy marihuana users.

9. *Poorer school performance is a common antecedent of subsequent initiation into illicit drugs.*

Low grades and high frequency of school absences or of classes cut have consistently been found to precede involvement in marihuana use, especially among high school students (Jessor, R., & Jessor, S. L., 1977; Jessor, R., et al., 1973; Johnston, 1973; Kandel et al., chap. 3; Mellinger et al., 1976; Smith & Fogg, chap. 4). Such relationships may not appear among college students (Johnston, 1973; O'Malley, 1975). Interestingly, Haagen (1970) found that, although students who started using marihuana in college, whether infrequently or frequently, had lower grades in high school and spent less time on their homework than persistent nonusers, they actually scored as high or even higher on aptitude and intelligence tests. The future users were no less gifted intellectually than the nonusers, but they were less interested and less willing to expend effort on academic pursuits.

10. *Delinquent and deviant activities precede involvement in illicit drugs.*

Extensive information on the relationship between delinquency and drug use is provided in Johnston's study of the Youth in Transition cohort, where participation in delinquent and criminal activities was assessed extensively prior to and concomitant with involvement in drugs (chap. 6). No other study of normal populations contains as rich a set of data on delinquency and criminal behavior. The authors conclude that: "The preponderance of the delinquency differences among the nonusers and various eventual drug-user groups existed *before* drug usage and thus could hardly be attributed to drug use" (p. 155). Criminal activities involving property, such as theft and vandalism, were more strongly related than interpersonal aggression to subsequent involvement in drug use. Similarly, Jessor and Jessor (chap. 2) found that greater "general deviant behavior," as indexed by lying, stealing, and aggression, was related to subsequent experimentation with marihuana.

The specific kind of delinquent activity can be predictive of different kinds of drug involvement. Among New York State high school students, participation in minor delinquency (such as cheating on a test, minor stealing, or driving too fast) predicted both hard-liquor and marihuana initiation. Dealing in drugs and participating in major delinquency (such as taking someone else's car, robbery, major stealing) predicted marihuana use and, especially, initiation into other illicit drugs (Kandel et al., chap. 3). Among the Vietnam veterans, the own-behavior scale, an index of prior participation in deviance (such as arrests, dropping out of or expulsion from school, truancy, and fighting) predicted use in and after Vietnam but not addiction liability after Vietnam. Addiction liability was lowest for those least and those most antisocial resulting from the fact that component elements of the scale had varying relationships to addiction liability (Robins et al., 1977).

11. *A constellation of attitudes and values favorable to deviance precedes involvement in illicit drugs.*

Not only deviant behaviors predict subsequent drug involvement. So do attitudes and values that are favorable to deviance and reflect lessened conformity to social institutions. Jessor and Jessor (chap. 2) found that initiation to marihuana was foretold by a lower value placed on academic achievement, a higher value on independence relative to achievement, lack of interest in goals of conventional institutions like church and school, criticism of existing society, and tolerance of deviance. Similar findings were reported by Smith and Fogg (chap. 4) and O'Malley (1975). Low scores on an index of conformity to adult expectations predicted initiation both to marihuana and to other illicit drugs among New York State high school students (Kandel et al., chap. 3). This same constellation of values measuring acceptance of various conventional values and beliefs was a most influential predictor of reduction in the heavy use of marihuana over time (Kessler et al., 1976).

12. *There is a process of anticipatory socialization in which youths who will initiate the use of drugs develop attitudes favorable to the use of legal and illegal drugs prior to initiation.*

Those adolescents who would start the use of marihuana had more favorable attitudes than their classmates toward smoking (Smith & Fogg, chap. 4). They had higher attitudinal tolerance of drug use (Lucas, Grupp, & Schmitt, 1975; Sadava, 1973b). They scored higher on an index that measures the positive, relative to the negative, functions of drinking and drug use (Jessor & Jessor, chap. 2; Sadava, 1973a). They were more likely to believe that casual, or even regular, use of marihuana is not harmful and that it should be legalized (Kandel et al., chap. 3). In fact, initiation to each of three forms of drug use—hard liquor, marihuana, and other illicit drugs—was preceded by beliefs that use of the specific drug in each case, especially casual use, was not harmful. Attitudes were especially important to predict subsequent initiation to marihuana. The cluster of variables indexing favorable attitudes toward drugs explained 11% of the variance in initiation into marihuana, while all the variables together explained a total of 20%. By contrast, beliefs and attitudes explained 9% of the variance for involvement in other illicit drugs, out of a total of 29% (Kandel et al., chap. 3).

13. *Drug behavior and drug-related attitudes of peers are among the most potent predictors of drug involvement.*

A most consistent finding of drug research is the strong relationship observed, at one time point, between an individual's drug behavior and the drug use of her or his friends, either as perceived by the individual or as reported by the friends themselves (Johnson, 1973; Kandel, 1973, 1974a, 1974b; Kandel et al., 1976; National Commission on Marihuana and Drug Abuse, 1972). Observations at one time point, however, leave the causal connection between friends' use and one's own unresolved. Friends may be similar in their drug use, either because of a process of interpersonal selection in which adolescents who share prior similarity in values and behaviors seek each other out as friends, or because of a socialization process in which one friend influences the behavior of another over time. Both processes, of course, can take place concurrently. The data derived from longitudinal studies indicate that a socialization process takes place. Extent of perceived drug use in the peer group, self-reported drug use by peers, and perceived peer tolerance for drug use are all very strong predictors of a youth's subsequent initiation into various forms of use. These peer influences appear to be more important at certain points of the process of involvement than at others.

Perceived extent of drug use in the peer group is an important precursor of involvement in marihuana and in other illicit drugs as well (Jessor & Jessor, chap. 2; Kandel et al., chap. 3; Lucas, Grupp, & Schmitt, 1975). Friends' use of hard liquor is less important for initiation into drinking, but perceived and self-reported peer attitudes favorable to drug experimentation are important for illicit drugs. In a multiple regression analysis in which 22 predictors of subsequent initiation to marihuana were considered among high school students who had already experienced alcohol, peer marihuana use and attitudes constituted a most important cluster of predictors. This cluster explained 10% of the variance in initiation of marihuana use and accounted for 50% of the total variance explained by all the predictors entered in the analyses (Kandel et al., chap. 3). These longitudinal results thus replicated multivariate analyses of cross-sectional data on the same sample (Kandel et al., 1976). Peer influences were not as important to the prediction of initiation to hard liquor and to other illicit drugs as they were for marihuana.

Although a socialization process takes place, a selection process in which people with similar attitudes select one another as friends is not excluded. Kandel (in press) provides preliminary answers to this question inasmuch as longitudinal sociometric data are available, not only on stable friendships over time, but also on friends-to-be and on former friends in changing friendships. It has been possible to examine the similarities or divergences in drug use among adolescents, not only while they are friends, but both before they select each other as friends and after they drop each other. The results indicate that selection (or assortative pairing) and socialization are approximately equal in importance.

Susceptibility to peer influences is accompanied by greater involvement in the peer subculture and by greater attachments to peers than to parents. Kandel,

Kessler, and Margulies (chap. 3) found that extensive participation in peer-related activities, such as getting together with friends outside of school, dating, attending parties, or driving around with friends, preceded initiation to hard liquor and to marihuana, although not to other illicit drugs. Extensive discussions of drugs with peers preceded initiation to all types of illicit drugs. Greater closeness to and reliance on peers as opposed to parents were also predictive of subsequent marihuana use (Kandel et al., chap. 3). Jessor and Jessor (chap. 2) found that future marihuana users reported less consensus between their parents and their friends in general expectations and values, and they attributed greater importance to friends' opinions than to parents' (Jessor & Jessor, chap. 2; Jessor, R., & Jessor, S. L., 1977; Jessor, R., et al., 1973).

Peers also have a role in stimulating increased involvement in marihuana. Detailed analyses of raw-change scores in frequency of current marihuana use over time indicate that peer influences, especially in the form of exposure to peers who use or supply marihuana, have a far greater impact on rates of increase than of decrease (Kessler et al., 1976).

14. *Parental behaviors, parental attitudes, and parental closeness to their children have differential importance at different stages of involvement in drugs.*

Two alternate social-learning processes have been posited to describe the influence of parents on their children:

1. *Imitation.* Youths model their own behaviors on parental behaviors by replicating the parental behaviors, or by transposing them into more acceptable forms. Adolescents may be more likely to start using hard liquor if their parents drink. They may also be more likely to use illegal drugs if their parents drink, smoke, or use a variety of psychoactive drugs, such as stimulants, tranquilizers, or barbiturates.
2. *Reinforcement.* Adolescents respond to specific parental norms and definitions of appropriate behaviors and values.

In addition to these two processes, the quality of the parent–child relationship, irrespective of parental behaviors and values, may have a positive effect in restraining youth from engaging in various deviant or delinquent activities (Hirschi, 1969; McCord, W., & McCord, J., 1959).

The data provided by Kandel, Kessler, and Margulies (chap. 3) address the issue of parental influences in detail (see also Kandel, 1974a, 1974b, for an earlier discussion of the issue). Parental models, in the form of use of hard liquor, predict adolescent initiation both to hard liquor and to other illicit drugs, although they do not predict marihuana use. Parental use of psychoactive drugs predicts initiation to other illicit drugs. Parents' specific rules against the use of drugs are ineffective, but parents' tolerance of marihuana use by their children or their belief in the harmlessness of various drugs favor subsequent drug use by their children. Lack of closeness between parents and children predicts subsequent initiation to marihuana and, especially, to other illicit drugs (Kandel et al., chap. 3). Analyses of changes in frequency of marihuana use over time indicate that although parents appear to be able to shield their children from initial involvement in heavy drug use, they do not have the ability to help their children give up a habit of heavy use once it is formed (Kessler et al., 1976). In this high school sample, parental influences were, however, of greatest importance in the third stage of drug involvement—the use of other illicit drugs.

Similarly, Robins found that parental behaviors such as divorce, arrest, drinking, or drug problems did not predict either use in Vietnam or continued use after Vietnam but were the strongest predictors of the third stage, liability to addiction after Vietnam (Robins et al., 1977).

15. *Sociodemographic variables hold little predictive power for initiation into marihuana.*

Most studies find that, both in absolute terms and relative to other factors, sociodemographic variables add very little to the explained variance of initiation into drugs, especially marihuana (Jessor & Jessor, chap. 2; Kandel et al., chap. 3; O'Malley, 1975). Robins, Davis, and Wish (1977), however, found inconsistent relationships between different demographic factors and different aspects of drug behavior. Inner-city residence, region (West Coast), age (young), and race (black) were correlated with preservice drug use. There was no correlation with father's occupation. Certain of the demographic variables predicted use of narcotics while in Vietnam and continuation of use after return but had a negative relationship to liability to addiction after Vietnam.

16. *Age of onset of drug use declines as degree of proneness to deviance increases.*

A large number of follow-up contacts permitted Smith and Jessor to determine not only which adolescents started using marihuana but at which point in high school they did so. The results consistently show that the higher the youngster's score on an item predictive of subsequent onset, the earlier the time of onset (Jessor & Jessor, chap. 2; Smith & Fogg, chap. 4) and the more extensive the involvement (Johnston et al., chap. 6). Similarly, Brill and Christie (1974) found that earlier onset was related to a greater likelihood of continued and heavy use. The concept of transition proneness was developed by Jessor and Jessor (chap. 2) to describe this process, namely, "a temporally prior pattern of attributes that constitutes a readiness to engage in transition-marking behavior . . . and that signals a higher likelihood of its onset" (p. 63).

The pattern of social-psychological attributes defining deviance or transition proneness includes

lower value on achievement and greater value on independence, greater social criticism, more tolerance of deviance, and less religiosity in the personality system; less parental control and support, more friends' influence, and more friends' models and approval for drug use in the perceived environment system; more deviant behavior, less church attendance, and lower school achievement in the behavior system (Jessor, R., 1976, p. 133).

The Jessors stress that the same constellation of attributes characteristic of transition proneness predicts not only the onset and time of onset of marihuana use but also other behaviors, such as drinking (Jessor, R., & Jessor, S. L., 1975) and sexual intercourse (Jessor, S. L., & Jessor, R., 1975).

17. *A social setting favorable to drug use reinforces and increases individual predisposition to use.*

Robins's study of a natural population exposed to very divergent social settings, as compared to a similar group without such experience, shows very dramatically the effect of the social setting on initiation to drug use. The experience in Vietnam was associated with a high rate of initiation for every one of the four classes of drug use investigated. Not only did the Vietnam experience accelerate the timing of initiation into certain drugs—the barbiturates and the amphetamines—but it also produced an important net gain in the number of users of marihuana and narcotics (Robins, chap. 8). The proportion of veterans who had ever tried narcotics was 48%, as against the expected 25% had the rates of initiation continued at pre-Vietnam levels. Vietnam provided a setting in which drugs of all kinds were easily available, and in which the restrictions against use were lowered. Heroin of a quality much superior to that in the United States was especially available. Soldiers with attributes indicative of a predisposition to use drugs were even more likely to begin such use in Vietnam than men without these characteristics: "In a setting greatly facilitating narcotic use, preexisting differences in predispositions were more fully expressed than they had been in a more inhibiting environment. . . . Rather than equalizing the drug experience of men from different social and behavioral backgrounds, easy access to narcotics in Vietnam seemed to increase their preexisting differences" (Robins, chap. 8, p. 195). Robins concluded that "a setting with greater opportunities to express deviant behavior *increases* the impact of prior predispositions to deviance" (p. 196). The strength of Robins's findings lies in the fact that she documented a striking temporal association between the introduction to the Vietnam setting and the change in drug-use patterns. Furthermore, the change in setting was "independent of influences either by actors themselves or by those who have influenced their sets of predispositions" (p. 180).

No other study has yet shown such striking contextual effects. Although geographical location (O'Malley, 1975) and kind of school attended (Kandel et al., chap. 3) predicted subsequent drug initiation, contextual effects of schools on drug use, beyond those that can be attributed solely to compositional effects, have not been documented.

Consequences of Drug Use

Much less attention has been directed to investigation of the consequences of drug use than to the determinants. Evidence on consequences is available in two areas: (1) criminal behavior, and (2) the amotivational syndrome, as indexed by academic performance. To anticipate our conclusions, the results available to date contradict widely held beliefs about the harmful consequences of marihuana use. Negative behaviors previously found to be associated with marihuana use at one time point would seem to precede use rather than to result from it.

18. *Nonaddictive illicit drug use has not been shown to lead to increased criminality.*

The potential effect of drug use in leading to criminal involvement has been a major concern, a concern that has focused mainly on heroin but has also been directed toward other illicit substances. As noted earlier, the data from Johnston's study include some of the richer and more complete information on the relationship between drug use and criminal activity. The evidence marshaled so far suggests that, in the population sampled, there are no potentiating effects of illicit drug consumption on criminal involvement (Johnston et al., chap. 6). A five-category index of drug behavior was related to two indexes of crimes: against property and against people. The index of theft and vandalism measured arson, car theft, minor and major theft, vandalism of school property, and trespassing. The interpersonal aggression scale included, among other items, "the use of a knife or gun . . . to get something from a person" and hitting an instructor or supervisor (Bachman et al.,

1967). Delinquency scores at five time points between 1966 and 1974 were plotted for the five groups of users defined in 1970 and 1974. Substantive differences in delinquency, especially crimes against property, anteceded drug use. Furthermore, the seriousness of drug involvement was directly related to the seriousness of prior delinquency, but changes in drug use were not related to parallel changes in delinquency. When initial patterns of drug use were controlled, those young people who increased their drug use over a 5-year period did not show a parallel increase in delinquency. Delinquency decreased over time among all groups. The rate of decrease was similar in groups of adolescents characterized by divergent patterns of drug use over the same period. Because a 4-year interval occurred between the last two follow-ups, the authors were careful to note that they could not identify any short-term effect of drug use on delinquency. They concluded that "the hypothesis that the association [between nonaddictive drug use and other forms of delinquency] exists because such drug use somehow causes other kinds of delinquency has suffered a substantial, if not mortal, blow" (p. 156). The association results from characteristics of the social environment in which drug users live and from the personality characteristics of the users. Johnston, O'Malley, & Eveland (chap. 6) have outlined the potential explanatory links:

> We think it quite possible that delinquents who, because of their delinquency, became part of a deviant peer group are more likely to become drug users because drug use is likely to be an approved behavior in such a peer group. We also suspect that the correlation between delinquency and drug use stems not only from such environmental factors but also from individual differences in personality. Both delinquency and drug use are deviant behaviors, and therefore both are more likely to be adopted by individuals who are deviance prone. The fact that other forms of delinquency tended to precede drug use (at least in this cohort) may simply reflect the fact that proneness toward deviance is expressed through different behaviors at different ages. (p. 156)

19. Drug use has not been shown to lead to the amotivational syndrome.

It is widely feared that the use of drugs by young people may lead to the amotivational syndrome, the "loss of interest in virtually all activities other than cannabis, with resultant lethargy, amorality, and social and personal deterioration" (National Commission on Marihuana and Drug Abuse, 1972, p. 64). If, indeed, the use of marihuana and other drugs led to such states, it would have very detrimental consequences, not only for the individuals involved, but for society as a whole. The evidence marshaled to date suggests that, although there is an association at one time point between indicators of the amotivational syndrome and drug use, such states precede the use of drugs. The association is also explained away by spurious factors that are simultaneously related to those states and to drug behaviors. By and large, drug use per se does not appear to have any adverse consequences on academic performance, clarity of occupational goals, or dropping out of school. Most of the documentation is provided by three studies: Mellinger and his associates' (1976a) study of male college freshmen at the University of California at Berkeley, Brill and Christie's (1974) study of undergraduates at the University of California at Los Angeles, and Johnston's (1973) follow-up of a cohort of 10th-grade high school boys. No differences in grade point average were observed by Brill and Christie (1974) either at one time point or over time in their sample of college students classified into six marihuana-use groups: never used, initiated, increased, remained stable, decreased, or stopped use. Other investigators report that users are more likely to drop out of school (Johnston, 1973; Mellinger et al., 1976), to have lower grades (Kandel et al., 1976), or to have greater difficulties in deciding on a career (Brill & Christie, 1974). Lowered academic performance tends to precede subsequent involvement in drugs (see also Haagen, 1970). Nonetheless, it would appear that low school performance does not lead to drug use, but rather that the same variables that lead to poor school performance are also related to involvement in drugs.

Whatever differences in drop-out rates or in indecision about career goals appeared among drug users among the Berkeley students in their junior year were eliminated in multivariate analyses that took into account the characteristics of these students when they entered college: family background, scholastic performance in high school, and academic values (Mellinger et al., 1976, also Mellinger et al., chap. 7). Exceptions involving very small groups of students were encoutered, however. The rate of dropping out of college was extremely high (53%) in a group ($N = 19$) of continuing multiple-drug users with low academic motivation at entrance to the University of California and with parents of low educational background. This contrasts with drop-out rates varying between 11% and 15% for other students with initially low academic motivation (Mellinger et al., 1976). Among another group of 22 men whose occupational goals were clear at Time 1 and who remained continuous multiple-drug (marihuana and other illicit drugs) users throughout the first $2\frac{1}{2}$ years of college, a larger proportion became undecided about their career goals. Also, an even smaller group of continuous multiple-drug users ($N = 12$) had lower grades at Time 2 than would be expected on the basis of their prior characteristics. This result, however, was not statistically significant (Mellinger et al., chap. 7).

Similarly, O'Malley (1975) found no significant changes in self-reported grades associated with drug use in the cohort of 10th-grade boys followed for 4 years after high school. Users of hard drugs had lower educational attainments than would be expected on the basis of their pre-drug use aspirations: The proportion aspiring to college dropped from 62% to 37% among those who began to use barbiturates or heroin, and from 76% to 50% among those who began to use hallucinogens. The reduction in aspirations for college tended, however, to precede, rather than to follow, the initiation into illicit drugs other than marihuana (O'Malley, 1975). Furthermore, the use of these illicit drugs had no effect on other motivational variables having to do with job attitudes and self-actualization.

DISCUSSION

This review of prospective longitudinal studies of normal populations has generated a number of propositions about patterns of involvement in various forms of illicit drugs and about some of the antecedents and consequences of drug use. There appear to be sequential stages in the initiation into drugs, such that involvement with alcohol or cigarettes almost always precedes involvement with illegal drugs. The notion of stages provides a useful strategy for pinpointing the role of specific factors in transitions in drug use. For example, peer factors are especially important for marihuana initiation, whereas intrapsychic factors and lack of closeness of family ties are most important for the later stages of involvement in other illicit drugs. Many of the dysfunctional factors found, in cross-sectional research, to be related to drug use, such as low academic performance, rebelliousness, depression, or criminal activity, precede the use of drugs. Few unfavorable outcomes of drug use, especially marihuana use, have been identified. Focusing on a population of addicts in a natural setting has shown that, without any intervention, remission in addiction is extremely high. In fact, remission in populations of Vietnam veterans is much higher than has been observed in populations of addicts exposed to various treatment modalities. A social environment highly conducive to deviance interacts with highly predisposed individuals to give rise to the highest rates of use. These findings and related propositions are only tentative at this time and are in need of further testing. Many conceptual and methodological issues remain to be solved. The parallel between the issues in longitudinal drug research and those in other areas of life history research is striking.

Need to Standardize

Better definitions and standardization of drug behavior are needed. Different investigators focus on different aspects of drug use and sometimes use different criteria to define seemingly identical behaviors. Recent efforts initiated by the National Institute on Drug Abuse to standardize criteria and predictor variables in drug research should help to bring about greater comparability among studies. A first report on the measurements of drug use has been issued (Elinson & Nurco, 1975).

Identification of Developmental Phases in Drug Behavior

In addition to standardization of measures, it will also be essential to redefine and subdivide drug behavior so as to specify the particular developmental phases involved. This specification has to be carried out for various social groups, because developmental patterns are likely to vary, not only with age, sex, ethnicity, and social class, but also within the ecological, cultural, and historical conditions. Thus, we know that whites are more likely to progress from marihuana to pills and psychedelics, whereas blacks are more likely to progress from marihuana to cocaine and to opiates, heroin in particular (Jessop et al., 1976). Ricks (1974) has pointed out that "the most valuable contributions of life history investigations are dynamic descriptions of sequential developmental patterns leading into the different psychopathological syndromes" (p. 351). We lack such systematic descriptions of drug use. More meaningful analyses require the decomposition of samples into appropriate groups at risk for involvement in the next phase in the sequence. Such partitioning, in turn, makes it possible to identify with accuracy the predictors and consequences of various patterns of use of specific drugs, and it also favors the development of optimal intervention strategies.

The range of drug behaviors under consideration also needs to be extended to include more serious forms of involvement. Most studies examine only the determinants of initiation into drug use, particularly marihuana. Few go on to examine the determinants of changing patterns of use, whether of increased use or abuse, or of decreased use or termination, although the determinants, as well as the consequences, of these various patterns of use are probably quite different from each other.

Panel Loss

Another major problem in large-scale longitudinal studies is panel loss. Although most studies start with a representative sample of normal adolescents and young adults, the attrition in these epidemiological field studies biases the resulting matched-panel samples available for longitudinal analyses, thereby weakening the results derived from analyses of these samples. Individuals most heavily involved in drugs at the initial interview and nonusers with attributes predictive of subsequent involvement are those most likely to drop out of the research. (For a review of panel loss in longitudinal drug research, see Josephson & Rosen, chap. 5.) A basic assumption underlying the analyses of the remaining samples is that the users who have been retained are similar to those who have been lost. Such assumptions may well be incorrect, although they cannot be accepted or rejected because of the very lack of data on those lost. For example, peer factors have been identified as among the strongest predictors of involvement in drugs; yet those future heavy users who drop out of a study and who are not included in the longitudinal analyses may be social isolates, with no peer contacts, for whom peer influences play no determining role in drug involvement. The problem of panel losses in large-scale longitudinal studies threatens to become even more serious in the future. Increasing concerns with the rights of research subjects impose increasingly restrictive requirements upon researchers dealing with human subjects. These requirements often preclude asking respondents to identify themselves by name. They also make continued contact with the sample extremely difficult. To link files over time, several recent studies (for example, Josephson & Rosen, chap. 5, and those of Kandel et al., chap. 3) had to rely on identification numbers self-generated by the subjects, which in part accounts for the high attrition rates in the resulting panel samples. It is especially important to attempt to keep sample attrition to a minimum to retain the very small proportion of a sample from a normal population that is most seriously involved in psychopathology or in deviance.

Span of Follow-up

The total follow-up period in these studies is very short, most often only 1 year, rarely longer than 4 years. Longer periods of the life cycle clearly need to be covered, for only in that way can the processes antecedent to, concurrent with, and resulting from drug involvement be adequately studied, if not through the life-span of an individual, at least through important developmental phases.

Interaction Effects and Relative Effects of Variables

The increasing popularity of multivariate techniques of analysis in the behavioral sciences is reflected in the longitudinal drug studies. Although these techniques are useful for controlling spurious factors and for specifying the contributions of a variable to the criterion of interest, they are for the most part based on linear mathematical models that assume additive effects of variables. This limits our understanding of drug behavior in two ways. First, it reduces the effectiveness of our predictions by not allowing for nonadditive interaction effects (Kaplan, 1975b). Although difficult to identify, such effects are likely to be very important. For instance, in a study of delinquency, Roff and Sells (Roff, 1972) showed that low status among peers was predictive of subsequent delinquency in all socioeconomic groups except the lowest. In the lowest social-class group, adolescents with highest peer status were as likely to become delinquents as those with lowest status. To understand the relationship between delinquency and peer status, the investigators needed to take social class into account.

Second, linear models provide little insight into dynamic processes of change. For example, we know that peers, parental closeness, and various intrapersonal attributes are important predictors of adolescent drug involvement, but none of the studies to date gives any understanding of how these factors interrelate and modify one another. Although peers are important predictors, not all adolescents with drug-using friends experiment with drugs. What factors, such as aspects of family functioning and intrapersonal characteristics, reinforce or mitigate peer influences? In our own work on interpersonal processes in adolescent drug use, I and my colleagues are currently investigating this set of questions.

Furthermore, detailed assessments of the relative impact of different classes of variables are seldom carried out, even though it is important for both theoretical and practical reasons to know the relative impact on drug use of social or inter-actional variables versus personality factors. Thus, Kandel and her colleagues (chap. 3) have shown that different classes of factors are important at different stages of involvement, but such analyses are hampered by the serious statistical problems in assessing the relative impact of clusters of variables and in adequately distributing the overlapping statistical effects with other clusters. Recent methodological developments (Coleman, 1976) provide a beginning to solutions of this problem.

Three Kinds of Changes

The cultural and historical conditions surrounding various kinds of drug behaviors should be taken into account. The predictors of drug involvement may be different for youths who start using drugs at a historical time when few in the total population are users than for youths who start at a time when the behavior is more prevalent and less deviant. Developmental psychologists (Baltes & Schaie, 1973; Nesselroade & Baltes, 1974; Schaie, 1965) and sociologists (Riley, 1973; Riley & Waring, chap. 10; Ryder, 1965) have sensitized us to the fact that three kinds of changes may be confounded in any longitudinal investigation based on a single cohort of respondents: (1) changes that reflect maturation; (2) those that result from historical changes, such as variations in the availability of drugs or cultural values about their use; and (3) peculiarities of a particular cohort. Baltes and Schaie (1973) suggest that sequential longitudinal studies be designed in which successive cohorts are selected and followed over time. The groundbreaking study, *Monitoring the Future,* initiated in 1975 by Johnston and Bachman, follows this design for a 5-year period (Johnston, Bachman, & O'Malley, 1977).

Need for Theory

In much existing drug research, scant attention is paid to theory and to systematic testing of causal models; yet in the absence of a guiding theoretical framework, sophisticated methodologies and statistical manipulations of the data will fail to increase significantly our understanding of drug behavior. The work by the Jessors (chap. 2) represents one of the most systematic attempts to develop a general theory of deviance, or problem-behavior theory, within which drug use becomes but a special case. In this system, three general classes of variables are considered: personality, perceived environment, and behavior. As noted by Jessor and Jessor, "Each system is composed of structures of variables interrelated and organized so as to generate a resultant: a dynamic state designated 'problem-behavior proneness' that has implications for a greater or lesser likelihood of occurrence of problem behavior" (p. 43). Concepts explicitly or implicitly derived from socialization theory constitute the most common theoretical underpinning of drug studies. The framework elaborated by Kandel and her colleagues (chap. 3) emphasizes the interaction between individual characteristics and the nature of the matrix of social relationships, especially parents and peers, in which adolescents are embedded. Much work, however, remains to be done before the findings derived from the various studies can be integrated into a unifying theoretical framework.

Consequences and Precursors

It has been argued here that much more attention has been paid to the antecedents, than to the consequences, of drug use. The consequences for health— especially the physiological, in contrast to the psychosocial, consequences—in normal populations in natural settings, have been almost completely ignored. An important exception is Brunswick's (1976) ongoing investigation of the health status of illicit drug users. The consequences of drug use, will, I hope, receive more attention in the near future. Furthermore, in examining health consequences, attention should be paid to potentially positive, as well as negative, effects. For example, Mellinger and his colleagues (1976) found that a small group of marihuana users obtained better grades than would be expected on the basis of their prior academic performance and social-class background. It has also been suggested that use of illicit drugs may be adaptive and may represent a form of self-medication used to deal with incipient psychopathology and to prevent severe forms of mental disorders. There is a suggestion in my own follow-up of high school students that illicit drugs are used to deal with depressive feelings and may, in fact, lessen depressive mood. We have found that depressive mood predicts onset of other illicit drug use and that continued use of these drugs by previously depressed users is related to a decrease in depression over time (Paton et al., 1977). Are there also possible health benefits to marihuana usage as there are thought to be for moderate use of alcohol?

Drug Behavior in Developmental Perspective

One of the most interesting findings to emerge from these studies is that the antecedents of drug use are similar in many respects to those linked with various forms of psychopathology (see the reviews by Garmezy, 1974; Lane & Albee, 1970; Robins, 1970a). Lack of interest in school work and poor academic performance, for example, predict susceptibility to schizophrenia and other mental disturbances (Ricks, 1974) as well as drug use. Poor relationships with parents are common precursors of character disorders (Robins, 1970a) or delinquency (McCord, J., & McCord, W., 1958) as well as use of illicit drugs other than marihuana. Future drug users, however, appear to differ from adolescents who will exhibit various forms of psychopathology in two important respects: Future drug users are of average, or perhaps even superior, intelligence, and they are peer oriented rather than isolated.

The research task, therefore, is to identify, within a commonality of findings, the combinations of factors that are predictive of specific behavioral states. Successful peer relationships, in combination with otherwise similar attributes, may differentiate the future heavy drug user from the future schizophrenic or delinquent adult. Environmental factors may play a particularly important role in determining the appearance of specific behaviors. For example, Cloward and Ohlin (1960) showed that, depending upon characteristics of the surrounding community, adolescent gangs focused their energies on either fighting, criminal activities, or drug use. A further basic question, of course, is why some individuals develop dysfunctional patterns of behaviors whereas others with similar attributes do not.

This last question suggests that drug use and related behaviors in all likelihood cannot be properly studied apart from concurrent developmental processes. To be meaningful, longitudinal studies of drugs must have a broader focus than drug usage. Involvement in drugs must be examined as one among several behavioral outcomes of developmental processes. The advantage of longitudinal studies that start with normal populations in natural settings is that they provide baseline data about normal development against which better to evaluate the aberrant development of those who get involved in drugs or exhibit other forms of disordered or deviant behaviors. Such studies should be broad in design and appreciate that behavior is the result of the interaction of biological and psychological, as well as social, factors.

REFERENCES

Bachman, J. G., Kahn, R. L., Mednick, M. T., Davidson, T. N., & Johnston, L. D. *Youth in transition,* Vol. 1, *Blueprint for a longitudinal study of adolescent boys.* Ann Arbor: Institute for Social Research, 1967.

Ball, J. C., & Chambers, C. D. *The epidemiology of opiate addiction in the United States.* Springfield, Ill.: Thomas, 1970.

Baltes, P. B., & Schaie, K. W. On life-span developmental research paradigms: Retrospects and prospects. In P. B. Baltes & K. W. Schaie (Eds.), *Life-span developmental psychology: Personality and socialization.* New York: Academic, 1973.

Brill, N. W., & Christie, R. L. Marihuana use and psychosocial adaptation. *Archives of General Psychiatry,* 1974, *31,* 713–719.

Brook, J. S., Lukoff, I. F., & Whiteman, M. Peer, family, and personality domains as related to adolescents' drug behavior. *Psychological Reports,* 1977, *41,* 1095–1102.

Brunswick, A. *Predicting drug use by Harlem youth: A feasibility study* (Final report to the National Institute on Drug Abuse, 1 RO1 DA 00852-01 NAD). New York: Columbia University, March 1976.

Cahalan, D., & Roizen, R. *Changes in drinking problems in a national sample of men.* Paper presented at the North American Congress on Alcohol and Drug Problems, San Francisco, December 1974.

Clark, W. B., & Cahalan, D. Changes in problem drinking over a four-year span. *Addictive Behaviors,* 1976, *1,* 251–259.

Cloward, R. A., & Ohlin, L. E. *Delinquency and opportunity: A theory of delinquent gangs.* New York: Free Press, 1960.

Coleman, J. S. Regression analysis for the comparison of school and home effects. *Social Science Research,* 1976, *5,* 1–20.

Davidson, S. T., Mellinger, G. D., & Manheimer, D. I. Changing patterns of drug use among university males. *Addictive Diseases,* 1977, *3,* 215–233.

Dunnette, M. D., & Peterson, N. G. *Causes and consequences of adolescent drug experiences: A progress report and research perspective.* Minneapolis: Personnel Decisions Research Institute, 1977.

Elinson, J., & Nurco, D. N. *Operational definitions in socio-behavioral drug use research 1975* (National Institute on Drug Abuse, Research Monograph Series 2). Washington: U.S. Government Printing Office, 1975.

Garfield, M., & Garfield, E. A longitudinal study of drugs on a campus. *International Journal of the addictions*, 1973, *8*, 599–611.

Garmezy, N. Children at risk: The search for the antecedents of schizophrenia: Pt. I, Conceptual models and research methods. *Schizophrenia Bulletin*, 1974, *8*, 14–90.

Goldstein, J. W., Gleason, T. C., & Korn, J. H. Whither the epidemic? Psychoactive drug-use career patterns of college students. *Journal of Applied Social Psychology*, 1975, *5*, 16–33.

Gorsuch, R. L., & Butler, M. C. Initial drug abuse: A review of predisposing social psychological factors. *Psychological Bulletin*, 1976, *83*, 120–137.

Gould, L., Walker, A. L., Crane, L. E., & Lidz, C. W. *Connections: Notes from the heroin world*. New Haven: Yale University Press, 1974.

Groves, W. E. Patterns of college student drug use and lifestyles. In E. Josephson & E. E. Carroll (Eds.), *Drug use: Epidemiological and sociological approaches*. Washington: Hemisphere, 1974.

Grupp, S. E. *The marihuana muddle*. Lexington, Mass.: Heath, 1973.

Gulas, I., & King, F. W. On the question of pre-existing personality differences between users and nonusers of drugs. *Journal of Psychology*, 1976, *92*, 65–69.

Haagen, C. H. *Social and psychological characteristics associated with the use of marihuana by college men*. Wesleyan University, 1970. (Available in mimeo.)

Haberman, P. W., Josephson, E., Zanes, A., & Elinson, J. High school drug behavior: A methodological report on pilot studies. In S. Einstein & S. Allen (Eds.), *Proceedings of the First International Conference on Student Drug Surveys*. Farmingdale, N.Y.: Baywood, 1972.

Hirschi, T. *Causes of delinquency*. Berkeley and Los Angeles: University of California Press, 1969.

Huba, G. J., Wingard, J. A., & Bentler, P. M. *Adolescent drug use and peer and adult interaction patterns*. University of California at Los Angeles, 1978. (Available in mimeo.)

Jessop, D. J., Kandel, D. B., & Lukoff, I. F. *Comparative analyses of stages of drug use in different ethnic groups*: Center cross-study 1, Bedford Stuyvesant and New York State. Columbia University, Center for Socio-Cultural Research on Drug Use, June 1976. (Available in mimeo.)

Jessor, R. Predicting time of onset of marijuana use: A developmental study of high school youth. *Journal of Consulting and Clinical Psychology*, 1976, *44*, 125–134.

Jessor, R., Collins, M. I., & Jessor, S. L. On becoming a drinker: Social-psychological aspects of an adolescent transition. In F. A. Seixas (Ed.), *Nature and nurture in alcoholism* (Annals of the New York Academy of Sciences, Vol. 197). New York: Scholastic Reprints, 1972.

Jessor, R., & Jessor, S. L. Problem drinking in youth: Personality, social, and behavioral antecedents and correlates. In M. E. Chafetz (Ed.), *Psychological and social factors in drinking: Proceedings of the Second Annual Alcoholism Conference* (National Institute on Alcohol Abuse and Alcoholism). Washington: U.S. Government Printing Office, 1973.

Jessor, R., & Jessor, S. L. Adolescent development and the onset of drinking: A longitudinal study. *Journal of Studies on Alcohol*, 1975, *36*, 27–51.

Jessor, R., & Jessor, S. L. *Problem behavior and psychosocial development: A longitudinal study of youth*. New York: Academic, 1977.

Jessor, R., Jessor, S. L., & Finney, J. A social psychology of marijuana use: Longitudinal studies of high school and college youth. *Journal of Personality and Social Psychology*, 1973, *26*, 1–15.

Jessor, S. L., & Jessor, R. The transition from virginity to nonvirginity among youth: A social-psychological study over time. *Developmental Psychology*, 1975, *11*, 473–484.

Johnson, B. D. *Marihuana users and drug subcultures*. New York: Wiley, 1973.

Johnston, L. D. *Drugs and American youth*. Ann Arbor: Institute for Social Research, 1973.

Johnston, L. D. Drug use during and after high school: Results of a national longitudinal study. *American Journal of Public Health*, 1974, *64* (Suppl.), 29–37.

Johnston, L. D., & Bachman, J. G. Monitoring the future: A continuing study of the lifestyles and values of youth. Ann Arbor: Institute for Social Research, 1975. (Descriptive brochure)

Johnston, L. D., Bachman, J. G., & O'Malley, P. M. *Highlights from: Drug use among American high school students 1975-1977*, Rockville, Md.: National Institute on Drug Abuse, 1977.

Josephson, E. Trends in adolescent marijuana use. In E. Josephson & E. E. Carroll (Eds.), *Drug use. Epidemiological and sociological approaches*. Washington: Hemisphere, 1974.

Kandel, D. B. Adolescent marihuana use: Role of parents and peers. *Science*, 1973, *181*, 1067–1070.

Kandel, D. B. Inter- and intra-generational influences on adolescent marihuana use. *Journal of Social Issues*, 1974, *30* (Special issue on generations and social change), 107–135. (a)

Kandel, D. B. Interpersonal influences on adolescent illegal drug use. In E. Josephson & E. E. Carroll (Eds.), *Drug use: Epidemiological and sociological approaches*. Washington: Hemisphere, 1974. (b)

Kandel, D. B. The measurement of "ever use" and "frequency-quantity" in drug use surveys. In J. Elinson & D. N. Nurco (Eds.), *Operational definitions in socio-behavioral drug use research 1975* (National Institute on Drug Abuse, Research Monograph Series 2). Washington: U.S. Government Printing Office, 1975. (a)

Kandel, D. B. Reaching the hard-to-reach: Illicit drug use among high school absentees. *Addictive Diseases*, 1975, *1*, 465–480. (b)

Kandel, D. B. Some comments on the relationship of selected criteria variables to adolescent illicit drug use. In D. J. Lettieri (Ed.), *Predicting adolescent drug abuse: A review of issues, methods and correlates* (National Institute on Drug Abuse). Washington: U.S. Government Printing Office, 1975. (c)

Kandel, D. B. Stages in adolescent involvement in drug use. *Science*, 1975, *190*, 912–914. (d)

Kandel, D. B. Homophily, selection and socialization in adolescent friendships. *American Journal of Sociology*, in press.

Kandel, D. B., & Faust, R. Sequence and stages in patterns of adolescent drug use. *Archives of General Psychiatry*, 1975, *32*, 923–932.

Kandel, D. B., Treiman, D., Faust, R., & Single, E. Adolescent involvement in legal and illegal drug use: A multiple classification analysis. *Social Forces*, 1976, *55*, 438–458.

Kaplan, H. B. Increase in self-rejection as an antecedent of deviant responses. *Journal of Youth and Adolescence*, 1975, *4*, 281–292. (a)

Kaplan, H. B. Understanding the social and social-psychological antecedents and consequences of psychopathology: A review of reports of invitational conferences. *Journal of Health and Social Behavior*, 1975, *16*, 135–151. (b)

Kellam, S. G., Ensminger, M. E., & Turner, J. Family structure and the mental health of children. *Archives of General Psychiatry*, 1977, *34*, 1012–1022.

Kessler, R. C., Kandel, D. B., & Margulies, R. Z. *Predicting changing involvement in marihuana use: A panel analysis.* Paper presented at the meetings of the Society for the Study of Social Problems, New York City, August 1976.

Lane, E. A., & Albee, G. W. Intellectual antecedents of schizophrenia. In M. A. Roof & D. F. Ricks (Eds.), *Life history research in psychopathology* (Vol. 1). Minneapolis: University of Minnesota Press, 1970.

Lucas, W. L., Grupp, S. E., & Schmitt, R. L. Predicting who will turn on. In S. E. Grupp (Ed.), *The marihuana muddle.* Lexington, Mass.: Lexington, 1973.

Lucas, W. L., Grupp, S. E., & Schmitt, R. L. Predicting who will turn on: A four-year follow-up. *International Journal of Addictions*, 1975, *10*, 305–326.

Lukoff, I. F., & Brook, J. S. A sociocultural exploration of reported heroin use. In C. Winick (Ed.), *Sociological aspects of drug dependence.* Cleveland: CRC, 1974.

Margulies, R. Z., Kessler, R. C., & Kandel, D. B. A longitudinal study of onset of drinking among high school students. *Quarterly Journal of Studies on Alcohol*, 1977, *38*, 897–912.

McCord, J., & McCord, W. The effects of parental role models on criminology. *Journal of Social Issues*, 1958, *14*, 66–76.

McCord, W., & McCord, J. *Origins of crime.* New York: Columbia University Press, 1959.

McGlothlin, W. H., Anglin, M. D., & Wilson, B. D. *An evaluation of the California Civil Addict Program: Preliminary report.* University of California at Los Angeles, Department of Psychology, 1976. (Available in mimeo.)

Mellinger, G. D., Somers, R. H., Davidson, S. T., & Manheimer, D. I. The amotivational syndrome and the college student. *Annals of the New York Academy of Sciences*, 1976, *282*, 37–55.

Mellinger, G. D., Somers, R. H., & Manheimer, D. I. Drug use and academic attrition among university men. Paper presented at the Conference on the Social Psychology of Drug Use, Los Angeles, 1975.

National Commission on Marihuana and Drug Abuse. *Marihuana: A signal of misunderstanding* (Appendix Vols. 1,2). Washington: U.S. Government Printing Office, 1972.

National Commission on Marihuana and Drug Abuse. *Drug use in America: Problem in perspective.* Washington: U.S. Government Printing Office, 1973.

Nesselroade, J. R., & Baltes, P. B. Adolescent personality development and historical change:

1970–1972. *Monographs of the Society for Research in Child Development,* 1974, *39*(1, Serial No. 154), 1–80.

Nurco, D. N., Bonito, A. J., Lerner, M., & Balter, M. B. The natural history of narcotic addiction: A first report. In *Problems of drug dependence.* Washington: National Academy of Sciences, 1975.

O'Donnell, J. A. *Narcotic addicts in Kentucky.* Washington: U.S. Government Printing Office, 1969.

O'Donnell, J. A. Lifetime patterns of narcotic addiction. In M. A. Roff, L. N. Robins, & M. Pollack (Eds.), *Life history research in psychopathology* (Vol. 2). Minneapolis: University of Minnesota Press, 1972.

O'Malley, P. M. *Correlates and consequences of illicit drug use.* Unpublished doctoral dissertation, University of Michigan, 1975.

Paton, S., & Kandel, D. B. Psychological factors and adolescent illicit drug use: Ethnicity and sex differences. *Adolescence,* in press.

Paton, S., Kessler, R. C., & Kandel, D. B. Depressive mood and illegal drug use: A longitudinal analysis. *Journal of Genetic Psychology,* 1977, *131*, 267–289.

Ricks, D. F. Life history research in psychopathology: Retrospect and prospect. In M. A. Roff & D. F. Ricks (Eds.), *Life history research in psychopathology* (Vol. 1). Minneapolis: University of Minnesota Press, 1970.

Ricks, D. F. Life history research: Retrospect and prospect 1973. In D. F. Ricks, A. Thomas, & M. A. Roff (Eds.), *Life history research in psychopathology* (Vol. 3). Minneapolis: University of Minnesota Press, 1974.

Riley, M. W. Aging and cohort succession: Interpretations and misinterpretations. *Public Opinion Quarterly,* 1973, *37*, 35–49.

Robins, L. N. Antecedents of character disorder. In M. A. Roff, & D. F. Ricks (Eds.), *Life history research in psychopathology* (Vol. 1). Minneapolis: University of Minnesota Press, 1970. (a)

Robins, L. N. Follow-up studies investigating childhood disorders. In E. H. Hare & J. K. Wing (Eds.), *Psychiatric epidemiology.* New York: Oxford University Press, 1970. (b)

Robins, L. N. *A follow-up of Vietnam drug users* (Interim Final Report, Special Action Office Monograph, Series A, No. 1). Washington: U.S. Government Printing Office, 1973.

Robins, L. N. *The Vietnam drug user returns* (Final Report, Special Action Office Monograph, Series A, No. 2). Washington: U.S. Government Printing Office, 1974.

Robins, L. N. Drug use among Vietnam veterans—Three years later. *Medical World News— Psychiatry,* 1975, 44–49.

Robins, L. N., Davis, D. H., & Nurco, D. N. How permanent was Vietnam drug addiction? *American Journal of Public Health,* 1974, *64* (Suppl.), 38–43.

Robins, L. N., Davis, D. H., & Wish, E. Detecting predictors of rare events: Demographic, family, and personal deviance as predictors of stages in the progression toward narcotic addiction. In J. S. Strauss, H. Babigian, & M. A. Roff (Eds.), *The origins and course of psychopathology: Methods of longitudinal research.* New York: Plenum, 1977.

Roff, M. A. A two-factor approach to juvenile delinquency and the later histories of juvenile delinquents. In M. A. Roff, L. N. Robins, & M. Pollack (Eds.), *Life history research in psychopathology* (Vol. 2). Minneapolis: University of Minnesota Press, 1972.

Ryder, N. B. The cohort as a concept in the study of social change. *American Sociological Review,* 1965, *30*, 843–861.

Sadava, S. W. Initiation to cannabis use: A longitudinal social psychological study of college freshmen. *Canadian Journal of Behavioral Science,* 1973, *5*, 371–384. (a)

Sadava, S. W. Patterns of college student drug use: A longitudinal social learning study. *Psychological Reports,* 1973, *33*, 75–86. (b)

Sadava, S. W., & Forsyth, R. Drug use and a social psychology of change. *British Journal of Addictions,* 1976, *71*, 335–342.

Schaie, K. W. A general model for the study of developmental problems. *Psychological Bulletin,* 1965, *64*, 92–107.

Schuckit, M. A., Halikas, J. A., Schuckit, J. J., McClure, J., & Rimmer, J. D. Drug use and psychiatric problems on the campus: I. Methods and drug use at onset. In D. F. Ricks, A. Thomas, & M. A. Roff (Eds.), *Life history research in psychopathology* (Vol. 3). Minneapolis: University of Minnesota Press, 1974.

Smith, G. M. *Antecedents of teenage drug use.* Paper presented at the meeting of the Eastern Psychological Association, Washington, D.C., May 1973, and at the 35th Meeting of the

Committee on Problems of Drug Dependence, National Academy of Sciences, National Research Council, Chapel Hill, May 22, 1973.

Smith, G. M., & Fogg, C. P. *Early precursors of teenage drug use.* Paper presented at the 36th Meeting of the Committee on Problems of Drug Dependence, National Academy of Sciences, National Research Council, Mexico City, 1974. (a)

Smith, G. M., & Fogg, C. P. *Teenage drug use: A search for causes and consequences.* Paper presented at the 82nd Annual Convention of the American Psychological Association, New Orleans, September 1974. (b)

Smith, G. M., & Fogg, C. P. High school performance and behavior before and after initiation of illicit drug use. *Federation Proceedings,* 1976, *35*(March 1), 564.

Stephens, R., & Cottrell, E. A follow-up study of 200 narcotic addicts committed for treatment under the Narcotic Addiction Rehabilitation Act (NARA). *British Journal of the Addictions,* 1972, *67,* 45–53.

Vaillant, G. E. A twelve-year follow-up of New York narcotic addicts: Some social and psychiatric characteristics. *Archives of General Psychiatry,* 1966, *15,* 599–609.

Waldorf, D. *Careers in dope.* Englewood Cliffs, N.J.: Prentice-Hall, 1973.

Weppner, R. S., & Agar, M. H. Immediate precursors to heroin addiction. *Journal of Health and Social Behavior,* 1971, *12,* 10–17.

II

THE HIGH SCHOOL YEARS

2

Theory Testing in Longitudinal Research on Marihuana Use

Richard Jessor
Shirley L. Jessor
Institute of Behavioral Science,
University of Colorado

In this chapter, we report some findings from a longitudinal study in which junior high school and college students were followed across four annual testings. Although the objectives of the study were broad and encompassed adolescent development in general, our concern here is focused primarily on the use of marihuana and on its personality, environmental, and behavioral antecedents, correlates, and consequences. Inasmuch as the strategy of longitudinal research is the unifying theme of this volume, a few comments about our own orientation to that theme may be helpful before turning to the study itself.

The uses of longitudinal or panel research are often too narrowly—and sometimes too optimistically—construed. Increasingly, one finds the same coda at the end of articles reporting on cross-sectional research findings: an exhortation that longitudinal study is needed to determine the causal structure of the obtained associations. The narrowness lies in the restriction of interest in longitudinal design to its relevance for causal inference only; the optimism lies in the rather naive notion that causal inference is easily attainable through mere temporal extension of observation. Neither perspective seems appropriate. In addition to their potential relevance to causal concerns, panel studies are uniquely important because of the *descriptive information* they can yield about process and change: descriptions of the course of human development, of the trajectories of psychosocial growth, or of the contour of behavioral trends. Descriptive data of this sort on youth are almost nonexistent at present, and their future accumulation depends entirely upon longitudinal study. It would indeed be unfortunate, as Wohlwill (1973) cautions, if we allowed traditional preoccupation with experimental paradigms to divert us from

This chapter, written for this volume, is Publication No. 168 of the Institute of Behavioral Science. We are much indebted to Dr. John E. Donovan for his assistance with the analyses. Figures 2-1 through 2-8 are reprinted and Tables 2-1 through 2-5 and 2-7 are either reprinted or adapted from R. Jessor and S. L. Jessor, *Problem Behavior and Psychosocial Development: A Longitudinal Study of Youth.* New York: Academic, 1977. Copyright © 1977 by Academic Press. Used with permission.

efforts to describe the natural course of individual change. Another unique use of longitudinal study is for assessing the adequacy of theories that contain propositions about development and change. Such dynamic formulations are obviously dependent upon time-extended research strategies.

The main contribution of panel design to causal inference itself would appear to derive from the temporal structure it imposes upon observation. Knowledge of temporal order and sequence does permit the rejection of certain alternative inferences. But causal inference depends ultimately on logic and theory rather than on an inevitable or automatic outcome of any research design. Causal inference is a presumption that, as Blalock (1964) points out, "can never be proved beyond all doubt no matter what the nature of one's empirical evidence" (p. 3). The problem remains the enduring, elusive, and general one of how to organize observations so they will have a coercive impact on inference, how to make a particular causal interpretation so compelling as to be almost inescapable. Generally, the compellingness of an inference increases as multiple lines of evidence converge upon it and as claims for alternative inferences can be empirically refuted or weakened. In an earlier work (Jessor, R., Graves, Hanson, & Jessor, S. L., 1968/1975, pp. 137–149), we discussed a variety of strategies in cross-sectional field research for *minimizing inferential ambiguity*. Longitudinal design is a particularly advantageous strategy toward that same end, but it would seem prudent to keep in mind that it is really only one more strategy in the armamentarium of inference.

In light of this perspective, our own longitudinal research was designed to make use of a variety of different strategies all of which, if convergent, might add an increment to the compellingness of interpretation: (1) the employment of a theoretical framework and of theory-derived measures; (2) a pervasive reliance on various kinds of replication—across time, across sex, across school levels, across cohorts within a school level, and across functionally related behaviors; (3) the demonstration of systematic cross-sectional relationships preliminary to examining time-extended ones; (4) the description of change over time in both "predictor" and "criterion" measures, with reliance on the logical implications of parallel change or concomitant variations; (5) the prediction, over time, of the onset of a new behavior, with reliance on the logical implications of successful forecasting of the initial occurrence of a behavioral event; and finally, (6) the demonstration of a systematic relation between time of onset of a behavior and variation in the course of psychosocial development, with reliance on the logical implications of such direct covariation. These various strategies provide the general structure for the chapter, and each is further elaborated to make its implications clearer; it should be noted, however, that only the last three depend uniquely upon the longitudinal design of the research.

A SOCIAL–PSYCHOLOGICAL FRAMEWORK
FOR THE STUDY OF PROBLEM BEHAVIOR

The investigation of drug use in our research was part of a larger interest in exploring the utility of a social-psychological theory of problem behavior and development in youth. Formulated initially to guide a study of deviance in a triethnic community (Jessor, R., et al., 1968/1975), the framework has since been modified and extended to bear on problem behavior among youth in contemporary American society—drug use, drinking and problem drinking, sexual experience, activist protest, and general deviance including stealing, lying, and aggression (Jessor, R., 1976; Jessor, R., Collins, & Jessor, S. L., 1972; Jessor, R., & Jessor, S. L., 1973a, 1973b, 1975; Jessor, R., Jessor, S. L., & Finney, 1973; Jessor, S. L., & Jessor, R., 1974, 1975; Rohrbaugh & Jessor, R., 1975; Weigel & Jessor, R., 1973). In addition, the logical implications of the framework for adolescent development and change have also been elaborated. Because theory can increase the relevance of the observations achieved to the inferences sought, it has played a central role in our overall strategy. By enabling a behavior such as drug use to be embedded in a network of concepts, theory also makes it possible to see the logical relation to other behaviors and to variation in personality and environmental characteristics.

Because of limitations of space and because the entire social-psychological framework is extensively discussed in R. Jessor and S. L. Jessor (1977), our presentation here is fairly brief. The conceptual structure of problem-behavior theory is schematized in Figure 2-1, and our discussion follows largely from it. In this chapter, we are concerned with the three boxes of variables labeled A, B, and C: the Personality System, the Perceived Environment System, and the Behavior System, respectively. The variables in all three of the systems lie at what is essentially a social-psychological level of analysis. The concepts that constitute personality, or the person system, (values, expectations, beliefs, attitudes, orientations toward self and others) are cognitive and reflect social meanings and social experience. The concepts that constitute the environment (supports, influence, controls, models, expectations of others) are those that are amenable to logical coordination with personality concepts and that represent environmental characteristics capable of being cognized or perceived; that is, they are socially organized dimensions of potential meaning for actors. Behavior, too, is treated from a social-psychological perspective, emphasizing its socially learned purposes, functions, or significance rather than its physical parameters. The occurrence of behavior is considered the logical outcome of the interaction of personality and environmental influence; in this respect, the formulation represents a social-psychological field theory, assigning causal priority neither to person nor to situation.

Each system is composed of structures of variables interrelated and organized so as to generate a resultant: a dynamic state designated "problem-behavior proneness" that has implications for a greater or lesser likelihood of occurrence of problem behavior. Instead of tracing the rationale for the selection of the particular variables and developing the reasoning that underlies their relation to problem behavior, it must suffice here just to list the characteristics of problem-behavior proneness in each system. In the Personality System, the main characteristics of proneness to problem behavior include lower value on academic achievement; higher value on independence; greater value on independence relative to value on achievement; lower expectations for academic achievement; greater social criticism and alienation; low self-esteem and orientation to an external locus of control; greater attitudinal tolerance of deviance; lesser religiosity; and more importance attached to positive, relative to negative, functions of problem behavior. The more these personality characteristics obtain for a person at a given point in time—the more they constitute a coherent pattern, constellation, or syndrome—the more personality proneness to problem behavior they theoretically convey.

Our conceptual focus in the environment system has been on the environment as perceived, the environment of socially learned significance, the environment constituted out of "definitions of the situation" (Thomas, 1928). Logically, the

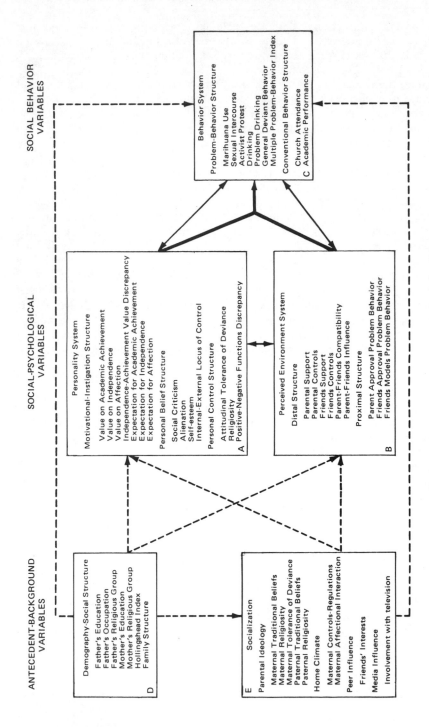

FIGURE 2-1 Conceptual structure of problem-behavior theory.

SOCIAL BEHAVIOR VARIABLES

Behavior System

Problem-Behavior Structure

Marihuana Use
Sexual Intercourse
Activist Protest
Drinking
Problem Drinking
General Deviant Behavior
Multiple Problem-Behavior Index

Conventional Behavior Structure

C Church Attendance
C Academic Performance

SOCIAL-PSYCHOLOGICAL VARIABLES

Personality System

Motivational-Instigation Structure

Value on Academic Achievement
Value on Independence
Value on Affection
Independence-Achievement Value Discrepancy
Expectation for Academic Achievement
Expectation for Independence
Expectation for Affection

Personal Belief Structure

Social Criticism
Alienation
Self-esteem
Internal-External Locus of Control

Personal Control Structure

Attitudinal Tolerance of Deviance
Religiosity
A Positive-Negative Functions Discrepancy

Perceived Environment System

Distal Structure

Parental Support
Parental Controls
Friends Support
Friends Controls
Parent-Friends Compatibility
Parent-Friends Influence

Proximal Structure

Parent Approval Problem Behavior
Friends Approval Problem Behavior
B Friends Models Problem Behavior

ANTECEDENT-BACKGROUND VARIABLES

Demography-Social Structure

Father's Education
Father's Occupation
Father's Religious Group
Mother's Education
Mother's Religious Group
Hollingshead Index
D Family Structure

E Socialization

Parental Ideology

Maternal Traditional Beliefs
Maternal Religiosity
Maternal Tolerance of Deviance
Paternal Traditional Beliefs
Paternal Religiosity

Home Climate

Maternal Controls-Regulations
Maternal Affectional Interaction

Peer Influence

Friends' Interests

Media Influence

Involvement with television

perceived environment is the one that should have the most invariant relation to behavior, as we have argued elsewhere (Jessor, R., & Jessor, S. L., 1973a). (In that same paper, incidentally, we have shown that the environment represented by demographic characteristics is conceptually so remote from behavior that the correlations of such measures with marihuana use, at least in our samples, are close to zero.) Within the perceived environment, we draw an important distinction between "regions," or structures, in terms of their proximal, versus distal, relation to behavior. Proximal variables (for example, peer models for marihuana use) directly implicate a particular behavior, whereas distal variables (for example, the degree of normative consensus between parents and peers) are more remote in the causal chain and therefore require theoretical linkage to behavior. Problem-behavior proneness in the Perceived Environment System consists of low parental support and controls; low peer controls; low compatibility between parent and peer expectations; and low parent, relative to peer, influence within the distal structure. In the proximal structure, problem-behavior proneness includes low parental disapproval of problem behavior and both high friends models for and high friends approval of engaging in problem behavior.

The Behavior System is differentiated into a problem-behavior structure and a conventional-behavior structure. *Problem behavior* refers to behavior socially defined either as a problem, as a source of concern, or as undesirable by the norms of conventional society or the institutions of adult authority; it is behavior that usually elicits some kind of social-control response. The latter, of course, may be as minimal as an expression of disapproval or as extreme as incarceration. The possibility that phenotypically very different behaviors (for example, smoking marihuana, engaging in sexual intercourse, or taking part in a peaceful demonstration) may all serve the same social-psychological function (for example, overt repudiation of conventional norms or expressing independence from parental control) is what underlies the notion of a structure of problem behavior. Research that is behavior specific, perhaps focusing on drug use alone, risks being theoretically parochial and ignores the important significance of the concept of problem behavior as one that may subtend functionally similar, mutually substitutable, even simultaneously learned, alternative social behaviors. The array of behaviors in the problem-behavior structure makes possible, not only an examination of their interrelations, but also—in providing multiple criterion variables—a more exhaustive appraisal of the explanatory capability of problem-behavior theory. Related to the making of such an appraisal is the conventional-behavior structure, which includes behaviors that should enable a demonstration of discriminant validity in the application of problem-behavior theory.

Thus far, our interest in Figure 2-1 has been cross-sectional. We have been concerned with describing problem-behavior proneness separately within the Personality and Perceived Environment Systems and, thereby, with separate linkages to the Behavior System, but as the heavy arrow connecting boxes A and B with C suggests, a further cross-sectional aim is to examine the *joint* relation between those two systems and behavior, that is, to take what we have termed the *field theoretical approach* to explanation.

Not dealt with as yet are the logical implications in problem-behavior theory for development and change, some comment on which is necessary. Although no time dimension is represented in Figure 2-1, implications for change over time can be drawn from the theory by the elaboration of the notions of age grading, age norms, and age expectations in relation to problem behavior (for a recent review of some of these considerations of age stratification and differentiation, see Elder, 1975; see also Riley, Johnson, & Foner, 1972). Neugarten and Datan (1973), in a very provocative essay, have pointed to the fact that "every society has a system of social expectations regarding age-appropriate behavior ... [and] ... individuals themselves are aware of age norms and age expectations in relation to their own patterns of timing" (pp. 59, 61). Much of what we have discussed as problem behavior is, of course, relative to age-graded norms; that is, the behavior may be permitted or even prescribed for those who are older, while being proscribed for those who are younger. Drinking, as one example, is proscribed for those under legal age but is permitted and even institutionally encouraged for those who are beyond that age; sexual intercourse, normatively acceptable for adults, is a normative departure for a young adolescent, and one that is likely to elicit social controls. Consensual awareness among youth of the age-graded norms for such behaviors carries with it, at the same time, the shared knowledge that occupancy of a more mature status is actually characterized by engaging in such behavior. Thus, engaging in certain behaviors for the *first* time can mark a transition in status from "less mature" to "more mature," from "younger" to "older," or from "adolescent" to "youth" or "adult."

Many of the important transitions that mark the course of adolescent development involve behaviors that depart from the regulatory age norms defining appropriate or expected behavior for that age or stage in life. It is important to emphasize that *behavior that departs from regulatory norms is precisely what problem-behavior theory is meant to account for,* and this becomes the basis for the systematic application of problem-behavior theory to developmental change in adolescence. By mapping the developmental concept of *transition proneness* onto the theoretical concept of *problem-behavior proneness*, it becomes possible to use problem-behavior theory to specify the likelihood of occurrence of developmental change through display of age-graded, norm-departing, transition-marking behaviors.

In summary, we have sketched out the structure and content of problem-behavior theory and its logical implications for both cross-sectional and longitudinal variation in problem behavior including the use of marihuana. Testing those implications leads us to examine both cross-sectional and panel data in accordance with the various strategies noted at the outset of the chapter. Before doing that, however, the general methodology of the research and the research design itself need to be described.

DESIGN OF THE RESEARCH

The larger research project included two parallel, but separate, short-term, longitudinal studies, one of high school youth and one of college youth. In each study, each participant was tested on four successive annual occasions so that there were four temporally ordered data points over an actual time span of 3 years. The initial data in the high school study were collected in April–May of 1969, and the final data were collected at the same point in the spring of 1972. The initial data in the college study were collected in April–May of 1970; final data, in the spring of 1973.

As part of a larger sampling design for the high school study, a random sample of 1,126 students, stratified by sex and grade level, was designated in grades 7, 8, and

9 of three junior high schools in a small city in the Rocky Mountain region. Students were contacted by letter and asked to participate in a 4-year study of personality, social, and behavioral development. Parents were also contacted by letter and asked for signed permission for their child's participation. Permission was received for 668 students and, of these, 589 (52% of the random sample) took part in the Year I testing in the spring of 1969. By the end of the Year IV testing in 1972, 483 students were still in the study, representing 82% retention of the Year I participants. Of these, there were 432 students (188 boys and 244 girls) for whom there was no missing year of data. It is this latter group that constitutes our high school core sample for longitudinal or developmental analyses, and it is this sample on which the high school data presented in this chapter are based. The sample is actually composed of six separate, sex-by-grade cohorts as of 1969: seventh-grade males ($N = 75$), seventh-grade females ($N = 96$), eighth-grade males ($N = 60$), eighth-grade females ($N = 82$), ninth-grade males ($N = 53$), and ninth-grade females ($N = 66$). By the final year in 1972, these students—initially all in junior high school—had reached senior high school and were in grades 10, 11, and 12.

The core sample, then, represents good retention (73%) of the initial-year participants over four annual testings; it provides a wide range of variation on all measures; and it is large enough to permit the kinds of breakdowns needed for the analyses reported later on in the chapter. Although generalization to the parent population is precluded by the fact that the core sample constitutes only 38% of the original random sample, the core sample is, nonetheless, satisfactory for the testing of hypotheses about variation in behavior and development. Demographically, the core sample is relatively homogeneous: almost entirely Anglo-American in ethnic background and middle class in socioeconomic status.

Data were collected in April–May of each year by an elaborate questionnaire, approximately 50 pages in length, requiring about an hour and a half to complete. The questionnaire consisted largely of psychometrically developed scales or indexes assessing the variety of personality, social, behavioral, and demographic variables shown in the conceptual framework in Figure 2-1. Although many of the measures derive from and were validated in previous work (for example, Jessor, R., et al., 1968/1975), prior to its present use, the entire questionnaire was pretested and scales were revised to increase their appropriateness for the student samples. The majority of scales were kept constant over the testing years, but modifications were made in some, and new ones were added at various times. Administration of the questionnaires took place in small group sessions outside of class, and strict confidentiality was guaranteed because questionnaires had to be signed to permit follow-up.

For the college study, a random sample of 497 freshman students was designated in the College of Arts and Sciences of a university in the same Rocky Mountain city. When contacted by letter in the spring of 1970 and asked to participate in the research over the next four years, 462 students were still in school. Of those contacted, 276 (60%) participated in the spring 1970 initial testing. By the end of the Year IV testing in 1973, 226 students were still in the study, and 205 of these had no missing year of data. The latter group (92 men and 113 women) constitutes the core developmental sample in the college study; the members represent 41% of the original random sample and 74% of the participants who had been tested in the freshman year.

Dropping out of school or moving away from the community were negligible in the high school study. In the college core sample, by 1973, 64% were still at the same university, 20% were at another university, and 16% had dropped out of school at some point and not returned, even though remaining in the study.

In the college study, data were also collected by questionnaires, administered in small group sessions, with confidentiality guaranteed. The questionnaire was very similar to that used in the high school, and many of the scales were, in fact, identical. Table 2-1 lists most of the major scales reported on in this chapter; it shows the number of items in each scale, the possible score range, Scott's homogeneity ratio (about .33 is considered optimal), and Cronbach's alpha reliability for both the high school and the college studies. For the most part, especially where scales have more than a few items, measurement properties are quite satisfactory.

Interest in the study was high among both the high school and the college students, and the quality of the questionnaire data is generally excellent. Participants seemed especially to appreciate the comprehensiveness of the questionnaire and its coverage of a wide range of content. Analyses of the attrition subsequent to the initial year of testing indicate that those who left the study were very similar on their initial-year data in both studies to those who stayed. Thus, selective dropout from the studies does not seem to be a source of additional bias beyond the original erosion from the designated random samples.

Several features of the research design are worth emphasizing in relation to the methodological orientation of the study as a whole. The first and most apparent one is the provision made for pervasive replication of observations and findings. For example, in both the high school study and the college study, there is opportunity to carry out four, separate, annual cross-sectional tests of the explanatory usefulness of the social-psychological framework. In addition, within any year, findings can be replicated across sexes, across age or grade groups, and across the two different school contexts. Considering the six sex-by-grade cohorts in the high school study and the two sex cohorts in the college study, there are actually eight independent subsamples in which any theoretical relationship may be separately examined. The possibility for such replication over time and across samples lessens the likelihood that findings would reflect the vicissitudes of a particular testing year or that the idiosyncrasies of a particular sample would be given more credence than deserved. Second, the previously noted descriptive interest in psychosocial development can obviously be pursued by following the cohorts through time with repeated measures. Third, the design makes possible the testing of the predictive implications of the theory by permitting the accumulation of data temporally antecedent to the event being predicted, for example, the initial use of marihuana among those who had not begun using it until after the Year I testing. The fourth and final feature worth mentioning, as it is not obvious in the structure of the design, is the role played by the theory in the content of the measures employed. Most of the major measures were theoretically derived to capture the logical properties of the concepts in the framework; as such, they make the data they yield germane to the testing of the theory in a way that ad hoc measures usually do not.

With this discussion in mind, we can turn to the presentation of specifically selected data from the overall longitudinal project. The presentation of data is organized around the several inferential strategies already listed. The strategy of reliance upon theory serves throughout as the background against which the data constitute the figure. The strategy of replication is illustrated in the context of the other strategies. Thus, we can begin with the first strategy that refers to a particular analytic mode: the analysis of cross-sectional relationships.

CROSS-SECTIONAL ANALYSIS AS PART OF A LONGITUDINAL STRATEGY

Because the appraisal of theoretical expectations on the basis of cross-sectional data is the conventional practice in most studies, a word should be said about our inclusion of this kind of analysis as part of a set of strategies in longitudinal research. If the research enterprise itself can be looked at as a developmental process through time, it might be argued that the establishment of cross-sectional relationships should be an ontogenetically prior stage to the investigation of time-extended relationships. The latter, precisely because of the time dimension involved, is likely to be a much more refractory and uncertain endeavor than the former. The prior demonstration that the relationships sought do indeed obtain at a cross section in time constitutes the kind of preliminary step to longitudinal inquiry that can provide the latter with both rationale and focus. Support for the cross-sectional utility of the theory serves, in short, to make its longitudinal appraisal a logical next step (and in any case, cross-sectional analyses offer the fringe benefit of giving the longitudinal researcher something to do while waiting for time to pass).

Our focus in this section is on a measure of increasing involvement with marihuana—the marihuana behavior involvement scale—and on marihuana user versus nonuser status. The marihuana behavior involvement scale includes four items:

1. Have you ever tried marihuana? (Never___ Once___ More than once___)
2. Have you ever been very high or stoned on marihuana to the point where you were pretty sure you had experienced the drug's effects? (Never___ Once___ More than once___)
3. Do you or someone very close to you usually keep a supply of marihuana so that it's available when you want to use it? (No___ Yes___)
4. Do you use marihuana a couple of times a week or more when it's available? (No___ Yes___)

Data on this measure from the 1970 testing in both the high school and college were reported in R. Jessor, S. L. Jessor, and Finney (1973); the data considered here are from the Year IV (1972) testing in the high school study, and they are presented in Tables 2-2 and 2-3.

The data in the first column of Table 2-2 are correlations of the measures in the three structures of the Personality System with the measure of marihuana behavior involvement, for males and females separately. Support for the hypothesized personality-behavior linkage (the arrow, in Figure 2-1, between box A and box C) is clear and quite pervasive. The strongest and most consistent relations between personality and marihuana involvement are those of the measures of the personal control structure, every one of which is significantly associated, and some of which are substantial in magnitude. Adolescents who are more intolerant of deviance and more religious have lesser involvement with marihuana. In the three areas of drinking, drug use, and sex, the more that importance is attached to positive, relative to negative, functions of these behaviors, the lower the control these functions exert and the greater the involvement with marihuana. Drug disjunctions, the most

TABLE 2-1 Scale Properties of the Year IV Measures in the High School Study (1972) and College Study (1973) Questionnaires

	High school study				College study			
Measures	Number of items	Score range	Scott's H.R.	Cronbach's alpha	Number of items	Score range	Scott's H.R.	Cronbach's alpha
	Personality System							
Motivational-instigation structure								
Value on academic achievement	10	0–90	.53	.91	10	0–90	.48	.90
Value on independence	10	0–90	.35	.84	10	0–90	.28	.78
Value on affection	10	0–90	.41	.87	10	0–90	.45	.89
Expectation for academic achievement	10	0–90	.57	.92	10	0–90	.49	.90
Expectation for independence	10	0–90	.36	.85	10	0–90	.21	.71
Expectation for affection	10	0–90	.42	.88	10	0–90	.48	.90
Personal belief structure								
Social criticism	9	9–45	.20	.69	13	13–52	.30	.85
Alienation	15	15–60	.23	.81	15	15–60	.23	.81
Self-esteem	10	10–40	.29	.80	10	10–40	.33	.83
Internal–external control	22	22–110	.13	.77	18	18–90	.15	.76
Personal control structure								
Tolerance of deviance	26	0–234	.36	.93	20	0–180	.36	.92
Religiosity	7	0–28	.55	.89	5	4–20	.49	.82

Perceived Environment System

Distal structure								
Parental support	2	2–10	.56	.71	2	2–10	.59	.74
Parental controls	2	2–10	.46	.62	2	2–10	.41	.58
Friends support	2	2–10	.52	.68	2	2–10	.59	.73
Friends controls	2	2–10	.16	.28	2	2–10	.34	.51
Parent–friends compatibility	3	3–15	.56	.79	3	3–15	.56	.79
Parent–friends influence	2	2–6	.47	.64	2	2–6	.44	.61
Proximal structure								
Parent approval problem behavior	4	a	.33	.66	4	a	.22	.53
Friends approval problem behavior	4	a	.28	.61	4	a	.26	.58
Friends models problem behavior	3	a	.45	.71	4	a	.27	.59

Behavior System

Problem-behavior structure								
Marihuana behavior involvement	4	0–8	.65	.88	4	0–8	.52	.81
General deviant behavior	26	26–104	.21	.85	20	20–80	.16	.74
Multiple problem-behavior index	5	0–5	.28	.66	5	0–5	.13	.43

[a] These scale scores are the sum of z scores from separate subscales. In the high school study, a constant of 11.0 was added to the z-score sums.

TABLE 2-2 Pearson Correlations between Personality System Measures and Selected Behavior System Measures in the High School Study, Year IV (1972)

Personality System measures	Behavior System measures					
	Marihuana behavior involvement		Deviant behavior in past year		Church attendance in past year	
	Male[a]	Female[b]	Male[a]	Female[b]	Male[a]	Female[b]
Motivational-instigation structure						
Value on academic achievement	−.27***	−.31***	−.21**	−.39***	.10	.24***
Value on independence	.09	.19**	.09	.13	−.21**	−.08
Value on affection	−.22**	−.19**	−.02	−.13	−.01	.17*
Independence-achievement value discrepancy	.31***	.39***	.24**	.44***	−.23**	−.27***
Expectation for academic achievement	−.16*	−.14*	−.28***	−.29***	−.04	.09
Expectation for independence	.06	.23***	.08	.11	−.21**	−.24***
Expectation for affection	−.12	.01	.02	−.05	−.12	.02
Personal belief structure						
Social criticism	.33***	.35***	.19*	.18**	−.11	−.21**
Alienation	.08	.08	.09	.14*	−.08	−.05
Self-esteem	.10	.08	.10	−.05	−.19*	−.04
Internal–external control	−.17*	−.06	−.27***	−.12	.03	.10
Personal control structure						
Tolerance of deviance	−.41***	−.40***	−.61***	−.57***	.18*	.22**
Religiosity	−.27***	−.31***	−.17*	−.27***	.58***	.48***
Drinking disjunctions	.16*	.18**	.22**	.31***	.02	−.10
Drug disjunctions	.58***	.64***	.27***	.44***	−.10	−.36***
Sex disjunctions	.28***	.38***	.35***	.37***	−.22**	−.32***

[a]$N = 188$.
[b]$N = 244$.
*$p \leqslant .05$.
**$p \leqslant .01$.
***$p \leqslant .001$.

proximal of the three functions-disjunction measures, has, as expected, the strongest relation to marihuana use. Of importance to note is the comparability of these personal-control findings for males and females.

Next in importance in accounting for involvement with marihuana are the motivational-instigation measures. The strongest correlation for both sexes is the independence-achievement value discrepancy; as expected, the more independence is valued relative to the value on academic achievement, the greater the involvement with marihuana. This finding is supported by the negative correlations with the measures of value on achievement and expectation for achievement, and also by the positive correlations (females only) with value on independence and expectation for independence. Finally, among the measures of personal beliefs, social criticism is positively associated with marihuana use, and consistently so for both sexes, but neither alienation nor self-esteem demonstrates any relationship at all.

Overall, as far as the link between personality and marihuana involvement is concerned, there is evidence for the conclusions that personality characteristics play a modest but significant role, and that the pattern of relations is similar for both males and females. Before turning to the perceived environment, it is of interest to examine the remaining data in Table 2-2. Another problem-behavior measure has been presented to illustrate the generality of the linkage between personality and problem behavior, and a measure of conventional behavior has been presented for discriminant validity. The measure of deviant behavior in the past year focuses on what might be called "conventional deviance," that is, lying, stealing, and aggression. None of the items has any reference at all to drug use, alcohol, sex, or protest. The pattern of findings is similar to that for the marihuana measure: The strongest relations are with the personal control measures (tolerance of deviance, now the most proximal to this criterion, has the largest correlation); the motivational-instigation measures, especially independence-achievement value discrepancy, are the next strongest; the personal belief measures are least related (interestingly, social criticism is substantially less associated with this criterion measure than it was with marihuana use). The pattern of relations is, once again, generally similar for both sexes. This introduction of another problem-behavior criterion measure makes it clear that the linkage between personality and marihuana use is not behavior specific, and this is a very important contribution to the explanatory effort.

The correlations in Table 2-2 with the frequency of church attendance in the past year add to our conviction about the adequacy of the measures and the theoretical formulation. The key personality measures relate to this measure of conventional behavior in a direction opposite to their relation to the two problem-behavior measures, as would be expected theoretically.

In Table 2-3, the high school data are presented for the measures of the Perceived Environment System in relation to the same three behavioral criteria. There is consistent and even substantial support for the hypothesized environment-behavior linkage (represented by the arrow, in Figure 2-1, between box B and box C). With respect to the marihuana involvement criterion, the expected prepotency of the proximal environment is apparent, with the two measures that refer to the peer reference group—friends approval for and friends models of problem behavior—having correlations of considerable magnitude for both sexes. The measures in the distal structure are also of interest; the more a supportive relation with parents is perceived, the less the involvement with marihuana. The measures of perceived compatibility or agreement between parents and friends and of the relative influence of these two different reference groups are particularly revealing: the less the compatibility and the greater the relative influence of friends, the greater the involvement with marihuana. Both of these measures suggest, other things being equal, that the developmental move out of the family context and into the peer context, either into incompatible peer expectations or into greater peer influence, is associated with an increase in behavior that departs from the norms of adult society, in this case, marihuana use.

The data for the deviant behavior and the church attendance measures play the same role they did in the preceding table. Relationships of the perceived environment measures to deviant behavior are comparable to their relationships with marihuana use, although not as strong, and are again similar for both sexes. With regard to church attendance, the expected opposite relations are apparent, especially in the proximal structure.

The cross-sectional data thus far presented have been correlational and focused

TABLE 2-3 Correlations between Measures of the Perceived Environment System and Selected Behavior System Measures in the High School Study, Year IV (1972)

Perceived Environment System measures	Behavior-system measures					
	Marihuana behavior involvement		Deviant behavior in past year		Church attendance in past year	
	Male[a]	Female[b]	Male[a]	Female[b]	Male[a]	Female[b]
Distal structure						
Parental support	−.31***	−.21**	−.28***	−.13	−.04	.11
Parental controls	−.15*	−.07	−.04	−.01	.18*	.09
Friends support	.00	.13	−.11	.14*	−.01	−.02
Friends controls	−.43***	−.35***	−.24**	−.22**	.19*	.20**
Parent–friends compatibility	−.31***	−.33***	−.25***	−.25***	.08	.17*
Parent–friends influence	.29***	.18**	.16*	.25***	−.02	−.19**
Proximal structure						
Parent approval problem behavior	.34***	.28***	.19*	.04	−.28***	−.29***
Friends approval problem behavior	.55***	.60***	.36***	.49***	−.32***	−.32***
Friends models problem behavior	.60***	.61***	.44***	.52***	−.22**	−.26***

[a]$N = 188$.
[b]$N = 244$.
*$p \leqslant .05$.
**$p \leqslant .01$.
***$p \leqslant .001$.

on a particular measure of marihuana involvement. That measure, marihuana behavior involvement, has been used throughout our research and in a national-sample survey of high school youth as well. As noted earlier, the measure includes items referring to getting high or stoned and to safeguarding a supply, as well as to frequency of use; in these respects, therefore, it differs from the use, versus nonuse, measure employed in most other research. The measure of marihuana behavior involvement has shown excellent Guttman-scale properties in both the present study and the national-sample study. Nevertheless, to make clear that the findings are stable and are not dependent on the particularities of a measure or statistic, another kind of analysis is presented in Tables 2-4 and 2-5. Here the participants in the high school study are divided by use status, *users* being those reporting at least more than once use of marihuana. Mean differences between nonusers and users on the various theoretical measures are evaluated by analysis of variance. An examination of the personality data in Table 2-4 and of the perceived environment data in Table 2-5 makes clear both their consistency with the correlational data on the somewhat different marihuana involvement measure presented earlier and their similarity for both sexes.

The final concern of the cross-sectional strategy is one that follows from the fact that the theoretical framework illustrated in Figure 2-1 is based upon a multivariate logic. The logic of each of the systems rests upon the joint operation of its component structures and variables, and the logic of the framework as a whole rests upon the joint contribution of the separate systems. To pursue these implications,

TABLE 2-4 Mean Scores of Nonusers and Users of Marihuana on Personality System Measures in the High School Study, Year IV (1972)

	Males		Females	
Personality System measures	Nonusers $(N = 117)$	Users[a] $(N = 68)$	Nonusers $(N = 148)$	Users[a] $(N = 95)$
Motivational-instigation structure				
Value on academic achievement	68.2	58.4***	67.6	53.7***
Value on independence	72.7	74.1	76.0	78.8*
Value on affection	66.4	59.0**	71.2	65.4**
Independence-achievement value discrepancy	94.5	105.6***	98.4	115.1***
Expectation for academic achievement	60.5	54.2*	59.2	51.0**
Expectation for independence	70.3	70.7	73.1	77.4**
Expectation for affection	58.3	54.3	60.5	59.9
Personal belief structure				
Social criticism	27.8	31.8***	29.7	32.7***
Alienation	34.6	36.1	35.3	36.6
Self-esteem	29.7	30.1	30.0	30.3
Internal–external control	61.7	58.4**	62.3	61.6
Personal control structure				
Tolerance of deviance	162.7	133.7***	176.9	151.8***
Religiosity	15.1	11.0***	17.4	12.5***
Drinking disjunctions	31.6	34.0	27.8	31.6*
Drug disjunctions	17.1	27.0***	15.5	28.4***
Sex disjunctions	18.9	21.1*	13.2	18.3***

[a]Asterisks refer to the level of significance of the difference between the nonuser and user mean scores by one-way analysis of variance, two-tail test.
*$p \leqslant .05$.
**$p \leqslant .01$.
***$p \leqslant .001$.

TABLE 2-5 Mean Scores of Nonusers and Users of Marihuana on Measures of Perceived Environment System in the High School Study, Year IV (1972)

	Males		Females	
Perceived Environment System measures	Nonusers $(N = 117)$	Users[a] $(N = 68)$	Nonusers $(N = 148)$	Users[a] $(N = 95)$
Distal structure				
Parental support	7.7	6.5***	7.8	7.1**
Parental controls	6.4	5.6**	6.0	5.5
Friends support	6.7	6.6	7.6	8.0
Friends controls	6.4	5.3**	6.7	5.7***
Parent–friends compatibility	8.5	7.3**	9.0	7.2***
Parent–friends influence	3.2	3.7**	3.4	3.9*
Proximal structure				
Parent approval problem behavior	10.4	12.4***	10.3	11.8***
Friends approval problem behavior	10.0	12.6***	9.8	13.1***
Friends models problem behavior	9.6	12.4***	10.0	13.2***

[a]Asterisks refer to the level of significance of the difference between the nonuser and user mean scores by one-way analysis of variance, two-tail test.
*$p \leqslant .05$.
**$p \leqslant .01$.
***$p \leqslant .001$.

we have relied upon multiple regression analyses carried out in what we have termed a *uniform multivariate analysis procedure*. This procedure involves a standard set of 14 multiple regressions run against each criterion measure for each sample in each study, both for a key data year and for a replication year. The 14 regressions are organized in sequential, cumulative sets to make possible an examination of the multivariate account achieved by each set of variables independently and prior to its inclusion with other sets of variables. In addition, not all the variables in the framework are used in the various sets and, as sets are cumulated, only certain variables of key theoretical interest are carried along, while others are dropped. Thus, the aims of the uniform multivariate analysis procedure are (1) to maintain the focus on the theoretical concerns by restricting the number of variables used and by examining the theoretical structures separately and (2) to appraise the magnitude of the variance in the criterion measures that can be accounted for by the joint influence of the components in the framework. Greater detail about the procedure and the specific variables used appears in R. Jessor and S. L. Jessor (1977, pp. 127–142). For present purposes, we rely on the information provided in Table 2-6.

The data in Table 2-6 are multiple correlations for the 14 separate runs against the marihuana behavior involvement scale. The table shows the replications of the multiple regressions across the two sexes and in both the high school study and the college study for their Year IV data. In parentheses are the comparable multiple correlations from the replications on the Year III data. From this array of replications, it is possible to get a sense of the stability and generality of the findings as well as some conviction about the general amount of variance for which the different sets of variables and the overall framework can account.

There is a great deal of information in Table 2-6, only a portion of which can be addressed in this context. Consider the males in the high school study for example. The Personality System run, which includes five variables, achieves an $R = .52$. This is an increase over the highest bivariate correlation of its best component, namely, the .41 correlation of tolerance of deviance with marihuana involvement. The run for the Perceived Environment System for the males yields an $R = .65$, which is higher than the .60 bivariate correlation of its strongest component, friends models for problem behavior. The field pattern, combining personality and environment, does not, in this case, yield a larger R than the environment alone. The overall set, a combination of 14 selected personality, perceived environment, behavioral, and socioeconomic-background variables (out of the 24 that are used in the procedure), yields a multiple R of .76, indicating that a substantial amount of variance in the marihuana involvement criterion—over 50%—is accounted for by the problem behavior framework.

The consistency of the major multiple Rs is noteworthy across sexes, across data years, and even across the two studies. For example, the eight separate multiple Rs for the overall set are all fairly close together. They all generate R^2s that account for about 50% of the criterion variance. Cross-sectional support for the utility of the framework, in relation to marihuana involvement, appears strong; but further strengthening comes from two additional considerations. First, when the uniform multivariate analysis procedure is applied, within the high school study, to the six sex-by-grade cohorts (rather than to the combined males and the combined females as in Table 2-6), the Rs for the overall set against the marihuana criterion are .81, .79, and .81 for 10th-, 11th-, and 12th-grade males, respectively, and .79, .85, and

TABLE 2-6 Multiple Correlations of the Theoretical Structures and Systems with Marihuana Behavior Involvement in the High School Study, Year IV (1972), and College Study, Year IV (1973)

	High school study		College study	
Multivariate run	Male $(N = 188)$	Female $(N = 244)$	Male $(N = 92)$	Female $(N = 113)$
1. Motivational-instigation	.31	.39	[g]	.25[h]
2. Personal belief	.35	.36	.40	.42
3. Personal control	.45	.44	.41	.36
4. Personality System[a]	.52 (.49)[f]	.54 (.45)	.40 (.48)	.43 (.51)
5. Distal structure	.42	.37	.22	.35
6. Proximal structure	.66	.66	.56	.64
7. Perceived Environment System[b]	.65 (.59)	.64 (.61)	.54 (.44)	.60 (.70)
8. Field pattern[c]	.65 (.60)	.68 (.59)	.57 (.55)	.61 (.70)
9. Aggregate set[d]	.70	.70	.69	.69
10. Functions discrepancy	.59	.64	.45	.56
11. Behavior	.60	.61	.49	.43
12. Functions-behavior	.72	.71	.56	.59
13. Socioeconomic background	[g]	.16	[g]	[g]
14. Overall set[e]	.76 (.71)	.77 (.70)	.67 (.70)	.68 (.77)

Note. All runs are stepwise regressions with an F-to-enter of 2.0 and an F-to-delete of 1.0. The names for the runs refer to the theoretical structures and systems shown in Figure 2-1.

[a]Run 4, Personality System, is a selection of the five theoretically most important variables from the nine variables in Runs 1, 2, and 3.

[b]Run 7, Perceived Environment System, is a selection of the four theoretically most important variables from Runs 5 and 6.

[c]Run 8, Field pattern, is a selection of six variables from those in Runs 4 and 7.

[d]Run 9, Aggregate set, includes all 16 of the variables used in Runs 1, 2, 3, 5, and 6, and thus it serves to maximize the R^2 as against the theoretically focused R^2 yielded by Run 8.

[e]Run 14, Overall set, adds selected behavior and functions and demographic measures to the variables included in Run 8 and reflects the contribution of more of the domains in the larger conceptual framework shown in Figure 2-1.

[f]Rs in parentheses are the comparable multiple correlations from the replication analyses of the Year III data in the high school and Year II data in the college.

[g]None of the variables in the set entered significantly.

[h]This multiple correlation does not reach an F value that is significant at the .05 level or better; all correlations without this symbol are significant at the .05 level or better.

.74 for the 10th-, 11th-, and 12th-grade females, respectively. Thus, the utility of the theory is apparent also at the specific cohort level. Second, when a different marihuana criterion is considered—a direct measure of frequency of use of marihuana in the past 6 months—the multiple Rs for the overall set are .63, .52, .63, and .48 for high school males, high school females, college males, and college females, respectively. Although considerably lower, these Rs are still significant and substantial, and they reflect a degree of robustness of the framework over alternative criterion measures in the drug use domain. It is of further interest in this regard to report the multivariate data from a recent national-sample survey of junior–senior high school youth that included many of our predictor measures. For a sample of over 6,000 males and over 6,000 females, the multivariate run equivalent to our overall set yielded multiple correlations against marihuana behavior involvement of .74 and .75, respectively (see Chase & Jessor, R., 1977).

The data in this section make a strong case for the cross-sectional utility of problem-behavior theory in relation to involvement with marihuana use. With these considerations serving as groundwork, it is now possible to turn to the first of three specifically longitudinal strategies for inference.

DESCRIPTION OF CHANGE AS PART
OF A LONGITUDINAL STRATEGY

The paucity of descriptive knowledge about the social-psychological growth of adolescents seriously limits efforts at understanding the nature of problem behavior. In our own work, considerable attention has been given to establishing how the variables in the theory change over time, to describing their trajectories, and to plotting "growth curves" of personality, environmental, and behavioral attributes during this developmental period. Establishing the fact that change takes place and the shape of its course, while important in its own right, has the additional advantage of providing a strategy, albeit an indirect one, for testing the developmental adequacy of problem-behavior theory. That strategy rests upon the theoretical expectation that there should be a *consonance* between the developmental changes occurring in the personality and the perceived environment measures—the "predictors"—on the one hand, and the behavior measures—the "criteria"—on the other. Such a developmental consonance, the congruence of theoretically parallel change, would constitute initial support for the relevance of the explanatory variables to behavioral development.

The implementation of this strategy can be accomplished by presenting, in graphic form, the changes on the measures of a few selected variables over the time span of the research. In Figure 2-2, the scores on the measure of value on academic achievement over the four annual testings are presented for the six sex-by-grade cohorts in the high school study. The most striking aspect of the six trajectories is their decline over the years; all the declines are statistically significant as indicated both by one-way analyses of variance across time and by matched-sample t tests of the difference, for each cohort, between its Year I and its Year IV mean score (the only exception is the ninth-grade female cohort, which declines significantly to 1971 but then increases). The consistency of these curves suggests a developmental lessening of the importance attached to academic achievement during the adolescent years. Given our theoretical interpretation of value on academic achievement as conventionally oriented motivation, this developmental trend is in a direction away from conventionality; it implies, instead, a higher problem-behavior proneness with development during adolescence.

The same data can be plotted against age to yield an age-related picture of the developmental changes in value on academic achievement in the various cohorts, over the age span of 13 to 18 in the high school study. This has been done in Figure 2-3, and the college study data have also been added to include the entire age range covered by our research. Looked at with a smoothing eye, there is a best-fitting line that suggests a clear developmental decline in value on academic achievement through the adolescent period from 13 to 18, with a possible leveling out near the end. Although the college sample is not really comparable to the high school samples, it is of interest to see that the college males and females start out not very different from where the high school cohorts finish, and they continue the leveling out suggested by the latter.

Plotting the data for value on independence would show a significant increase

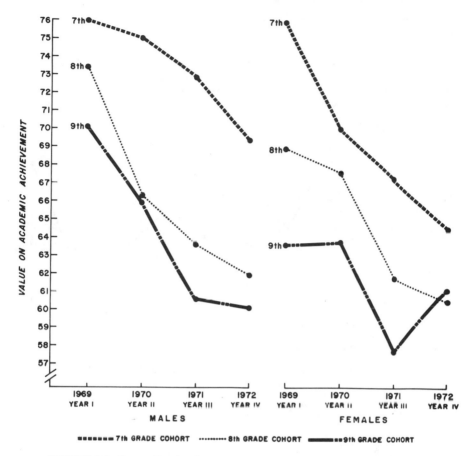

FIGURE 2-2 Personality development during adolescence in the high school study.

for the cohorts over time. Because higher value on independence is, theoretically, a problem-prone motivational orientation, these changes are also in the direction of an increased likelihood of problem behavior with adolescent development. Thus, the decline in value on academic achievement and the increase in value on independence are consonant in their implications for problem behavior. The developmental changes in attitudinal tolerance of deviance (a variable in the personal control structure) show a consistent decline in intolerance for both sexes. This increased acceptance of transgression is also theoretically consonant with the directions of the two previously discussed personality attributes.

Turning to the perceived environment, we have argued elsewhere (Jessor, R., & Jessor, S. L., 1973a) that it makes sense to conceive of growth curves for attributes of the perceived environment in the same way as for attributes of personality or ability. A similar point has been made by Nesselroade and Baltes (1974) in relation to their concept of *environmental ontogeny*. We have selected one attribute from the proximal structure to illustrate development in the perceived environment. In Figure 2-4, the data on perceived friends models for drinking are plotted for the combined high school males and the combined high school females. A highly signifi-

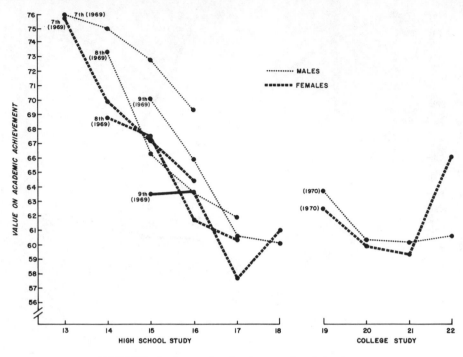

FIGURE 2-3 Personality development in relation to age.

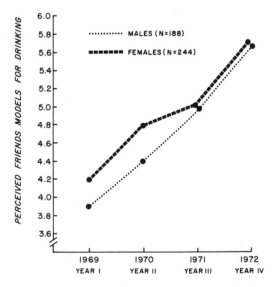

FIGURE 2-4 Perceived environment development
during adolescence in the high school study.

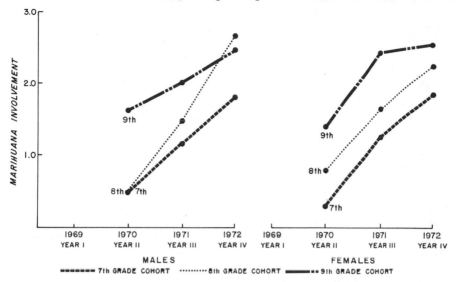

FIGURE 2-5 Behavior development during adolescence in the high school study.

cant increase in the perceived prevalence of drinking among friends is evident in the curves for both sexes over the four measurements. This measure and others suggest that, ontogenetically, the proximal environment becomes more approving of problem behavior and provides more models for it over time. Such environmental changes are, theoretically, in the direction of greater proneness toward problem behavior. These environmental trends are, therefore, fully consonant with those discussed earlier for personality.

In order to examine whether these trends are actually consonant with the expected increase in problem behavior during adolescence, we have plotted the marihuana behavior involvement scores for each cohort over the three years in which it was measured. Figure 2-5 clearly shows that a significant increase in marihuana involvement does occur for all cohorts. The same data are plotted against age in Figure 2-6, and the college study data are also included. Once again,

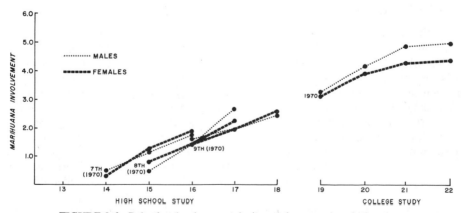

FIGURE 2-6 Behavior development during adolescence in relation to age.

an age-related developmental trend toward increased involvement with marihuana seems very apparent. These developmental increases in marihuana use are entirely consonant, theoretically, with the developmental changes noted above in the personality and perceived environment predictors. The marihuana-use changes are themselves supported by other behavioral trends not illustrated here, for example, a significant developmental increase in deviant behavior and a significant developmental decline in church attendance.

There are two issues relevant to the interpretation of these changes that are discussed in detail in our book (Jessor, R., & Jessor, S. L., 1977) but which can only be noted here. First, there is the question of the adequacy of the measures for representing developmental change. Stability coefficients were computed for all measures over the three 1-year intervals and over the one 3-year interval; in general, temporal stability is satisfactory for a time interval of the length of a year, especially where scales have more than a few items. Second, there is the question of whether the changes simply reflect a repeated testing effect. In the absence of an untested control group, we have to seek to minimize this alternative inference on other grounds. Of interest here is the fact that Nesselroade and Baltes (1974), in a recent related study, did employ such a control; and they conclude for their data that "by and large, the longitudinal gradients of personality dimensions are not contaminated by . . . testing . . . effect" (p. 38). Further, the actual content of the developmental changes they observed are, in several instances, comparable to those reported here, for example, a decrement in superego strength and in achievement and an increase in independence.

Description of change as part of a longitudinal strategy for inference appears to permit the following conclusion: There is an evident developmental consonance between the changes observed in the personality and perceived environment systems on the one hand, and in the behavior system on the other. These theoretically parallel changes would seem to provide support, although indirect, for the developmental utility of problem-behavior theory. At the same time, and more specifically, they call attention to the variables that are likely to be relevant to changes in marihuana involvement.

FORECASTING OF ONSET AS PART
OF A LONGITUDINAL STRATEGY

In the preceding strategy, it was possible to establish that changes do occur over time on the variables in the framework and to establish the direction of those changes, but it was not possible to establish a time lag between any of the changes. It is toward the latter objective that the present strategy is directed. Forecasting is a procedure that does incorporate a time lag, inasmuch as a temporally subsequent event is predicted on the basis of temporally antecedent information. A particularly compelling implementation of such a procedure would seem to be the forecasting of the initial appearance of an event or, in our terms, the onset of a new behavior. In the present context, we consider the onset of marihuana use.

The approach pursued was to establish three groups of students on the basis of their status as users or nonusers of marihuana in Years III and IV of the high school study. One group consisted of nonusers in Year III who remained nonusers in Year IV, that is, a no-onset group; a second group consisted of nonusers in Year III who became users by the Year IV testing, that is, an onset group; and a third group consisted of those who were users already in Year III, that is, a group that had experienced onset previously. By comparing the first two groups on their data in Year III when both were nonusers, it is possible to ascertain whether they differ in what we have defined as "transition proneness," namely a temporally antecedent pattern signaling a readiness to engage in transition-marking behavior. In evaluating differential transition proneness in the two groups, a reference standard is provided by the group that had begun use prior to Year III. The high school study data relevant to this analysis are presented in Table 2-7.

There is clear support in Table 2-7 for the predictive utility of the theoretical concept of transition proneness, and in that regard, these findings replicate an earlier analysis made of the Years I–II onset and described in R. Jessor, S. L. Jessor, & Finney (1973). The results are stronger and more consistent for the females than for the males, though support is present for both sexes. Those females who were nonusers in Year III, but who began marihuana use by Year IV, differ from the nonusers in Year III who remained nonusers by Year IV on a variety of theoretical attributes measured in Year III. They had significantly lower value on academic achievement; higher value on independence; higher value on independence relative to value on achievement; higher expectations for independence; higher alienation; greater tolerance of deviance; greater positive, relative to negative, functions for drinking, drugs, and sex; less parental support; less parent–friends compatibility; greater friends, relative to parents, influence; greater friends approval of and friends models for problem behavior; and greater general deviant behavior. Several other measures, for example, expectations for academic achievement and religiosity, while not significantly different, yield mean scores that are also in the theoretically expected direction. The pattern is pervasive and consistent. The Year-III mean scores of the group that will initiate in the subsequent year are, in almost every case, intermediate between the mean of the group that will not initiate and the mean of the group that had previously initiated. For the high school females, then, this analysis indicates the existence of a temporally prior pattern of attributes that constitutes a readiness to engage in transition-marking behavior, in this case the use of marihuana, and that signals a higher likelihood of its onset. The content of the pattern is similar to the content that emerged from the cross-sectional analyses of the differences between marihuana users and nonusers reported earlier in Tables 2-4 and 2-5.

The results for the high school males, while considerably weaker than they were for the previously reported Years I–II analysis, do indicate transition-proneness differences in the personal-control structure and, especially, in the proximal structure of the perceived environment. Similar analyses for the onset of other behaviors, such as beginning to drink and engaging in sexual intercourse, also provide strong evidence that measures antedating onset are predictive of its prospective occurrence among high school youth. When multiple regression analyses were run for the overall set of predictors in Year III against the dichotomous criterion of onset, versus no onset, of marihuana use by Year IV, the Rs for females and males were .41 and .33, respectively. Though not accounting for very much of the variance, they are nevertheless significant.

TIME OF ONSET AND COURSE OF DEVELOPMENT
AS PART OF A LONGITUDINAL STRATEGY

The final strategy we discuss briefly, for it has been reported previously for both the onset of drinking (Jessor, R., & Jessor, S. L., 1975) and the onset of marihuana

TABLE 2-7 Year III (1971) Mean Scores on Personality, Perceived Environment, and Behavior System Measures for Marihuana Nonusers Who Remain Nonusers by Year IV, for Marihuana Nonusers Who Begin Use by Year IV, and for Users in Both Years, in the High School Study

Measure	Males (N = 188)					Females (N = 244)				
	NU3–NU4 (N = 115)	NU3–U4 (N = 24)	U3–U4 (N = 44)	Onset t	F	NU3–NU4 (N = 147)	NU3–U4 (N = 22)	U3–U4 (N = 73)	Onset t	F
Personality System										
Motivational-instigation structure										
Value on academic achievement	69.8	68.2	57.2	0.4	7.6***	69.1	57.2	52.3	2.3*	19.4***
Value on independence	72.0	69.9	76.1	0.7	2.3†	73.4	77.8	75.4	−1.8†	1.3
Value on affection	65.1	64.3	59.2	0.2	1.8	71.0	67.3	63.4	0.9	5.2**
Independence achievement value discrepancy	92.1	91.7	108.9	0.1	13.4***	94.2	110.5	113.1	−3.0**	25.9***
Expectation for academic achievement	58.8	56.9	50.6	0.5	2.8†	59.4	54.5	47.3	0.9	10.2***
Expectation for independence	66.3	62.4	68.4	1.4	1.6	68.8	74.9	71.0	−2.3*	2.4†
Expectation for affection	56.1	57.9	53.6	−0.6	0.7	60.6	60.4	58.1	0.0	0.7
Personal belief structure										
Social criticism	28.6	29.0	32.8	−0.4	11.9***	30.3	30.4	32.7	−0.1	6.3**
Alienation	35.6	36.1	36.8	−0.5	0.7	35.1	38.4	36.2	−2.2*	3.1*
Self-esteem	29.6	29.1	29.7	0.7	0.2	29.4	30.7	29.6	−1.6	1.3
Personal control structure										
Tolerance of deviance	168.2	152.3	130.2	2.0†	18.5***	179.1	155.1	148.9	2.5*	16.3***
Religiosity	13.1	12.1	9.9	0.9	9.2***	14.4	12.3	10.9	1.7†	17.3***
Drinking disjunctions	29.8	33.2	34.6	−1.6	4.0*	27.7	32.4	33.1	−1.7†	6.4**
Drug disjunctions	15.6	21.7	27.8	−2.8**	28.4***	15.5	23.6	28.6	−4.2***	55.1***
Sex disjunctions	17.4	17.7	22.2	−0.2	8.2***	11.9	17.1	16.5	−4.6***	12.6***

Perceived Environment System

Distal structure										
Parental support	7.5	6.9	6.6	1.7†	4.7*	7.5	6.7	6.7	1.7†	4.6*
Parental controls	6.3	6.5	5.6	−0.7	3.0†	6.1	6.1	5.9	0.1	0.3
Friends support	6.1	6.4	6.5	−0.9	1.4	7.4	7.5	7.9	−0.2	1.8
Friends controls	5.8	5.8	5.4	0.0	2.0	6.3	5.9	5.5	1.3	6.7**
Parent-friends compatibility	8.4	8.0	6.8	0.8	7.9***	9.1	7.4	6.5	3.0**	28.2***
Parent-friends influence	3.1	3.2	4.0	−0.5	12.6***	3.3	4.2	4.2	−3.2**	17.8***
Proximal structure										
Parent approval problem behavior	10.7	10.9	11.9	−0.4	4.2*	10.3	10.0	11.5	0.6	4.7**
Friends approval problem behavior	10.0	12.2	12.8	−4.7***	29.3***	9.8	11.7	12.8	−3.9***	38.0***
Friends models problem behavior	9.5	10.7	12.3	−3.6***	46.5***	10.2	11.1	12.9	−2.8**	56.9***
Behavior System										
General deviant behavior	35.6	40.1	45.8	−3.1**	37.6***	34.0	39.4	42.8	−3.1**	42.4***
Church attendance, past year	27.3	20.8	11.9	1.3	6.2**	32.3	33.8	14.8	−0.2	10.4***
Grade-point average	3.0	3.0	2.8	−0.5	1.8	3.1	2.8	2.7	1.5	11.0***

Note. All t tests are two tailed.
†$p \leq .10$.
*$p \leq .05$.
**$p \leq .01$.
***$p \leq .001$.

use (Jessor, 1976) among high school youth. The aim of the strategy is to show a further connection between changes in the theoretical attributes and the occurrence of problem behavior, in this case, marihuana use. More specifically, the strategy seeks to demonstrate that the course of social-psychological development during adolescence varies systematically, depending on whether and on when marihuana use begins. For this purpose, four groups of students were constituted: (1) *nonusers* ($N = 258$; 113 males and 145 females)—those students who reported no use of marihuana over the study years; (2) *initiates 1971-1972* ($N = 45$; 24 males and 21 females)—those relatively late-onset students who began use of marihuana in the final year of the study; (3) *initiates 1970-1971* ($N = 48$; 18 males and 30 females)—those relatively early-onset students who began use of marihuana a year earlier than the preceding group; and (4) *users* ($N = 69$; 26 males and 43 females)—those previous-onset students already using marihuana before the 1970 testing. Groups 1, 2, and 3 were all nonusers at the 1970 testing; Groups 2, 3, and 4 were all current users in 1972. When the developmental curves for the theoretical attributes are plotted for the four groups separately, it is possible to see the relation between time of onset of marihuana use and the course of social-psychological development.

In Figure 2-7, the curves for the development of attitudinal tolerance of deviance over the four testing years in the high school study are presented (the higher the score, the greater the intolerance). The course of development of this attribute of the personal control structure varies as a function of whether and when marihuana onset took place. The nonusers were most intolerant in 1969 and remained most intolerant throughout; though declining in intolerance significantly over the years, they nevertheless were still less tolerant in 1972 than any of the

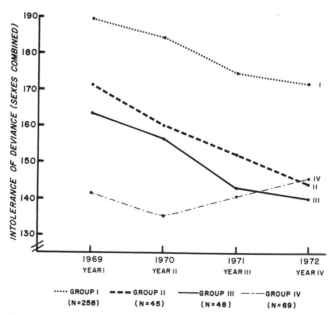

FIGURE 2-7   Development of attitude toward deviance and the onset of marihuana use.

other groups had been in 1969. The users were most tolerant of deviance in 1969, and they show no significant change on this measure over the years. The two groups that make the transition from nonuse to use are intermediate in tolerance of deviance at the outset, and both become significantly more tolerant by the end. What is especially interesting is that the two initiate groups, significantly more intolerant of deviance than the users in 1969, converge upon the users so that, by 1972, there is no difference between the means of the three groups, and all three means are significantly different from the mean of the nonusers in that year.

What this figure and others not shown here (see Jessor, R., 1976; Jessor, R., & Jessor, S. L., 1975, 1977) illustrate is a systematic relation between marihuana use and social-psychological development. The curves represent interindividual differences in intraindividual developmental change as a function of time of onset of marihuana use. Unlike the logic of theoretically parallel change dealt with in an earlier section, the present developmental curves are tied directly to variation in behavior. Temporal priority here remains uncertain, however, although in many of the figures there is evidence of anticipatory psychological change in the year preceding the onset of marihuana use.

DISCUSSION

It is apparent that a general strategy for longitudinal research may have a variety of components. We have emphasized six that have played a role in our own work, only three of which are uniquely dependent upon time-extended data, and there are others that will be mentioned in a moment. The rationale for this proliferation rests upon the point made earlier, that the compellingness of inference is largely a function of the convergence of multiple lines of evidence. In this chapter, we have introduced both cross-sectional and longitudinal lines of evidence—three kinds of the latter: descriptive, predictive, and associative. The convergence among these alternative analytic methods has been notable, providing considerable support for the relevance of problem-behavior theory as an explanatory framework for variation in marihuana use. The convergence is strengthened by the replications carried out across various samples at different times as well as by the fact that the measures employed were derived from the theory being tested.

It is only fair to say, however, that the causal texture of the relationships we have been dealing with remains very much a matter of presumption. None of our strategies, not even the prediction of onset where a time lag was involved, can do more than document an association and the temporal order of the events or processes involved. That the subsequent events were "produced" by those that were antecedent still eludes direct demonstration, and even if demonstrated, the possibility of the reverse direction in other samples at other times cannot be ruled out. For social-psychological concerns, such as those dealt with here, this latter point is of special importance. Given the nature of the processes involved, it would be strange indeed if causal influence could not in fact operate in different directions in different instances, for example, becoming more tolerant of deviance influencing the exploration of marihuana in one case, and the exploration of marihuana influencing a more tolerant attitude toward deviance in another. It may be that the preoccupation with univocal directionality of cause is an unwarranted legacy from experimental method in the physical sciences. In behavioral science, it may be preferable to adopt a network model of causal influence, with the possibility of traversing from one point to another by a variety of pathways and in alternative directions. In such a perspective, the critical question becomes the relevance of the network.

In establishing the relevance of a network, we have dealt with data obtained from several different procedures. More might have been mentioned. For example, an additional longitudinal strategy we employed focused on the socialization process that links parent with adolescent child. Although the actual data from parent and child were collected at the same time, the focus of the parent interview was on an earlier time than the measure of the child's behavior, and thus a longitudinal time interval was "constituted" between the two sets of data (see Jessor, S. L., & Jessor, R., 1974). A further strategy one of our colleagues has begun to explore with our data is the procedure of cross-lagged panel correlation. Because this is a developing strategy of interest, we present from Finney's work the cross-lagged panel correlations for the relation between attitudinal tolerance of deviance (a variable of the personal control structure in the Personality System) and marihuana behavior involvement. Because Kenny (1975) has suggested that a cross-lagged difference should ideally replicate across different time lags and different groups of subjects, the data in Figure 2-8 are three-wave data for the high school males and females separately. The data suggest that the causal direction is from personality variable to behavior, from tolerance of deviance to marihuana involvement (results not supported, incidentally, at the college level). They provide one more indication of the relevance of the variables in the problem-behavior framework to marihuana involvement, that is, one more convergent strategy.

The emphasis on inference, whether to causality or to relevance, ought not to divert our attention from the importance of the sheerly descriptive information yielded by the time-extended observations. The data suggest important developmental regularities through the adolescent period in personality, the perceived environment, and behavior—regularities that reflect a developmental move away from conventionality. These regularities may, of course, be restricted to these samples or to this period of history; no claim is being made for them as developmental invariants. On the other hand, the trends observed are not at all inconsonant with descriptions of adolescence that transcend the most recent period of time. The general point we wish to stress is the value of longitudinal study for purposes of describing the natural course of psychosocial growth and development per se.

In the content of our findings, there is quite impressive coherence, whether considering the cross-sectional differences between marihuana users and nonusers, or the longitudinal predictive differences between those likely to begin use in the near future and those not, or the developmental convergence of new users with the characteristics of those already using. If a single summarizing dimension underlying the differences in personality were sought, it might be termed *conventionality-unconventionality*. The adolescent less likely to engage in marihuana use is one who values and expects to attain academic achievement, who is not much concerned with independence, who treats society as unproblematic rather than as an object for criticism, who maintains a religious involvement and a more uncompromising attitude toward normative transgression, and who sees little attraction in problem behavior relative to its negative consequences. The adolescent more likely to be involved with marihuana shows an opposite pattern: a concern with personal autonomy, a lack of interest in the goals of conventional institutions like church and school, a jaundiced view of the larger society, and a more tolerant view of transgression.

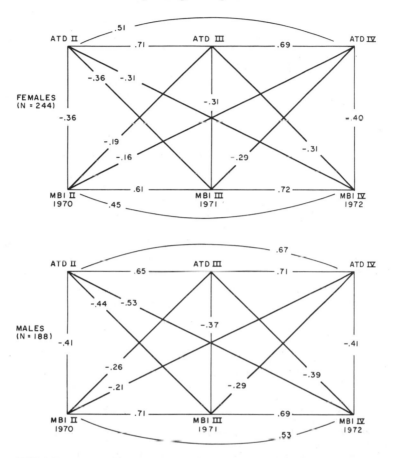

FIGURE 2-8 Cross-lagged panel correlations for attitudinal tolerance of
deviance (ATD) and marihuana behavior involvement (MBI) for Years II, III,
and IV in the high school study.

In the environment, the youth likely to be involved with marihuana perceives
less parental support, less compatibility between parents' and friends' expectations,
greater influence of friends relative to parents, and greater friends support of and
models for drug use. These variables reflect both the importance of whether the
reference orientation of a youth is toward parents or peers and the models and
reinforcements available in the peer context (see also Kandel, 1973; Sadava, 1971).
With respect to behavior, the adolescent likely to use marihuana is one likely to be
more involved in other problem behaviors as well and to be less involved in conventional behavior than his or her non-drug-using counterpart.

The distinctions listed in the preceding paragraphs are not intended to be valua-
tive. As a matter of fact, it is important to emphasize that the characteristics
associated with use of marihuana in these samples of normal youth tend to be
attributes associated with greater developmental maturity, for example, greater
value on independence, greater tolerance of transgression, greater orientation to
peers than parents.

The findings have been generally similar for both males and females, a fact worthy of emphasis. The similarity between high school and college youth, however, is attenuated, particularly in the Personality System and in the distal structure of the Perceived Environment System, suggesting that development is not homogeneous throughout the early-to-late stages of adolescence and youth. For college youth, among which the prevalence rate of drug use is relatively high, the important factors in marihuana use appear to be the immediate peer context. Personality factors, important for the adolescent at the high school level, play a far less important role among older youth. Of course, all of the generalizations we are making need to be restricted to our samples and not applied casually to the larger population from which they were drawn.

Overall then, problem-behavior theory has emerged as a useful explanatory framework both for marihuana use and for problem behavior more generally. The various research strategies reported in the chapter have yielded convergent support for the social-psychological formulations. They have documented their ability to account, in our samples, for a sizable portion of the variance in youthful drug use. While this convergence does strengthen our conviction about the relevance of the theoretical network, it still is not enough to sustain a claim for directly demonstrated causal influence. Such a causal claim, rather than following from strong tacit conviction, would seem to require a certain measure of hubris.

REFERENCES

Blalock, H. M., Jr. *Causal inferences in nonexperimental research*. Chapel Hill: University of North Carolina Press, 1964. (Originally published, 1961.)

Chase, J. A., & Jessor, R. *A social-psychological analysis of marijuana involvement among a national sample of adolescents* (Contract No. ADM 281-75-0028). Washington, D.C.: National Institute on Alcohol Abuse and Alcoholism, January 1977, pp. 1–99.

Elder, G. H., Jr. Age differentiation and the life course. In A. Inkeles, J. Coleman, & N. Smelser (Eds.), *Annual Review of Sociology*, Vol. 1. Palo Alto, Calif.: Annual Reviews, 1975.

Jessor, R. Predicting time of onset of marijuana use: A developmental study of high school youth. *Journal of Consulting and Clinical Psychology, 1976, 44*, 125–134.

Jessor, R., Collins, M. I., & Jessor, S. L. On becoming a drinker: Social-psychological aspects of an adolescent transition. In F. A. Seixas (Ed.), *Nature and nurture in alcoholism* (Annals of the New York Academy of Sciences, Vol. 197). New York: Scholastic Reprints, 1972.

Jessor, R., Graves, T. D., Hanson, R. C., & Jessor, S. L. *Society, personality, and deviant behavior: A study of a tri-ethnic community*. New York: Holt, 1968; reprinted, Huntington, N.Y.: Krieger Publishing Co., 1975.

Jessor, R., & Jessor, S. L. The perceived environment in behavioral science: Some conceptual issues and some illustrative data. *American Behavioral Scientist, 1973, 16*, 801–828. (a)

Jessor, R., & Jessor, S. L. Problem drinking in youth: Personality, social, and behavioral antecedents and correlates. In M. E. Chafetz (Ed.), *Psychological and social factors in drinking: Proceedings of the Second Annual Alcoholism Conference* (National Institute on Alcohol Abuse and Alcoholism). Washington: U.S. Government Printing Office, 1973. (b)

Jessor, R., & Jessor, S. L. Adolescent development and the onset of drinking: A longitudinal study. *Journal of Studies on Alcohol, 1975, 36*, 27–51.

Jessor, R., & Jessor, S. L. *Problem behavior and psychosocial development: A longitudinal study of youth*. New York: Academic, 1977.

Jessor, R., Jessor, S. L., & Finney, J. A social psychology of marijuana use: Longitudinal studies of high school and college youth. *Journal of Personality and Social Psychology, 1973, 26*, 1–15.

Jessor, S. L., & Jessor, R. Maternal ideology and adolescent problem behavior. *Developmental Psychology, 1974, 10*, 246–254.

Jessor, S. L., & Jessor, R. Transition from virginity to nonvirginity among youth: A social-psychological study over time. *Developmental Psychology, 1975, 11*, 473–484.

Kandel, D. B. Adolescent marihuana use: Role of parents and peers. *Science*, 1973, *181*, 1067–1070.

Kenny, D. A. Cross-lagged panel correlation: A test for spuriousness. *Psychological Bulletin*, 1975, *82*, 887–903.

Nesselroade, J. R., & Baltes, P. B. Adolescent personality development and historical change: 1970–1972. *Monographs of the Society for Research in Child Development*, 1974, *39*(1, Serial No. 154).

Neugarten, B. L., & Datan, N. Sociological perspectives on the life cycle. In P. B. Baltes & K. W. Schaie (Eds.), *Life-span developmental psychology: Personality and socialization*. New York: Academic, 1973.

Riley, M. W., Johnson, M. E., & Foner, A. *Aging and society*, Vol. 3, *A sociology of age stratification*. New York: Russell Sage, 1972.

Rohrbaugh, J., & Jessor, R. Religiosity in youth: A personal control against deviant behavior. *Journal of Personality*, 1975, *43*, 136–155.

Sadava, S. W. A field-theoretical study of college student drug use. *Canadian Journal of Behavioral Science*, 1971, *3*, 337–346.

Thomas, W. I. *The child in America*. New York: Knopf, 1928.

Weigel, R. H., & Jessor, R. Television and adolescent conventionality: An exploratory study. *Public Opinion Quarterly*, 1973, *37*, 76–90.

Wohlwill, J. F. *The study of behavioral development*. New York: Academic, 1973.

3

Antecedents of Adolescent Initiation into Stages of Drug Use: A Developmental Analysis

Denise B. Kandel
New York State Psychiatric Institute,
and School of Public Health
and Department of Psychiatry, Columbia University

Ronald C. Kessler
Center for Policy Research, New York City

Rebecca Z. Margulies
School of Public Health, Columbia University

The use of drugs by adolescents provides a unique opportunity for studying processes of socialization, whereby individuals learn values and behaviors. There are few well-studied examples of socialization, in part because its beginning and end points are often difficult to define. Socialization occurs over time, is determined by a series of repeated interactions between an individual and others, and therefore is best studied by longitudinal analyses. Moreover, because interpersonal influences often originate from more than one person, information is needed about the various sources of influence as well as about the persons being influenced. Drug use is a behavior with a clear onset and involves the resolution of conflicting social influences. To study it effectively, we have obtained independent data from the two major sources of influence in adolescence, parents and peers, and have assessed the impact of these interpersonal influences over time.

A conceptualization of drug behavior as involving clear-cut stages underlies our analyses and defines a developmental approach for which a longitudinal research design is particularly well suited. Stages in adolescent drug behavior were established in earlier analyses in which we found that very few adolescents who had used

Names are listed alphabetically. A slightly revised version of this paper appears in the *Journal of Youth and Adolescence,* 1978, 7, pp. 13–37. This research is supported by research grant DA-00064 from the National Institute on Drug Abuse and by the Center for Socio-Cultural Research on Drug Use, Columbia University. The untiring assistance of Stephanie Paton and Rozanne Marel in running the computer analyses is gratefully acknowledged. We also benefited greatly from critical comments made by Donald Treiman and Robert Hauser on earlier versions of the paper.

drugs at a particular stage had not also used drugs at the preceding stage or stages (Kandel, 1975c; Kandel & Faust, 1975). In advancing the notion of stages, we do not imply a causal sequence such that the use of a drug at a prior level causes the progression to the next, nor do we assume that, once started with the first drug, adolescents will necessarily progress through the entire sequence. These stages characterize the behaviors of particular cohorts studied in a particular sociocultural setting and at a particular historical period.

This chapter focuses on the antecedents of *entry* into three specific stages of drug use in a cohort of high school students followed over the course of 1 school year, namely: hard liquor, marihuana, and other illicit drugs. Within any one stage or drug class, experimental users do not necessarily continue their use, and continuing users can go on to exhibit various patterns of use, culminating for some in abuse or compulsive use. In this chapter, the focus is on *initiation*, that is, on the first experience with a particular drug. We show that different factors are related to initiation at different stages: Prior involvement in minor delinquent activities is most important for hard-liquor initiation; beliefs and values favorable to the use of marihuana, and association with marihuana-using friends are most important for marihuana initiation; parental factors, feelings of depression, and contact with drug-using peers are most important for initiation into other illicit drugs.

Our basic assumption is that the acquisition of behaviors and values is in large part determined by the matrix of social relationships in which individuals are embedded and that it is crucial to consider the various members of this network simultaneously in order to understand socialization processes (Kandel & Lesser, 1972). The values, attitudes, and behaviors of the parental and peer generations, which differ on many issues, are especially divergent concerning the use of illicit drugs. Most adults disapprove of the use of illegal drugs and do not themselves use these drugs [Abelson & Atkinson, 1975; National Commission on Marihuana and Drug Abuse (NCMDA), 1972, 1973]. In our sample, the overwhelming majority of parents report that they actively discourage or forbid their children to use illicit drugs. In comparison, many adolescents use a variety of illicit drugs, and only a minority (21%) report strong disapproval of illicit drug use among their friends. Indeed, almost half the students have been offered marihuana by at least one friend. Parental and peer attitudes on the use of hard liquor are less divergent than on marihuana use, although the differences remain substantial. A majority of the parents (68%) in our sample discourage or forbid the use of liquor by their children. Many of these same parents, however, report frequent use of hard liquor themselves.

It is not clear, a priori, which of these sources of influence, peers or parents, will be the most important in leading to adolescent drug use. Indeed, while it is commonly held that contact with members of one's own age group increases sharply in adolescence as attachment to parents declines (Bowerman & Kinch, 1959; Floyd & South, 1972), this view is not without its critics (Curtis, 1974; Kandel & Lesser, 1972). Some feel that the separation between same and older age groups is almost absolute and that attachment to peers implies rejection of parental values, whether these are intellectual interests (Coleman, 1961), general life values (Mead, 1970), or the development of delinquent activities (Cohen, 1955; Hirschi, 1969; Miller, 1958). Others argue that peer-group values do not always stand in opposition to those of adults (Berger, 1963), that youths can be close to both parents and peers and can be influenced simultaneously by both groups (Kandel & Lesser, 1972) (see note on p. 96).

We assume that interpersonal influences can exert themselves in three basic ways: (1) *Directly*, when one person influences the behavior of another by setting an example, by providing social reinforcement, or as the result of the quality of the relationship between that individual and the focal respondent. Thus, friends may provide the drugs and teach how to recognize and enjoy their effects (Becker, 1953). (2) *Indirectly*, when one individual influences the development of another's values, attitudes, or behaviors, including the formation of interpersonal ties, which in turn determine the behavior of interest. (3) *Conditionally*, when one source of influence modifies a person's susceptibility to the influence of another.

The direct effects of interpersonal influences are those most often discussed in the socialization literature, with two alternate social-learning processes posited (Bandura & Walters, 1963; Maccoby, 1968): (1) *Imitation*, in which youths model their own behavior on the behavior of valued others. For example, adolescents may be more likely to start using hard liquor if their parents drink, or they may be more likely to use marihuana if their friends use it than if they do not. (2) *Reinforcement*, in which adolescents respond to what parents and peers define as appropriate behaviors and values concerning specific issues. For example, adolescents may be partially dissuaded from marihuana use if their parents are vocal in their views that the child should not be using the drug. Thus, behaviors on the one hand and values on the other are important components of interpersonal influence.

It has also been proposed that irrespective of the particular standards of behavior or values upheld by parents, the quality of the bond between parent and child may have in itself a direct positive effect in restraining youth from engaging in various deviant or delinquent activities (Glueck & Glueck, 1950; Hirschi, 1969; McCord & McCord, 1959; Nye, 1958). Furthermore, parents and peers may have an indirect effect on adolescent behavior. For example, adolescents from a loving home may be less likely to become delinquent, not because of the direct influence of the parental bond, but because youths from such homes will tend to associate with certain kinds of friends less prone to delinquent activities. It is these friends, in turn, who directly influence the adolescent.

Finally, the extent to which each of the two learning processes will take place is determined in part by the general quality of the relationship between the focal respondent and the source of influence, partly by characteristics of the focal respondent and partly by more specific situational factors (Clausen, 1968). We would expect parents to be more influential on children who feel close to their parents rather than distant and who respect their parents as sources of information rather than ignore them (Clausen, 1968; Smith, 1970). Similarly, we would expect peers to be less influential on a youth deeply committed to personal values and behaviors than on one without personal standards of conduct.

In this chapter, we limit our attention to the effects of the interpersonal influences of parents and peers on drug use. Methodologically, this means that we can treat the effects of the two as additive sources of influence in a multiple regression analysis. In a subsequent paper, we will treat individual, interactive effects and address the question: Under what conditions are youths more or less likely to respond to the influences of parents and peers? In summary, our aims in this analysis are to determine (1) the relative influence of parents and peers at each of three stages of drug use and (2) the extent to which these two sources of influence overlap with each other, as well as other factors, such as characteristics of the focal respondent and the quality of the relationship between the focal respondent and the source of influence.

DATA AND METHOD

Samples

The analyses are based on a two-wave panel sample of adolescents and relational subsamples of dyads of adolescents matched to parents and best schoolfriends at Time 1. A multiphasic random sample of adolescents representative of public secondary students in New York State was contacted in fall ($N = 8,206$) and spring of the same academic year (1971–1972), at an interval of 5–6 months, depending on the school. The two-stage sampling procedure entailed selection of a stratified sample of 18 high schools and subsequent cluster sampling of homerooms within schools. Structured self-administered questionnaires were given to selected homerooms in 13 schools and to the entire student body in 5 schools, making it possible in the latter to collect data from a student's best schoolfriend. Because in 79% of the cases, an adolescent's best friend in school is also the best friend outside of school, the data permit inferences about the role of best friends in general. Questionnaires were mailed, 2 or 3 weeks after each of the 18 schools was surveyed, to one parent (alternately mother or father) of each student. Usable questionnaires were obtained from 61% of the parents ($N = 5,574$). At Time 1, both student and parent samples were weighted to reflect the variable probabilities of selection of schools and homerooms and to correct for different absentee and nonparticipation rates among students in each school and for nonresponse rates among parents in each community. The sample is restricted to regular high school students; it does not include school absentees and dropouts, who exhibit higher rates of drug use than regular students (Johnston, 1973; Kandel, 1975b) and who are most likely to progress to serious drug involvement.

Because of concern with the protection of the rights of the participants in the study, no respondent signed any of the questionnaires. Identification and linkage of records were accomplished through the use of self-generated identification code numbers (Kandel, 1973), leading to a substantial loss in cases. The student panel sample ($N = 5,423$) represents 66% of the students surveyed at Time 1; the student–parent dyads ($N = 3,988$) include 49% of the adolescents at Time 1; student–best schoolfriend dyads at Time 1 ($N = 1,879$) represent 38% of the eligible cases in the five schools. (In a previous study not dealing with drugs, in which names were used [Kandel & Lesser, 1972], 93% of adolescents could be matched to their best schoolfriend. With an overall return rate of 70% to a mailed parental questionnaire, 59% of the students were matched to a parent.)

The elimination of certain respondents from our relational and panel samples constitutes an important source of bias. Students who cannot be matched, either to themselves over time or with a parent or friend at one time point, exhibit consistent differences from those matched. The most important difference involves the underrepresentation of drug users in the matched samples, a consistent finding in longitudinal drug surveys (see Cahalan & Roizen, 1974; Fillmore, 1974). Thus, 24% of the students who could be matched to themselves at Time 2 reported marihuana use at Time 1 compared with 41% of those not matched; 7% and 16%, respectively, reported use 40 or more times. Further differences observed at Time 1 between students matched and unmatched to themselves at Time 2 include: 62% and 72% respectively have used hard liquor; 28% versus 47% are residents of New York City; 44% versus 61% rarely go to church; 35% versus 47% get together with friends everyday; 11% versus 25% have been absent from school 16 or more days since the beginning of the term; 63% versus 47% are A and B students. Similar differences appear between students matched and unmatched to a friend, a parent, or both at Time 1. Furthermore, the higher the frequency of marihuana use at Time 1, the greater the likelihood that the adolescent will start using other illicit drugs by Time 2. To correct somewhat for these biases, the $T1-T2$ student panel sample was weighted to reproduce the frequency distribution of marihuana use observed at Time 1 in the total adolescent sample. The loss of cases in the panel samples must be recognized as a serious problem even though the samples were used, not to estimate incidence or prevalence rates of drug use in the New York State population, but to analyze interrelationships among variables.

Partitioning of Panel Sample according to Stage in Drug Use

The identification of cumulative stages in drug behavior has important methodological implications for studying the factors that relate to drug use. Users of a particular drug must be compared, not to all nonusers, but only to nonusers among the restricted group of respondents who have already used drug(s) at preceding stage(s). Otherwise, the attributes identified as apparent characteristics of a particular class of drug users may actually reflect characteristics important for involvement in drugs at the preceding stages. In order to isolate the determinants of passage from one stage to another, we created cohorts by partitioning our two-wave panel sample on the basis of initial Guttman patterns of use at Time 1 and their subsequent initiation or continued abstention from the next step of use at Time 2. The definition of stages allowed us to define a population at risk and to isolate, within that population, those individuals who succumbed to this risk within a specified time interval.

We focused on three stages: initiation into hard liquor; marihuana, and other illicit drugs. Initiation to beer and wine was not analyzed because most adolescents in the sample (82%) had already used these substances by Time 1. The groups compared are: (1) among Time 1 nonusers of hard liquor ($N = 1,936$), those who started to use hard liquor by Time 2 (30%) and those who remained nonusers (70%); (2) among adolescents who had used hard liquor or cigarettes more than twice ($N = 1,947$), those who started using marihuana (17%) and those who did not (83%) (students who had used hard liquor only once or twice were excluded because they are similar to the nonusers of hard liquor, and their probability of starting to use marihuana is close to zero); and (3) among adolescents who had used one legal drug (alcohol, cigarettes, or both) and marihuana but no other illicit drugs by Time 1 ($N = 523$), those who started using other illicit drugs by Time 2 (24%) and those who did not (76%).

Measurement of Variables

Adolescent Drug Use

At both time periods, adolescents were asked how many times they had ever used for nonmedical reasons each of the following 12 substances: hard liquor; marihuana; hashish; LSD; other psychedelics [psilocybin, mescaline, peyote, dimethyl tryptamine (DMT), DOM (STP)]; methedrine; other amphetamines

(Dexedrine, Benzedrine, Dexamyl), barbiturates (Seconal, Nembutal, Tuinal, phenobarbital); tranquilizers (Equanil, Miltown, Librium, Valium, Thorazine); cocaine; heroin; other opiates (opium, morphine, Dolophine, methadone, Demerol, Darvon); and inhalants (glue, freon, Carbona). Extent of current use was asked for beer and wine and for cigarette smoking, the alternative "never used" being available to respondents. Following current practice in epidemiological drug studies (Kandel, 1975a; NCMDA, 1972), an adolescent was defined as a user of a particular drug if she or he used it at least once. Responses to the questions about drug use appear to be reliable (Single, Kandel, & Johnson, 1975). Substances other than cigarettes, alcohol, or marihuana were classified as other illicit drugs.

Independent Variables

In line with the theoretical assumptions that guided our study, 14 subclusters of variables were defined to characterize the three major concepts of interest: (1) parental influences, (2) peer influences, and (3) adolescent intrapersonal characteristics. The complete list of independent variables for each stage, with a specification of the sources of data, appears in Table 3-2. For both parents and best schoolfriends, three groups of independent variables indicated the significant others' frequency of drug use, drug-related attitudes, and quality of the relationship with the focal respondent. These indicators were elicited, not only separately from parents (either mothers or fathers) and peers, but also by asking the focal respondent to report on the characteristics of both of these others. (We avoided asking adolescents to report on the specific drug use and attitudes of the youths they had identified as their best friends in school for fear that such questions would severely reduce the cooperation of our respondents and their willingness to identify their friends.) The parental items could be specific to mothers or fathers, or about both parents jointly. A fourth subcluster under peer influences measured the availability of illicit drugs.

For focal respondents, we included seven separate sets of possible predictors of subsequent change in drug use: intrapsychic states, academic orientation, life-style values, drug-related attitudes (including reasons for using or not using certain drugs), delinquent involvement, prior drug use, and demographic characteristics.

Whenever possible, the same variables were used throughout, although some items were either not applicable or not available for certain of the stages. A total of 66 predictor variables were used for hard liquor, 100 for marihuana, and 93 for other illicit drugs. The questionnaires included many items about reasons for using illicit drugs, accounting for the discrepancy in the number of variables in the hard-liquor analyses as compared to the other two. The variables are either responses to single questionnaire items or scales created by summation of questionnaire-item scores, the specific items having been selected on the basis of exploratory factor analysis. All indicators, with the exception of demographic factors, are assumed to be linear or are coded as dummy (0, 1) variables. Demographic variables are treated as categorical, and the coefficients calculated represent weighted nonlinear composites (Heise, 1972).

Analytical Procedures

The analyses are based on multiple regressions with dummy dependent variables for continued abstention and initiation. At each stage, we began with the subsample of individuals who were homogeneous in their drug use as of Time 1 and predicted initiation to the next drug in the sequence of Guttman-scale drugs by Time 2. Initiation and continued abstention were coded as a dummy variable (0 = continued abstention, 1 = initiation). Predictions were made on the basis of Time-1 data reported by the focal respondent, his or her mother or father, and the best schoolfriend. In no case, however, did we have complete data from all these sources for every adolescent. Data were available from only one parent for each student, and for best schoolfriends in only 5 of the 18 schools. In no case did we have complete data from the focal respondent, parents, and the best schoolfriend. The correlations are based on the largest number of cases with relevant information for that variable. In Table 3-1, we list the four subfiles used in each case.

For each stage, we created an estimated correlation matrix by substituting correlations from the subfiles of data when they were not available for the entire sample. This merging procedure was justified by our assumption that the coefficients obtained from the restricted samples would not differ from those that might have been obtained had the full set of data been available for each adolescent in the basic sample. Coefficients of determination between predictors of the added variables were similar for each added item taken from a restricted sample and for items available in both the restricted and the basic samples. This finding suggests, although it does not prove, that any biases present in the restricted samples do not affect the covariance and variance estimates taken from these samples.

The total set of variables was reduced by entering each of the 14 subclusters of independent variables into a stepwise multiple regression equation and retaining for further analyses only those predictors within each series and for each of the three subsamples separately that explained at least 1% of the variance in the criterion, independent of other variables in the same series. The original number of variables was reduced to 14, 22, and 23, respectively, for the three analyses of hard liquor, marihuana, and other illicit drugs.

This procedure allowed us to select a small subset from the various indicators of each conceptual influence that could be easily manipulated in further analyses but that would retain the major predictive power of the larger set. We do not imply that

TABLE 3-1 Number of Cases Included in Panel Analyses of Adolescent Initiation at Three Different Stages of Drug Use

Nature of sample	Starting hard liquor (N)	Starting marihuana (N)	Starting other illicit drugs (N)	Total included in analyses (N)	Total in initial sample[a] (N)	Retained in analysis (col.4:col.5) (%)
Adolescents T1–T2 panel sample	1,936	1,947	523	4,406	5,423	81
Best schoolfriends matched to adolescents at T1	537	526	202	1,265	1,879	67
Mothers matched to adolescents at T1	659	669	209	1,537	2,395	64
Fathers matched to adolescents at T1	483	460	156	1,099	1,593	69

[a]Number of cases in total T1–T2 adolescent panel sample and T1 dyads.

each of the 14 conceptual clusters represents a single underlying causal influence. Indeed, the exploratory factor analyses used to create the indicators indicate that many of the indicators contained in the same cluster are independent of each other. The meaning of each of the 14 clusters derives from the relative sizes of the zero-order correlations of predictors with the criterion.

Assessment of Relative Importance of Clusters of Variables

In order to establish clearly the relative importance of various classes of factors as predictors of initiation within and across each stage of drug use, the significant predictors were grouped into four summary conceptual clusters: (1) parental influences (including behaviors, attitudes-values, and the quality of parent–adolescent relations), (2) peer influences (including behaviors, attitudes-values, quality of adolescent–best friend relations, and drug availability), (3) adolescent beliefs and values, and (4) adolescent involvement in a variety of behaviors. These retained the major emphasis on the two separate sources of interpersonal influences and divided the adolescent intrapersonal characteristics into behaviors and attitudes. The relative effect of each cluster was indexed by the total variance accounted for by each summary cluster considered alone as well as by the increments to the total explained variance contributed by each successive cluster entered sequentially in a hierarchical order.

FINDINGS

The results of two different analyses are presented: (1) the predictive values of (a) single predictors and (b) 14 subclusters of predictors at each of three different stages of drug use and (2) comparisons of the relative predictive values of the four summary clusters of predictors for each of the three stages. Analyses are presented for boys and girls together. Throughout, it must be kept in mind that we are dealing with the earliest phases of involvement in any of the stages, namely, starting to use each of the three types of drugs.

General Considerations

In Table 3-2, we present, grouped under the 14 conceptual subclusters of interest, all the predictors entered in the analyses and those retained on the basis of the stepwise regression for each stage separately. The table lists the observed zero-order correlation of each predictor with the criterion score and, with the exceptions specified below, two coefficients of multiple determination for each of the 14 subclusters separately with the criterion score, including: (1) all the predictors $(R^2 T)$ and (2) only those retained $(R^2 *)$. The three parental clusters include three coefficients, because separate statistics are presented for the predictors obtained from mothers and from fathers. Only one coefficient $(R^2 T)$ is presented when the total cluster has no single item that correlates with the criterion at the minimal level of $r = .10$, for example, parental behaviors in relation to starting to use marihuana. These summary coefficients represent the predictive power of each subcluster separately, although indicators from different subclusters may be correlated with each other.

Certain statistical features of the results common to all three analyses can be

TABLE 3-2 Pearson Correlations between Time 1 Predictors and Initiation by Time 2 to Hard Liquor, Marihuana, and Other Illicit Drugs; Two Coefficients of Multiple Determination for Each of 14 Subclusters of Variables, Including Total Set of Predictors (R^2T) and Restricted Set of Starred Items (R^2*) Selected by Stepwise Multiple Regressions

		Time 2 initiation to		
Time 1 predictors[a]	Data source[b]	Hard liquor	Marihuana	Other illicit drugs
Parental influences				
Parental drug behaviors:				
Father's hard-liquor use	A	*.197	.051	.096
	Fa	.127	.083	*.118
Father's psychoactive use (past 12 months)	A	.066	.049	.100
	Fa	−.023	.012	.076
Mother's hard-liquor use	A	.176	−.006	.077
	Mo	.098	.015	.039
Mother's psychoactive use (past 12 months)	A	.021	.023	*.135
	Mo	.006	−.029	.011
R^2T (with mother self-reports)		*.048*	*.009*	*.030*
R^2T (with father self-reports)		*.049*	*.012*	*.035*
R^2*		*.039*		*.028*
Parental drug-related attitudes:				
Is tolerant of child's hard-liquor use	A	.054		
	Pa	.085		
Is tolerant of child's marihuana use	A		*.126	.066
	Pa		.024	−.013
Considers casual hard-liquor use harmful	A	.002	.026	
	Pa	*.106	−.092	
Considers casual marihuana use harmful	A		−.056	−.073
	Pa		−.048	.066
Rules against cigarettes, liquor, drugs	A	.034	.021	.026
	Pa	.043	.017	.050
Thinks marihuana should be legalized	Pa		.096	−.076
Is against marihuana use because it (no–yes):	Pa			
May cause harm			−.007	
May cause addiction			−.067	
Is illegal			−.007	
Interferes with academic work			−.046	
R^2T		*.026*	*.040*	*.023*
R^2*		*.011*	*.016*	
Quality of parent–adolescent relations:				
Closeness to father index	A	−.038	*−.143	*−.278
	Fa	−.095	−.049	−.046
Closeness to mother index	A	−.088	−.078	−.106
	Mo	−.029	−.052	.009
Father–child decision making[c]	A	−.003	.004	−.006
	Fa	−.010	.022	*−.070
Mother–child decision making	A	.008	.027	.019
	Mo	−.020	−.010	−.042
Parental rules about friends (no–yes)	A	.034	.027	.014
	Pa	.041	−.063	*.104
Family intactness	A	.006	−.094	−.051
Relative closeness to parents–peers index	A	*.112	.088	.167

(Note: See page 85 for footnotes)

TABLE 3-2 Pearson Correlations between Time 1 Predictors and Initiation by Time 2 to Hard Liquor, Marihuana, and Other Illicit Drugs; Two Coefficients of Multiple Determination for Each of 14 Subclusters of Variables, Including Total Set of Predictors (R^2T) and Restricted Set of Starred Items (R^2*) Selected by Stepwise Multiple Regressions (*Continued*)

Time 1 predictors[a]	Data source[b]	Hard liquor	Marihuana	Other illicit drugs
Parental influences (*Continued*)				
Quality of parent–adolescent relations (*Continued*):				
Parental disagreement about child	Pa	.065	.007	.109
Consistency of punishment	A	−.025	−.004	−.029
Parental anticipated reaction to child's marihuana use (no–yes):	Pa			
Reason with child		−.007	.023	−.070
Take away rights and privileges		.021	.020	.025
R^2T (with mother self-reports)		*.021*	*.038*	*.118*
R^2T (with father self-reports)		*.027*	*.038*	*.121*
R^2 *		*.013*	*.021*	*.091*
Peer influences				
Peer drug behaviors:				
Perceived number of friends who use:				
Hard liquor	A	*.187		
	Bf	*.160		
Marihuana	A		*.222	*.154
	Bf		*.232	.092
Other illicit drugs	A			.126
	Bf			.110
Cigarette use[c]	Bf	.026	.122	.072
Beer/wine use[c]	Bf	.076	.098	.069
Frequency of hard-liquor use (ever)	Bf	.139	.058	*.150
Frequency of marihuana use (ever)	Bf		.104	.146
Frequency of other illicit-drug use (ever)	Bf			*.194
R^2T		*.051*	*.088*	*.065*
R^2 *		*.046*	*.077*	*.062*
Peer drug-related attitudes:				
Considers casual hard-liquor use harmful	Bf	*−.137		
Considers regular hard-liquor use harmful	Bf	−.006		
Considers casual marihuana use harmful	Bf		−.087	*−.132
Considers regular marihuana use harmful	Bf		−.112	−.085
Considers casual heroin use harmful	Bf			−.115
Thinks marihuana should be legalized	Bf		.127	.052
Perceives peer approval of drug use	A		*.182	.098
R^2T		*.019*	*.043*	*.033*
R^2 *		*.019*	*.033*	*.017*
Quality of peer–adolescent relations:				
Degree of peer-activity index[c]	A	*.206	*.148	.039
Degree of general peer conversation	A	.052	.012	−.020
Degree of peer conversation about drugs	A		*.132	*.186
Intimacy of friendship with best schoolfriend	A	.051	−.014	*−.093
R^2T		*.043*	*.038*	*.050*
R^2 *		*.042*	*.034*	*.045*

TABLE 3-2 Pearson Correlations between Time 1 Predictors and Initiation by Time 2 to Hard Liquor, Marihuana, and Other Illicit Drugs; Two Coefficients of Multiple Determination for Each of 14 Subclusters of Variables, Including Total Set of Predictors (R^2T) and Restricted Set of Starred Items (R^2*) Selected by Stepwise Multiple Regressions (*Continued*)

Time 1 predictors[a]	Data source[b]	Time 2 initiation to		
		Hard liquor	Marihuana	Other illicit drugs
Peer influences (*Continued*)				
Availability:				
Perceived number of people who might supply:				
Marihuana	A		.173	*.160
Speed	A			.085
Heroin	A			*.185
Has been offered marihuana (no–yes)	A		*.224	
R^2T			.056	.052
R^2*			.050	.046
Adolescent values and life-styles				
Intrapsychic states:				
Depression index	A	.075	.064	*.158
Normlessness index	A	.061	.050	.092
Self-image (negative-positive)	A	−.040	−.005	−.030
Personal-growth index[c]	A	.046	.027	.043
R^2T		.009	.006	.029
R^2*				.025
Academic orientation:				
Number of classes cut	A	*.152	*.127	.099
Grade average	A	−.051	*−.122	.016
Number of days absent	A	.054	.102	.066
Educational expectations	A	.030	−.018	−.048
R^2T		.028	.033	.019
R^2*		.023	.026	
Life-style values:				
Conformity-to-adult-expectations index[c]	A	−.065	*−.137	*−.149
Participation in politics	A	*.159	*.104	.056
Political attitudes (conservative-liberal)	A	.090	.107	.020
Church attendance	A	−.074	−.067	.015
Materialistic career-orientation index[c]	A	.014	−.025	−.063
R^2T		.036	.038	.028
R^2*		.025	.030	.022
Adolescent drug-related attitudes:				
Considers casual hard-liquor use harmful	A	*−.119		
Considers regular hard-liquor use harmful	A	−.030		
Considers casual marihuana use harmful	A		−.167	−.032
Considers regular marihuana use harmful	A		*−.206	−.082
Considers casual heroin use harmful	A			*−.117
Thinks marihuana should be legalized	A		*.272	.017
Didn't use marihuana at $T1$ because of (no–yes):	A			
No desire to experience effects			*−.158	
Fear of psychological dependence			−.134	
Illegality			−.049	

TABLE 3-2 Pearson Correlations between Time 1 Predictors and Initiation by Time 2 to Hard Liquor, Marihuana, and Other Illicit Drugs; Two Coefficients of Multiple Determination for Each of 14 Subclusters of Variables, Including Total Set of Predictors (R^2T) and Restricted Set of Starred Items (R^2*) Selected by Stepwise Multiple Regressions (*Continued*)

		Time 2 initiation to		
Time 1 predictors[a]	Data source[b]	Hard liquor	Marihuana	Other illicit drugs

Adolescent values and life-styles (*Continued*)				
Adolescent drug-related attitudes (*Continued*):				
Didn't use marihuana at T1 because of (no–yes) (*Continued*):				
Disapproval by parents			−.055	
Unavailability			.065	
Fear of addiction			−.103	
Disapproval by peers			−.066	
Interference with academic work			−.074	
Used hard liquor at T1 because of desire to (no–yes):	A			
Increase self-understanding			.024	
Decrease depression			.042	
Go along with friends			.011	
Relax			.018	
Use with friends			.054	
Intense feelings			.077	
Pleasure			*.127	
Rebellion			.042	
Fun			.064	
Forget troubles			.074	
Used marihuana at T1 because of desire to (no–yes):	A			
Increase self-understanding				*.175
Decrease depression				*.137
Go along with friends				−.057
Relax				.041
Use with friends				.100
Intense feelings				.101
Pleasure				.111
Rebellion				.025
Fun				.057
Forget troubles				.081
R^2T		*.014*	*.126*	*.076*
R^2*		*.014*	*.112*	*.053*
Delinquent involvement:				
Minor delinquency index	A	*.243	*.168	.066
Major delinquency index	A	.080	.062	*.112
Dealing in drugs[c]	A		*.123	*.134
R^2T		*.060*	*.040*	*.029*
R^2*		*.059*	*.040*	*.028*
Prior drug use:				
Cigarette use[c]	A	*.285	*.171	.046
Beer/wine use[c]	A	*.310	*.115	*.118
Frequency of hard-liquor use (ever)	A		.068	.082
Frequency of marihuana use (ever)	A			*.246

TABLE 3-2 Pearson Correlations between Time 1 Predictors and Initiation by Time 2 to Hard Liquor, Marihuana, and Other Illicit Drugs; Two Coefficients of Multiple Determination for Each of 14 Subclusters of Variables, Including Total Set of Predictors (R^2T) and Restricted Set of Starred Items (R^2*) Selected by Stepwise Multiple Regressions (*Continued*)

		Time 2 initiation to		
Time 1 predictors[a]	Data source[b]	Hard liquor	Marihuana	Other illicit drugs
Adolescent values and life-styles (Continued)				
Prior drug use (*Continued*):				
R^2T		*.136*	*.043*	*.077*
R^2*		*.136*	*.039*	*.077*
Demographic characteristics:				
Race (effect proportional scaling)[c]	A	.048	.071	.049
Religion (effect proportional scaling)[c]	A	.084	.077	.097
School (effect proportional scaling)[c]	A	*.143	*.199	*.323
Family income	A	.063	.059	−.007
Father's education	A	.008	.015	.030
Year in school	A	.001	*−.112	−.030
Sex (male = +)	A	.097	.012	.010
R^2T		*.046*	*.057*	*.133*
R^2*		*.020*	*.045*	*.105*
Total N	A =	(1936)	(1947)	(523)
	Bf, P ⩾	(537)	(526)	(202)

Note. The criterion for selection of the starred items is 1% of the added variance in each subcluster.
[a]The direction of the predictor variables is from low to high, from unfavorable to favorable, or from negative to positive. More detailed descriptions of certain variables appear in the Appendix.
[b]A = adolescent report; Pa = parent report; Fa = father report; Mo = mother report; Bf = best-friend report.
[c]A detailed description of the variable appears in the Appendix.

noted. The subsets of variables chosen by the stepwise regression analysis appear to express adequately the predictive relationship between each subcluster and the dependent variable, inasmuch as the subsets extract the major part of the variance explained by the total set of items in each cluster. The sizes of the coefficients of multiple determination are relatively small, in only a few instances as high as .10, indicating that none of the subclusters nor their individual component variables are strong predictors of the behaviors under consideration. In part, these low values result from the highly skewed distribution of the criterion variables. No satisfactory solution is available to correct for such skew (Goodman, 1975; Knoke, 1975; Netter & Maynes, 1970). In interpreting these results, it is critical that one examine the order of entry of predictors in light of the zero-order correlations of each independent variable with the criterion. Indeed, when predictors are approximately equal in size, the selection of one as an indicator of the influence of the total set is a somewhat arbitrary result of the stepwise procedure.

In the following discussion, we first discuss for each stage separately the specific indicators within each of the 14 conceptual subclusters retained by the stepwise analyses. This is followed by a comparison of the relative impact of summary clusters of variables on initiation into each of the stages.

Starting to Use Hard Liquor

It is as role models that parents influence adolescent initiation to hard liquor. Frequency of use of hard liquor by either fathers ($r = .197$) or mothers ($r = .176$) is a moderately good predictor. By comparison, indicators of the quality of parent-child relationships and parental attitudes and values are unimportant. To the extent that parents' attitudes and values have any impact, it is in pointing out the negative consequences of the activity (parental attitude about harm of casual liquor use, $r = -.106$) rather than in setting strict rules and limits ($r = .043$). An appeal based on reasoning appears to be more successful than one based exclusively on controls.

The behaviors of peers are also important in predicting adolescent hard-liquor use. The important items are the adolescents' and their friends' perceptions of how many of their friends are using hard liquor; the friends' use of other legal drugs (tobacco, beer, wine) is of less importance. The perceptions of friends' alcohol use are more strongly correlated with the criterion ($r = .187$ with adolescent's perceptions, $r = .160$ with best friend's perceptions) than with the best friend's actual self-reported frequency of use of hard liquor ($r = .139$) (see Table 3-2). Inasmuch as perceptual reports are to some degree projections of the perceiver's behaviors and values (Kandel, 1974), adolescents who will start using a particular drug in the near future may also exaggerate somewhat the consumption of that drug in their social environment. The example provided by the specific use of hard liquor by friends is the most important peer factor for the focal adolescent. The relative predictive power of the various indicators of peer behaviors suggests that drug use in the peer group as a whole may be a more important source of influence than use by a single best friend.

Best friends' attitudes about the harmfulness of using hard liquor restrain the adolescents from starting to drink hard liquor. Finally, an important factor in initiation to the use of hard liquor is the degree of adolescent involvement in peer activities, such as frequency of getting together with friends, dating, attending parties, hanging around with a group of friends, or driving around ($R^2 = .042$).

Thus, parental and peer influences on adolescent involvement in hard liquor exert themselves in very similar ways. There is a modeling effect, in which the adolescent imitates the behaviors of significant others who are using hard liquor, the influences of the behaviors of parents and peers being approximately equal in importance ($R^2 = .039$ and $.046$, respectively). There also is a less important cognitive reinforcing effect, in which the expression by significant others of their attitudes concerning the potential harmfulness of alcohol use has a restraining effect. Peers have an additional nonspecific effect that is generated when adolescents are actively engaged in many social activities involving other adolescents ($R^2 = .042$ for quality of peer–adolescent relations).

Characteristics of the focal adolescent are far more important predictors of initiation, however, than is either kind of interpersonal influence. Of primary importance are prior behaviors, including the extent of use of other drugs, such as beer, wine, and tobacco, and participation in forms of minor delinquent activity. By comparison, attitudes and values are of minor importance, with the exception of the specific belief that the use of liquor is harmful. Finally, indicators of various intrapsychic states, such as depression and normlessness, are poor predictors of onset.

The kind of school attended is significantly related to probability of starting to use hard liquor. Because our sample is a stratified sample of 18 high schools in the state of New York, this effect may reflect compositional differences among schools, as well as true contextual effects of schools. In preliminary analyses not reported in this chapter we were unable to document any consistent school-climate effects in the form of statistical interactions between selected predictors and schools on the three separate criteria. Consequently, we assume that the observed predictive power of school indexes compositional effects.

In summary, the onset of hard-liquor use is influenced by both example and individual predisposition. Examples can come both from parents and from peers. The attributes of adolescents that predict initiation do not indicate a need to rebel or psychological problems; they are, rather, behaviors of the same order as alcohol use, mild forms of deviation from socially prescribed behavior for individuals of this age.

Starting to Use Marihuana

Parental influences on adolescent marihuana use are quite small. To the extent that these effects exist, they do not result from parental drug behaviors, such as liquor or psychoactive drug use, as was observed for initiation into hard-liquor use. Indeed, among youths who have used hard liquor, initiation into marihuana is virtually unrelated to any type of drug use on the part of the parent. Rather, parental influences on marihuana use seem to derive from parental attitudes and the closeness of the relationship with their children. Adolescents who report that their parents "positively discourage or forbid the use of marihuana as best they can" are less likely to start using the drug than those who report more permissive parental attitudes, such as leaving the decision regarding use up to the adolescent. This finding, however, appears to reflect selective perception on the part of the adolescent, inasmuch as these same attitudes as reported by the parent are not significant predictors of initiation.

Peer influences, by comparison, are substantial and varied. Perceptions (by the adolescent and her or his best friend) of marihuana use in their peer groups are relatively strong predictors ($r = .187$ and $r = .160$, respectively) as are the adolescent's perceptions of peer approval of the use of drugs ($r = .182$). As was true for initiation to hard liquor, the friends' perceptions of their friends' behaviors are more important ($r = .232$) than the friends' self-reported use ($r = .104$) (Table 3-2). These findings suggest that overall extent of use of a particular substance in the peer group is a more important source of influence than use by a single friend, although, as we noted earlier, perceptions reflect to an unknown degree of adolescent's own values and behaviors. General extent of exposure to peer influences and the availability of marihuana in the peer group are also of importance ($R^2 = .034$ and $R^2 = .050$, respectively). Each of the four kinds of peer influences is substantially higher than each of the influences of parents.

Marihuana use, unlike the use of liquor, is a behavior associated primarily with the young generation. It is of interest that so many aspects of peer influence are important in predicting marihuana in comparison to hard-liquor initiation. Peer behaviors and the general extent of involvement in activities with peers are the important components of peer influence on hard-liquor use. For initiation into marihuana, being offered marihuana, together with the attitudes and values held by peers, or perceived to be held by peers, are also important. This supports the interpretation that exposure to peers provides access to illegal drugs and is a source of socialization. Youths are more likely to be initiated into the use of marihuana when their friends use, when their friends espouse values and attitudes conducive to use, and when the drugs are made available.

Finally, certain adolescent activities and favorable attitudes toward the use of marihuana (such as the beliefs that marihuana use is not harmful or that marihuana should be legalized) are most important predictors of initiation. These behaviors and attitudes are strikingly similar to those found to predict hard-liquor use: frequency of use of drugs lower in the sequence of drug involvement (beer, wine, cigarettes, or hard liquor), minor delinquent activities, cutting classes, low grades in school, political behaviors, and liberal political orientation. Political orientation, which was not selected by the stepwise procedure, has as high a correlation with the criterion ($r = .107$) as does actual participation in political activities ($r = .104$). Prior dealing in drugs ($r = .123$) predicts initiation to marihuana, indicating that a number of youths are selling drugs before using drugs themselves. They may get involved in illicit drugs as a result of marketing activities (Goode, 1969; Johnson, 1973). Lack of conformity to adult expectations, which was not significant for starting to use hard liquor, has some importance for initiating the use of marihuana. Finally, citing pleasure as the main reason for prior use of liquor and expressing the desire to experience the effects of marihuana are both significant predictors of initiation.

Overall, these findings are consistent with the interpretation that there is a process of anticipatory socialization in which the adolescent who holds certain attitudes favorable to marihuana is more likely subsequently to start using it. In addition to participating in a variety of minor delinquent activities, adolescents who start using marihuana are more likely than those who do not start to be characterized by an anticonformist ideology with respect to the values of the larger society.

Among the demographic variables, year in school and kind of school are the only significant factors. As in the case of hard liquor, we concluded (on the basis of analyses not reported here) that the school represents a compositional effect. The negative correlation with year in school indicates that the rates at which adolescents start using marihuana in the course of a school year decrease in the later years of high school, as the pool of potential users becomes smaller (Hughes, Schaps, & Sanders, 1973). Thus, the increasing number of users consistently observed in the higher grades of high school (NCMDA, 1972) represent greater stability among the users rather than higher rates of conversion of nonusers into users. (See also Kandel, Single, & Kessler, 1976.)

Starting to Use Illicit Drugs Other than Marihuana

Parental influences on initiation into the use of illicit drugs other than marihuana are strong, especially the quality of the adolescent–parent relationship. Among the items in that subcluster, lack of closeness to parents is a particularly important predictor, with adolescents reporting highest closeness least likely to start using other illicit drugs ($r = -.278$ for father, and $r = -.106$ for mother). A second important factor is the extent of control exercised by the parent. The greater the control, as indexed by rules about friends and by unilateral decisions, the greater the tendency for the child to start using other illicit drugs (Table 3-2). It is possible that adolescents prone to deviance elicit stricter controls from their parents. Amount of parental disagreement about disciplining the child is important ($r = .109$), although the item was not selected in the stepwise procedure. Finally, adolescent's feelings of greater closeness to parents than to peers is a deterrent to initiation to hard liquor ($r = .167$). Thus, two components of the parent–child relationship, warmth as well as control, have some importance, warmth being more important than control.

Although parental attitudes toward drugs are unrelated to adolescent initiation into other illicit drugs, parental drug use is an important predictor. Parents who use hard liquor and psychoactive drugs (tranquilizers, stimulants, or barbiturates) are more likely to have children who initiate the use of other illicit drugs. A parallel finding was noted for initiation into hard-liquor use, where adolescents imitate parental drinking. For illicit drugs other than marihuana, the father's impact is especially important insofar as he uses hard liquor, the mother's impact insofar as she uses psychoactive drugs. These sex-related differences in the influence of parental drug use are particularly important for substantiating the argument that parents provide role models for their children's use of illicit drugs. Indeed, Parry, Cisin, Balter, Mellinger, and Manheimer (1974) have documented that, when faced with life crises, adult men are more likely to use hard liquor and women more likely to use psychoactive drugs as coping mechanisms. As we will see, adolescents appear to be using illicit drugs partly to cope with feelings of depression. This suggests that, although adolescents may not specifically imitate the use of the particular drugs used by their parents, they learn methods of coping with psychological stress from their parents, one such method being the use of mood-changing drugs. The importance of parental factors may, however, decrease for those who begin the use of other illicit drugs at a later age after high school (Halikas & Rimmer, 1974).

Among peer influences, best friend's use of all types of drugs is an important predictor of an adolescent's initiation into the use of other illicit drugs. In contrast to the relationships observed in connection with alcohol and marihuana use, the *self-reported uses* of other illicit drugs by the specific best friend are more important than either the adolescent's or the best friend's perceptions of drug use in the peer group as a whole. Peer influences on the use of these harder drugs may reflect a more specific kind of peer influence than the group influence suggested for alcohol or marihuana initiation. This interpretation is substantiated by the finding that the general level of peer activity, which was significant for both marihuana and hard liquor, has no importance for initiation into other illicit drugs. Intimacy of friendship with the best friend, which had no impact on starting to use either hard liquor or marihuana, is, however, negatively related to initiation into other illicit drugs ($r = -.093$). Youths who start using other illicit drugs, although greatly influenced by association with individual drug users, may be youths who have been unable to develop intimate and meaningful ties with their peers.

Among the intrapersonal variables, the most important is extent of prior use of marihuana. The heavier the use, the greater the likelihood that the adolescent will progress to other illicit drugs ($r = .246$). In addition, the future user of other illicit

drugs exhibits signs of depression ($r = .158$) and is more likely to have used marihuana earlier to overcome depression. Academic orientation and life-style values,
with one exception, do not differentiate those who begin using other illicit drugs
from those who do not. Conformity to adult expectations, however, deters the use
of harder drugs. Among reasons given for prior use of marihuana, those significantly
related to subsequent use of harder illicit drugs indicate personal, rather than social,
incentives for drug use. Thus, increasing self-understanding ($r = .175$) and reducing
depression ($r = .137$) are important as predictors, whereas going along with friends
is not. In the delinquent subcluster, involvement in major delinquency and dealing
in drugs are two important predictors. For the prior two stages, involvement in
minor delinquency was more important than major delinquency.

In summary, poor relations with parents, lack of intimacy with the best schoolfriend, extensive use of marihuana, use of illicit drugs by the best schoolfriend, and
feelings of depression are among the most important predictors of adolescent initiation into the use of other illicit drugs.

Relative Effect of Various Clusters at Different Stages

The preceding analyses describe in some detail the predictive power of each of
various subsets of variables. For theoretical purposes, however, it is important to
assess within and across the three stages the relative overall importance of variables
that represent conceptually different classes of predictors. Those considered in the
present analyses include interpersonal and intrapersonal factors. As noted earlier,
four summary clusters were created: parental influences, peer influences, adolescent's values and attitudes, and adolescent behaviors. The items selected as
significant in the stepwise multiple regression analyses for each stage were grouped
into one of these four summary clusters. The specific number of items included in
each summary cluster varied for each stage (see footnote to Table 3-3). The relative

TABLE 3-3　Total Variance Explained and Increments in Variance Explained by Each of
Four Successive Clusters of Time 1 Predictors for Adolescent Initiation to Hard Liquor,
Marihuana, and Other Illicit Drugs

Variance by cluster	Hard liquor	Marihuana	Other illicit drugs
Total variance due to each cluster alone			
Parental influences	.047	.028	.115
Peer influences	.089	.102	.106
Beliefs-values	.012	.113	.086
Behaviors	.156	.085	.122
Added variance due to each cluster			
Parental influences	.047	.028	.115
Peer influences	.070	.096	.094
Beliefs-values	.004	.051	.042
Behaviors	.086	.023	.036
Total R^2	.207	.198	.287

Note. Clusters of Time 1 predictors are based on 13 predictors for hard liquor, 19 predictors
for marihuana, and 22 predictors for other illicit drugs. Parental influences cluster includes 3
items for hard liquor, 2 for marihuana, and 5 for other illicit drugs. Peer influences cluster
includes 4 items for hard liquor, 5 for marihuana, and 8 for other illicit drugs. Beliefs-values
cluster includes 1 item for hard liquor, 5 for marihuana, and 4 for other illicit drugs. Behaviors
cluster includes 5 items for hard liquor, 7 for marihuana, and 5 for other illicit drugs. (See items
starred in Table 3-2.) Table 3-1 gives the number of cases in each sample.

effect of each cluster, within and across stages of drug use, was indexed by the total variance accounted for by each summary cluster considered alone, as well as by the increments to the total explained variance contributed by each successive cluster to the variance already accounted for by the preceding clusters (see Table 3-3). Although there are arguments for alternative sequences, we felt it most plausible to assume the causal priority of parental influences, followed by peer influences, with beliefs and values reflecting the socialization by these significant others, and these beliefs and values, in turn, predisposing the adolescent toward certain acts. In interpreting the results, one must be careful to keep in mind the "asymmetry" of the coefficients (Coleman, 1975). Whenever there is overlap among the clusters, the common part of the variance explained by two or more of these clusters is attributed entirely to the cluster or clusters entered first in the causal sequence. The coefficient for the first cluster indicates the total predictive effect of that cluster on the dependent variable. The effect of each successive cluster, however, is the direct effect of each particular cluster controlling for the preceding clusters in the sequence and is dependent upon the specified causal order and the position of a particular cluster in the assumed causal sequence. With one exception, the results are identical whether one examines the total variance explained by each cluster or the increment to the variance contributed by each cluster (Table 3-3). To facilitate comparisons across stages, the increment in variance explained by each cluster was displayed as a percentage of the total explained variance for each stage (Figure 3-1). In principle, neither the R^2s presented in Table 3-3 nor the correlation coefficients in Table 3-2 lend themselves to a precise comparison of the relative influence of different factors over the three stages of involvement in drug use. Their size may reflect, not only differences in the strength of the relationship, but also differences in the composition of the subsample on which these separate analyses are based, inasmuch as they are affected by the sample-specific standard deviations of the predictors. It is to facilitate comparisons across stages that the increment in variance explained was computed as a proportion of the total explained variance for each stage.

For initiation into hard liquor, involvement in a variety of activities contributes most to the explained variance, whether one considers the total effect of the cluster by itself ($R^2 = .152$) or its incremental effect, having controlled for the effect of all other clusters. Controlling for all prior influences (those of parents, peers, and values and beliefs), prior activities of the adolescent still account for 41% of the total variance in initiation into hard liquor explained by all the factors considered in the present analysis. Interpersonal influences, by comparison, are small. The influence of peers ($R^2 = .089$) is greater than that of parents ($R^2 = .047$).

The clusters of adolescent beliefs and values and of peer influences by themselves have the largest total explained variance in initiation into marihuana ($R^2 = .113$ and $R^2 = .102$, respectively). Once parental and peer influences have been taken into account, however, the predictive power of beliefs and values is very much reduced. The relative importance of parental and peer influences differ from initiation into hard-liquor use, with peers relatively more important in starting marihuana than in starting hard liquor. This difference is partially accounted for by the lesser importance of parental behaviors in serving as models for their children in the use of marihuana. The importance of parental influences for initiation into hard-liquor use is not necessarily explained by the earlier age of beginning hard-liquor use, because parental influences are also very important at a later stage of

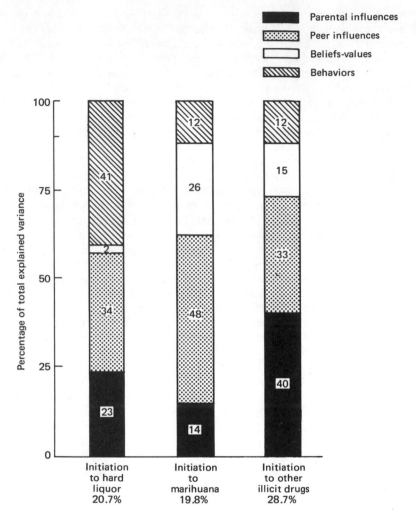

FIGURE 3-1 Percentage of explained variance accounted for by each successive cluster.

drug use, that is, initiation into the use of other illicit drugs. Another important difference in predicting initiation to marihuana, compared to initiation into hard-liquor use, is the much lesser importance of precipitating activities relative to the importance of adolescent beliefs and values, once the effects of all three other clusters have been taken into account. Adolescent behaviors account for 41% of the total explained variance in initiation to hard liquor, but only for 12% in initiation to marihuana. Comparable proportions for beliefs and values are 2% and 26%, respectively. The acceptance of attitudes about the lack of harmfulness of marihuana use, attitudes that are less widely agreed upon by adolescents than are similar attitudes about hard liquor, are critical conditions for initiation to the use of marihuana.

Each of the four clusters by itself has approximately the same predictive power for initiation into other illicit drugs, with a slightly smaller effect of beliefs and values. Compared to the other two stages, parental factors explain a much greater proportion of the total explained variance, 40% compared to 23% for initiation into hard liquor and 14% for marihuana. Once interpersonal influences have been taken into account, beliefs and values and prior behaviors are relatively unimportant.

DISCUSSION AND CONCLUSION

With the notion that adolescent drug use involves sequential stages, we have combined a longitudinal research design in which the population at risk for initiation into each of the stages can be clearly identified so that we could assess the relative importance of various factors for predicting initial transitions into various types of drug behaviors. We can now begin to specify which of the variables associated with different types of drug use in cross-sectional studies actually precede the use of these drugs.

Before reviewing our findings and their implications, it is important to keep in mind two among the several limitations of the research. First, the severe loss in the number of cases included in our panel and relational samples may have biased to an unknown degree the nature of our findings. Second, because only two waves of data were collected, it is difficult to establish a clear causal order for more than two variables at a time. One advantage of the longitudinal design is that it allowed us clearly to define a population at risk and to obtain measurements of variables predicting the change in behavior. These longitudinal data, however, are no better than cross-sectional data in permitting us to determine the causal order among the various predictors measured at Time 1, prior to the transitions of interest. We cannot say whether a certain kind of parental relationship leads to certain kinds of interactions with peers, or whether involvement with peers determines the quality of relationships with parents. Furthermore, the short interval between the waves may not have allowed for certain processes to manifest themselves, especially those involving interpersonal influence, which may have a longer time lag.

We have found that each of four clusters of variables—parental influences, peer influences, adolescent's beliefs and values, and involvement in certain activities—assumes differential importance for each of three stages of drug use. Furthermore, within the same conceptual cluster, important similarities as well as differences emerge in the relative importance of single predictors for the different stages. Overall, for initiation into hard liquor, the most important class of predictors is involvement in minor forms of deviant behavior. For initiation into marihuana, peer influences and the adolescent's beliefs and values have most importance. For initiation into other illicit drugs, the dominant factors are parental influences, especially the quality of the parent–child relationship. The documentation that different factors are important for different drugs provides additional supports for the claim, developed on the basis of Guttman-scale analyses, that drug involvement proceeds through discrete stages. In considering the results, however, the reader is reminded of the biases in our sample, which may limit the generalization from our findings. The use of a high school sample that does not include absentees and dropouts probably eliminates young people who are heavily involved in drugs.

Within the limitations of our sample, these longitudinal data support and further refine a developmental model of involvement in drug use that was first proposed on the basis of cross-sectional data (Kandel, Treiman, Faust, & Single, 1976). At the earliest levels of involvement, adolescents who have engaged in a number of minor delinquent or deviant activities, who enjoy high levels of sociability with their peers, and who are exposed to peers and parents who drink, start to drink. The relationship with parental use of hard liquor suggests that these youths learn drinking patterns from their parents. The use of marihuana is preceded by acceptance of a cluster of beliefs and values that are favorable to marihuana use and in opposition to many standards upheld by adults, by involvement in a peer environment in which marihuana is used, and by participation in the same minor forms of deviant behaviors that precede the use of hard liquor. By comparison, use of illicit drugs other than marihuana is preceded by poor relationships with parents, by exposure to parents and peers who use a variety of legal, medical, and illegal drugs, by psychological distress, and by personal characteristics somewhat more deviant than those of the novice marihuana or hard-liquor user.

The longitudinal data indicate that many of the factors that have been previously found to be associated with various kinds of drug behaviors at one time point (Kandel, Treiman, Faust, & Single, 1976) actually precede the use of these drugs. Involvement in delinquent activities precedes the use of hard liquor; association with drug-using peers precedes the use of marihuana; depression is antecedent to the use of illicit drugs other than marihuana. There may be continuous processes going on whereby these intrapersonal characteristics change further as a consequence of drug use. Jessor, Jessor, and Finney (1973) have shown that involvement in delinquent activities, which predicted the use of marihuana, progressed with continued use of the drug.

Several of our findings, in particular the change in the structure of influences across various stages of drug use, have general implications for issues related to understanding adolescent socialization and involvement in increasingly deviant behaviors.

Role of Interpersonal Influences
in Adolescent Socialization

The finding that parental and peer influences on initiation into marihuana use are completely independent of each other provides important insights into the relations between the generations. In particular, it throws doubt on the view that, in earlier work (Kandel & Lesser, 1972), we have labeled the "exclusive" or "hydraulic theory" of interpersonal influence. The assumption that the stronger the rejection of adult standards, the stronger the acceptance of peer standards or vice versa is too simplified. We propose an alternate model, that of *generalized social interaction* according to which adolescents could display different levels of responsiveness to social influences. There may be areas of behavior in which adolescents will show high reliance on parents and low reliance on peers, or vice versa, that is, they will behave according to an *exclusive theory*. In other domains of behavior and under different social or cultural conditions or both, adolescents will display high reliance on both parents and peers, that is, they will confirm a theory of generalized social interaction. The data presented here for marihuana suggest that, even in the case of domains relevant to the immediate needs and life-styles of youth, both sources of influence can exert themselves independently of one another.

For different kinds of behaviors, not only are there different sources of influence, but there are also differences in the aspects of those interpersonal influences that are of importance. In the early stage of drug use, parental behavior seems to be critical in leading the youth to experiment with hard liquor. In later phases of initiation, the quality of the parent–child relationship becomes important. Similarly, there is evidence that a generalized peer influence, which is important in predicting initiation to legal drugs and marihuana, is partially supplanted by the influence of a single best friend in leading to the initiation of other illicit drugs. Findings of this kind point to the importance of examining profiles of interpersonal influences over a series of behaviors, values, and attitudes, in order better to understand their processual nature. Thus, if one accepts the notion that a continuum of progressively more serious involvement in drugs underlies the stages we have outlined, the data suggest that the more serious the behavior, the greater the relative importance of the specific role model provided by one friend in contrast to the same behavior by the whole group. The nature of peer influences changes from being generalized and nonspecific to representing the influence of a particular group and, in the last stage, to emanating principally from a single individual with whom the adolescent need not be intimate. The individual who progresses to the use of other illicit drugs may, as a result of his or her drug-related behavior, factors of availability, or family difficulties, move away from long-term friendships and seek less intimate relationships with others who share his or her attitudes, behaviors, and problems.

The drug behaviors of parents and peers are consistently more important than their drug-related beliefs and values as predictors of transitions in adolescent drug use. This suggests that adolescent socialization may take place more through a modeling effect than through social reinforcement, although values and prescriptions do play some role. Adolescents are more likely to initiate a certain behavior if those around them hold values and attitudes defining the behavior in favorable terms.

Quality of the parent–child relationship is important only at the last stage of drug use, with closeness to parents shielding adolescents from involvement in the most serious forms of drug use. Furthermore, at that stage, closeness and warmth are more important than the extent of control exercised by the parent. It remains to be seen what differences would obtain in families with various combinations on these two dimensions (Elder, 1968; Maccoby, 1968; Martin, 1975; Straus, 1964); closeness and control may prove to be most effective. The quality of interaction with fathers consistently assumes greater importance than the quality of interaction with mothers. This obtains for boys as well as for girls (data not presented). Controversy exists about the relative influence of mothers and fathers on the development of children's delinquent activities, some arguing for the greater importance of fathers (Gold, 1963; Nye, 1958); others, for mothers (McCord & McCord, 1959); still others, for similar impact of both parents (Hirschi, 1969). Those who argue for the greater importance of fathers suggest that this comes about because of the greater differentiation of adolescents' relationships to fathers as compared to mothers (Nye, 1958). This interpretation could account for our results, because the adolescents' reports of closeness to their parents are more positively skewed for mothers than fathers. Thus, 62% of all the adolescents surveyed at Time 1 report being "extremely" or "quite" close to their mothers, compared to 51% for their fathers; 47% report that their mothers provide positive encouragement several times a week, compared to 34% for fathers.

Involvement in Increasingly Deviant Behaviors

Many theories of drug dependence make some conception of individual pathology a primary explanation, whereas others stress social factors. Each of these conceptualizations may apply to different stages of the process of involvement in drug behavior, social factors playing a more important role in the early stages and psychological factors in the later ones. Cahalan and Room (1974) have suggested that psychological factors may become important only in the later phases of problem drinking. Similarly, psychological factors may become important in later stages in the overall sequence of involvement in drug use.

Participation in various deviant behaviors is most relevant for starting to use alcohol, least for illicit drugs. The less serious the drug, the more its use or nonuse may depend on situational factors. At the earliest stage, an adolescent user does not hold different beliefs and values from a nonuser. Users of hard liquor would conform to those youths described by Matza (1964) who become involved in a number of deviant behaviors without having made a conscious decision to deviate, simply by drifting into such behaviors as part of casual sociability in a group of peers. Users of other illicit drugs, by contrast, present an image of seekers (Lofland, 1969) who are using drugs consciously for a reason having to do with intrapsychic pressures of some sort or another. Users of marihuana would fall in between the two. While they do not report greater psychic stress than nonusers and do not mention personal or family problems that could serve as an impetus to the use of drugs for escape, marihuana users are not drifters either. Prior to starting to use the drug, the values and beliefs of these adolescents undergo important transformation.

The findings we have presented have implications beyond the area of drug use per se. They draw attention to the fact that the acquisition of a particular social behavior should be seen as a process and that, in various phases of this process, different influences are involved. Situational and interpersonal factors are most important for initiation into a behavior. Intrapsychic factors are most important for increased involvement or participation in that behavior.

Note added in proof. Findings from earlier drug studies suggest that adolescents use a variety of substances in response to interpersonal influences both from peers and from parents. Peer influences have been reported for drinking (Alexander & Campbell, 1967; Jessor, Collins, & Jessor, 1972; Wechsler & Thum, 1973; Cahalan & Room, 1974), smoking (Williams, 1971), and using marihuana (Becker, 1953; Brook, Lukoff, & Whiteman, 1977; Goode, 1969; Jessor & Jessor, 1977; Jessor, Jessor, & Finney, 1973; Johnson, 1973; Kandel, 1973, 1974), as well as other illicit drugs (Kandel, 1974). Parental influences have been claimed for all of these substances: cigarettes (Williams, 1971), liquor (Cahalan, Cisin, & Crossley, 1969; Bacon & Jones, 1968; Cahalan & Room, 1974), and illicit drugs (Smart & Fejer, 1972; Kandel, 1974). There are both similarities and differences in the nature of individual characteristics found to be associated with alcohol and illicit drugs. Low levels of academic interests (Mellinger, Somers, Davidson, & Manheimer, 1976; Smith & Fogg, 1975, 1977), school absences, or involvement in delinquent activities have been found to be associated with use of marihuana or other illicit drugs (Jessor & Jessor, 1977; Jessor, Jessor, & Finney, 1973; Johnson, 1973; Suchman, 1968) and of alcohol (Jessor, Collins, & Jessor, 1972; Wechsler & Thum, 1973). Depression (National Commission on Marihuana and Drug Abuse, 1972) and alienation (Mellinger, Somers, & Manheimer, 1975) have been stressed as important factors in the use of marihuana and other illicit drugs. Rebelliousness, which has been reputed to be a good predictor of illicit drug use (Smith & Fogg, 1975, 1977), has been especially emphasized as a factor in drinking (Bacon & Jones, 1968). Radical political ideology and lack of religiosity have been associated with use of illicit drugs (Jessor, Jessor, & Finney, 1973; Johnson, 1973) and of alcohol (Maddox & McCall, 1964; Cahalan, Cisin, & Crossley, 1969). However, the absence of proper partitioning of the samples in prior studies, whether at one point in time or over time, may have obscured some differences and confounded some findings.

APPENDIX

Description of Selected Predictor Variables

Parent–child Decision Making: ranges from "parent makes all decisions for adolescent" to "adolescent makes all decisions for himself" (5 categories)

Degree-of-peer-activity Index: measures frequency of getting together with friends outside of school, dating, attending parties, hanging around with a group of kids, and driving around with friends (5 items) [reliability measured by omega = .69 (Heise & Bohrnstedt, 1970)]

Personal-growth Index: based on importance to adolescent of discovering new ways to experience things and of finding a purpose and meaning to his or her life (2 items) (omega = .58)

Conformity-to-adult-expectations Index: based on importance to adolescent of getting into college, of getting along with her or his parents, and of learning as much as possible in school (3 items) (omega = .60)

Materialistic-career-orientation Index: based on importance to adolescent of making a lot of money and of having a job with security and prestige (3 items) (omega = .69)

Dealing in Drugs: five categories ranging from "neither buys nor sells any drugs" through "buys marihuana only," "sells marihuana only," "buys other illicit drugs" to "sells other illicit drugs"

Cigarette Use: six categories, from "never smoked" through "only smoked once or twice ever," "used to smoke, but stopped," "smoke occasionally," "smoke less than a pack a day," to "smoke a pack a day or more"

Beer/wine Use: seven categories, from "never" through "less than once a month," "about once a month," "2 or 3 times a month," "about once a week," "several times a week," to "every day"

Race: four categories, black, white, Puerto Rican, and other

Religion: five categories, Roman Catholic, Protestant, Jewish, other, and no religion

School: 18 high schools sampled

REFERENCES

Abelson, H. I., & Atkinson, R. B. *Public experience with psychoactive substances* (National Institute on Drug Abuse). Princeton: Response Analysis Corporation, 1975.

Alexander, C., & Campbell, E. Peer influences on adolescent drinking. *Quarterly Journal of Studies on Alcohol,* 1967, *28,* 444–453.

Bacon, M., & Jones, M. *Teen-age drinking.* New York: Crowell, 1968.

Bandura, A., & Walters, R. H. *Social learning and personality development.* New York: Holt, 1963.

Becker, H. S. Becoming a marihuana user. *American Journal of Sociology,* 1953, *59,* 235–242.

Berger, B. Adolescence and beyond: An essay review of three books on the problems of growing up. *Social Forces,* 1963, *10,* 394–408.

Bowerman, C. E., & Kinch, J. W. Changes in family and peer orientation of children between the 4th and 10th grades. *Social Forces,* 1959, *37,* 206–211.

Brook, J., Lukoff, I., & Whiteman, M. Correlates of adolescent marijuana use as related to sex, age, and ethnicity. *Yale Journal of Biological Medicine,* 1977, *50,* 383–390.

Cahalan, D., Cisin, I., & Crossley, H. *American drinking practices.* New Haven: College and University Press, 1969.

Cahalan, D., & Roizen, R. *Changes in drinking problems in a national sample of men.* Paper presented at the North American Congress on Alcohol and Drug Problems, San Francisco, December 1974.

Cahalan, D., & Room, R. G. W. *Problem drinking among American men* (Monograph No. 7). New Brunswick, N.J.: Rutgers Center of Alcohol Studies, 1974.

Clausen, J. A. (Ed.). *Socialization and society*. Boston: Little, Brown, 1968.

Cohen, A. *Delinquent boys*. New York; Free Press, 1955.

Coleman, J. S. *The adolescent society*. New York: Free Press, 1961.

Coleman, J. S. Methods and results in the IEA studies of effects of school on learning. *Review of Educational Research*, 1975, *45*, 355–386.

Curtis, R. Parents and peers: Serendipity in a study of shifting reference groups. *Social Forces*, 1974, *52*, 368–375.

Elder, G. H., Jr. Adolescent socialization and development. In E. F. Borgatta & W. W. Lambert (Eds.), *Handbook of personality theory and research*. Chicago: Rand McNally, 1968.

Fillmore, K. M. Drinking and problem drinking in early adulthood and middle age: An exploratory 20-year follow-up study. *Quarterly Journal of Studies on Alcohol*, 1974, *35*, 819–840.

Floyd, H. H., & South, D. R. Dilemma of youth: The choice of parents or peers as a frame of reference for behavior. *Journal of Marriage and the Family*, 1972, *34*, 627–634.

Glueck, S., & Glueck, E. *Unraveling juvenile delinquency*. New York: Commonwealth Fund, 1950.

Gold, M. *Status forces in delinquent boys*. Ann Arbor: Institute for Social Research, 1963.

Goode, E. Multiple drug use among marihuana smokers. *Social Problems*, 1969, *17*, 48–64.

Goodman, L. A. The relationship between modified and usual multiple-regression approaches to the analysis of dichotomous variables. In D. R. Heise (Ed.), *Sociological methodology 1976*. San Francisco: Jossey-Bass, 1975.

Halikas, J. A., & Rimmer, J. D. Predictors of multiple drug abuse. *Archives of General Psychiatry*, 1974, *31*, 414–418.

Heise, D. R. Employing nominal variables, induced variables, and block variables in path analysis. *Sociological Methods and Research*, 1972, *1*, 147–174.

Heise, D. R., & Bohrnstedt, G. W. Validity, invalidity and reliability. In E. G. Borgatta & G. W. Bohrnstedt (Eds.), *Sociological methodology 1970*. San Francisco: Jossey-Bass, 1970.

Hirschi, T. *Causes of delinquency*. Berkeley and Los Angeles: University of California Press, 1969.

Hughes, P. H., Schaps, E., & Sanders, C. R. A methodology for monitoring adolescent drug abuse trends. *International Journal of the Addictions*, 1973, *8*, 404–419.

Jessor, R., Collins, M. I., & Jessor, S. L. On becoming a drinker: Social-psychological aspects of an adolescent transition. In F. A. Seixas (Ed.), *Nature and nurture in alcoholism* (Annals of the New York Academy of Sciences, Vol. 197). New York: Scholastic Reprints, 1972.

Jessor, R., & Jessor, S. L. *Problem behavior and psychosocial development: A longitudinal study of youth*. New York: Academic, 1977.

Jessor, R., Jessor, S. L., & Finney, J. A social psychology of marijuana use: Longitudinal studies of high school and college youth. *Journal of Personality and Social Psychology*, 1973, *26*, 1–15.

Johnson, B. D. *Marihuana users and drug subcultures*. New York: Wiley, 1973.

Johnston, L. D. *Drugs and American youth*. Ann Arbor: Institute for Social Research, 1973.

Kandel, D. B. Adolescent marihuana use: Role of parents and peers. *Science*, 1973, *181*, 1067–1070.

Kandel, D. B. Interpersonal influences on adolescent illegal drug use. In E. Josephson & E. E. Carroll (Eds.), *Drug use: Epidemiological and sociological approaches*. Washington: Hemisphere, 1974.

Kandel, D. B. The measurement of "ever use" and "frequency-quantity" in drug use surveys. In J. Elinson & D. N. Nurco (Eds.), *Operational definitions in socio-behavioral drug use research 1975* (National Institute on Drug Abuse, Research Monograph Series 2). Washington: U.S. Government Printing Office, 1975. (a)

Kandel, D. B. Reaching the hard-to-reach: Illicit drug use among high school absentees. *Addictive Diseases*, 1975, *1*, 465–480. (b)

Kandel, D. B. Stages of adolescent involvement in drug use. *Science*, 1975, *190*, 912–914. (c)

Kandel, D. B., & Faust, R. Sequence and stages in patterns of adolescent drug use. *Archives of General Psychiatry*, 1975, *32*, 923–932.

Kandel, D. B., & Lesser, G. S. *Youth in two worlds*. San Francisco: Jossey-Bass, 1972.

Kandel, D. B., Single, E., & Kessler, R. C. The epidemiology of drug use among New York State high school students: Distributions, trends and change in rates of use. *American Journal of Public Health*, 1976, *66*, 43–53.

Kandel, D. B., Treiman, D., Faust, R., & Single, E. Adolescent involvement in legal and illegal drug use: A multiple classification analysis, *Social Forces*, 1976, *55*, 438–458.

Knoke, D. A comparison of log-linear and regression models for systems of dichotomous variables. *Sociological Methods and Research*, 1975, *3*, 416–434.

Lofland, J. *Deviance and identity*. Englewood Cliffs, N.J.: Prentice-Hall, 1969.

Maccoby, E. E. The development of moral values and behavior in childhood. In J. A. Clausen (Ed.), *Socialization and society*. Boston: Little, Brown, 1968.

Maddox, G., & McCall, B. *Drinking among teen-agers*. New Brunswick, N.J.: Rutgers Center of Alcohol Studies, 1964.

Martin, B. Parent–child relations. In F. Horowitz (Ed.), *Review of child development research* (Vol. 4). Chicago: University of Chicago Press, 1975.

Matza, D. Position and behavior patterns of youth. In R. Faris (Ed.), *Handbook of modern sociology*. Chicago: Rand McNally, 1964.

McCord, W., & McCord, J. *Origins of crime*. New York: Columbia University Press, 1959.

Mead, M. *Culture and commitment*. Garden City, N.Y.: Doubleday, 1970.

Mellinger, G. D., Somers, R. H., Davidson, S. T., & Manheimer, D. I. The amotivational syndrome and the college student. *Annals of the New York Academy of Sciences*, 1976, *282*, 37–55.

Mellinger, G. D., Somers, R. H., & Manheimer, D. I. Drug use research items pertaining to personality and interpersonal relations. In D. J. Lettieri (Ed.), *Predicting adolescent drug abuse: A review of issues, methods and correlates* (National Institute on Drug Abuse). Washington: U.S. Government Printing Office, 1975.

Miller, W. Lower class culture as a generating milieu of gang delinquency. *Journal of Social Issues*, 1958, *14*, 5–19.

National Commission on Marihuana and Drug Abuse. *Marihuana: A signal of misunderstanding* (Appendix Vols. 1, 2). Washington, D.C.: U.S. Government Printing Office, 1972.

National Commission on Marihuana and Drug Abuse. *Drug use in America: Problem in perspective*. Washington, D.C.: U.S. Government Printing Office, 1973.

Netter, J., & Maynes, E. On the appropriateness of the correlation coefficients with a 0, 1 dependent variable. *Journal of American Statistical Association*, 1970, *65*, 501–509.

Nye, F. *Family relationships and delinquent behavior*. New York: Wiley, 1958.

Parry, H., Cisin, I., Balter, M., Mellinger, G. D., & Manheimer, D. I. Increased alcohol intake as a coping mechanism for psychic distress. In R. Cooperstock (Ed.), *Social aspects of the medical use of psychotropic drugs*. Toronto: Alcoholism and Drug Addiction Research Foundation of Ontario, 1974.

Single, E., Kandel, D. B., & Johnson, B. D. The reliability and validity of drug use responses in a large scale longitudinal survey. *Journal of Drug Issues*, 1975, *5*, 426–443.

Smart, R. G., & Fejer, D. Drug use among adolescents and their parents: Closing the generation gap in mood modification. *Journal of Abnormal Psychology*, 1972, *79*, 153–160.

Smith, G. M., & Fogg, C. P. Teenage drug use: A search for causes and consequences. In D. J. Lettieri (Ed.), *Predicting adolescent drug abuse: A review of issues, methods and correlates* (National Institute on Drug Abuse). Washington: U.S. Government Printing Office, 1975.

Smith, G. M., & Fogg, C. P. Psychological antecedents of teenage drug use. In R. L. Simmons (Ed.), *Research in community and mental health: An annual compilation of research* (Vol. I). Greenwich, Conn.: JAI Press, 1977.

Smith, T. Foundations of parental influence upon adolescents: An application of social power theory. *American Sociological Review*, 1970, *35*, 860–873.

Straus, M. Power and support structure of the family in relation to socialization. *Marriage and Family Living*, 1964, *26*, 318–326.

Suchman, E. The "hang-loose" ethic and the spirit of drug use. *Journal of Health and Social Behavior*, 1968, *9*, 146–155.

Wechsler, H., & Thum, D. Teen-age drinking, drug use, and social correlates. *Quarterly Journal of Studies on Alcohol*, 1973, *34*, 1220–1227.

Williams, T. Summary and implications of review of literature related to adolescent smoking. Bethesda, Md.: U.S. Department of Health, Education and Welfare, National Clearinghouse for Smoking and Health, 1971.

4

Psychological Predictors of Early Use, Late Use, and Nonuse of Marihuana among Teenage Students

Gene M. Smith
Harvard Medical School, and
Massachusetts General Hospital

Charles P. Fogg
College of Basic Studies, Boston University

In seeking a better understanding of the psychodynamics of teenage drug use, investigators have defined comparison groups variously in terms of whether subjects have ever used, frequency of use, precocity of use, reasons for use, consequences of use, and patterns based on such classification criteria considered in complex combinations (for examples, see Block, Goodman, Ambellan, & Reverson, 1973; Gergen, Gergen, & Morse, 1972; Goode, 1972; Groves, 1974; Hogan, Mankin, Conway, & Fox, 1970; Jessor, Jessor, & Finney, 1973; Johnson, 1971; Johnston, 1973; Josephson, Haberman, Zanes, & Elinson, 1972; Kandel, 1975; McGlothlin, Jamison, & Rosenblatt, 1970; Mellinger, Somers, & Manheimer, 1975; Naditch, 1975; Robins, Darvish, & Murphy, 1970; Sadava, 1972; Segal, 1974; Smart, Fejer, & White, 1970; Smith, 1973; Smith & Fogg, 1975; and Whitehead, Smart, & Laforest, 1972). The questions that most often orient such studies are: Who uses illicit drugs? Which drugs are used? How often? Why? With what effects?

The study that generated the results presented here is a 5-year longitudinal study of nine cohorts from each of six participating school systems that seeks information concerning both the causes and the consequences of teenage drug use. The present analysis predicts precocity of marihuana use in a sample of 651 students from one of our six school systems. They were 7th or 8th graders in 1969 and were 11th or 12th graders in 1973. All 651 reported that they were nonusers of marihuana in

This work was supported by research grant DA00065 from the National Institute on Drug Abuse. We are pleased to acknowledge the assistance of Frederick T. Schwerin in preparing the data for analysis and the advice of our statistical consultants, William G. Cochran and Richard A. Labrie. We also wish to thank Ira H. Cisin for reading the report and for making numerous helpful suggestions.

1969. Those referred to hereafter as "early users" are 128 students who initiated marihuana use as 9th graders or earlier. Those called "late users" are 317 who did so as 10th graders or later. Those called "nonusers" are 206 who remained nonusers through the fifth year of the study. Thus, the comparisons are among junior high school initiates, high school initiates, and students who remained nonusers of marihuana through the 5-year period of our study. The questions posed are: Which pre-use psychosocial variables differentiate those three groups, and how successfully can they be differentiated?

To place this analysis in context, it is necessary to describe the larger study briefly. Approximately 12,000 to 14,000 students in grades 4 to 12 were studied each year for 5 years between 1969 and 1973 in six suburban school systems in the greater Boston area. Students were mostly from white, middle-income families. Each year, the participants were recruited on a school-wide basis and were asked to identify their questionnaires to permit longitudinal linkage. Each year, we lost the preceding year's 12th graders and gained a new group of 4th graders. Participation in the study was voluntary. Each year, some sample attrition resulted from absences, noncooperation, and scheduling problems. Typically, for cohorts of the age range used in the present analysis, about 90 to 95% of the enrolled students were present on the day of testing, and approximately 75 to 85% of those students completed questionnaires that were identified and were acceptable for analysis.

In 1969, information was collected on personality, grade-point average, cigarette smoking, and attitudes toward cigarette smoking. Personality traits were measured both by a 400-item questionnaire and by peer rating procedures described in detail below. Information concerning grade-point average was obtained from school records. Cigarette smoking and attitudes toward cigarette smoking were measured with self-report questionnaires. In 1970, the same information, except for the peer ratings, was collected again. In the 1971, 1972, and 1973 testings, the cigarette attitude questionnaire was deleted, and drug questionnaires were added. Thus, information concerning drug use was sought for the first time in Year 3 of the 5-year study. Retrospective questions were asked concerning drug use that year, and each year thereafter, to help identify time of onset of drug use. Three questions were asked regarding use of marihuana and hashish: How many times have you used it in your lifetime (never, only once, 2–5 times, 6–10 times, 11–25 times, more than 25 times)? As of 1 year ago, how many times had you used it? As of 2 years ago, how many times had you used it?

The analysis presented in this chapter compares the three groups (nonusers, late users, and early users) on 37 variables measured at a time when none of the 651 students had begun using drugs.

THE PREDICTOR VARIABLES

The items in the 400-item personality questionnaire are intended to measure personal competence and social responsibility, viewed from the perspective of desires and expectations of parents who hold traditional middle-class values. Factor analytic studies have led to the development of the following eight scales:

1. *Obedient, Law-abiding*: obeys rules, laws, parents, and other authorities; is motivated to be conscientious and trustworthy
2. *Works Hard and Effectively*: is diligent, thorough, and persistent in work and

study; is orderly and well organized; has well-directed effort; works ener-
getically; takes pride in effort and accomplishment
3. *Feels Capable*: is confident when facing challenges and problems; is optimistic
about self; feels capable and competent
4. *Confident Academically*: feels smarter than average; is confident regarding
academic success
5. *Self-sufficient*: relies on self; is not dependent
6. *Likes School and Intellectual Activities*: likes mental challenge and activities
requiring intellectual effort; enjoys thinking and problem solving; likes school;
values education and strives for intellectual attainment
7. *Ambitious*: sees instrumental value of effort; is ambitious
8. *Feels Valued and Accepted*:   feels valued and accepted by peers, teachers, and
other people

The peer ratings of personality were obtained with procedures described previously (Smith, 1967b). Each student in a homeroom of 20 to 30 students was asked
to rate each of the other students on each of the 20 traits identified in abbreviated
form in Table 4-2. When the peer rating procedure was administered, each trait was
defined in bipolar terms. For example, peer Variable 9 was defined as follows:

Obedient: obeys and cooperates with parents and teachers without arguing; feels it is important to obey rules	versus	*Disobedient*: doesn't always obey parents and teachers, especially if he thinks they are wrong; does not cooperate; doesn't mind breaking rules

A rater was asked to examine each bipolar personality trait and select the four
members of his or her peer group most like the left-hand pole and the four most
like its opposite on the right. Selections on the left were considered positive
nominations, and those on the right were considered negative. The positive and
negative nominations a ratee received were scored +1 and −1, respectively. Failure
to be nominated was scored 0. Thus, in a peer group of 25, a ratee's score on any
trait could range from +24 to −24.

The peer rating procedure was used in the present study for two reasons. First,
our earlier studies had shown that such information has excellent analytic resolving
power (Smith, 1967a, 1967b, 1969). Second, the peer rating information augments
that obtained with the self-report personality questionnaire, thus making it possible
to test conclusions based on self-report data using information having an instrumental origin that is distinctly different and independent.

The grade-point averages included in our data base have been standardized ($\bar{X} = 0$;
$SD = 1$). Cigarette-smoking status was scored in terms of response to the question:
About how often do you smoke cigarettes (never; only a few in my whole lifetime;
one or two a week; one or two each day; several each day but less than half a pack
each day; about half a pack each day; about a pack each day; more than a pack
each day; more than two packs each day)? Cigarette attitudes were scored on the
basis of answers to items in a 182-item questionnaire. Results obtained with three
of seven scales derived from that questionnaire by factor analysis are reported in
Tables 4-3 through 4-5. For all seven scales, high scores indicated negative attitudes
toward cigarette smoking, toward cigarette smokers, or both.

RESULTS

Table 4-1 reports point biserial correlation coefficients between drug-use classification status and scores on each of the eight self-report measures of personality, analyzed both with the sexes combined and with the sexes separated. The first three columns report results obtained with a sample involving nonusers (coded 0) and early users (coded 1). The next three columns are for nonusers (coded 0) and late users (coded 1). The last three are for late users (coded 0) and early users (coded 1). Point biserial correlations provide an efficient method of comparing pairs of groups because a single signed number and its associated probability level give information concerning the direction, magnitude, and level of statistical significance of each comparison between two groups. For example, the value $-.50$ ($p = .001$), which is the first result in column 1 of Table 4-1, indicates that nonusers scored higher on the variable "obedient, law-abiding" than did early users, that the correlation is significant at the .001 level, and that 25% of the variance in this scale is accounted for by group membership.

All 24 of the correlations in columns 1–3 of Table 4-1 have negative signs, and all 24 are statistically significant. Quite clearly, each of the eight self-report measures of personality obtained in Year 1 of the study significantly predicts which students will begin using marihuana early (before grade 10) and which will remain nonusers. (Late users are not involved in analyses presented in columns 1–3.)

The 24 correlations in columns 4–6 of Table 4-1, which compare nonusers with late users, and the 24 in columns 7–9, which compare late users with early users, are smaller than those in columns 1–3; but they are all negative in sign, and 32 of the 48 are statistically significant. The fact that the signs in columns 4–9 are consistently negative indicates that nonusers score higher than late users and that late users score higher than early users on all eight self-report measures of personality.

Table 4-2 reports point biserial correlations for the 20 peer rating measures of personality. In the age group that provided the data reported here, factor analysis of the 20 peer variables typically reveals one large factor, defined by 18 of the 20 peer variables, which we call "Socialization." Variable 5 (emotional) and Variable 10 (sociable) are treated as specific variables. The upper portion of Table 4-2 presents results for the nine positively oriented peer variables of the Socialization factor. Immediately below those correlations are the ones for the nine negatively oriented measures of that factor. Results for the peer variables "emotional" and "sociable" appear at the bottom of Table 4-2.

Of the 81 correlations involving the positively oriented measures of socialization, 80 have minus signs and 69 are statistically significant. Of the 81 correlations involving its negatively oriented measures, 79 have plus signs and 63 are statistically significant. Thus, as evaluated by the 18 nonindependent peer variables that measure the factor we call Socialization, nonusers score highest, early users score lowest, and late users are intermediate. These results are highly consistent internally, and they are conceptually concordant with those based on the self-report measures reported in Table 4-1.

For males, and for the total sample, early users are rated as being more emotional (Variable 5) than late users or nonusers. A similar tendency is seen for females, but it is not statistically significant. For both sexes, nonusers are rated as being significantly less sociable (Variable 10) than either late users or early users.

TABLE 4-1 Point Biserial Correlations between Self-report Personality Variables Measured in Grades Seven and Eight and Drug Status Measured 2–4 Years Later

Variable	Nonusers versus early users[a]			Nonusers versus late users[b]			Late users versus early users		
	Total	Males	Females	Total	Males	Females	Total	Males	Females
1. Obedient, law-abiding	-.50***	-.51***	-.49***	-.26***	-.27***	-.26***	-.26***	-.24***	-.27***
2. Works hard and effectively	-.35***	-.37***	-.33***	-.14**	-.19**	-.11	-.20***	-.17*	-.21**
3. Feels capable	-.23***	-.24**	-.22**	-.08	-.13*	-.04	-.14**	-.10	-.18**
4. Confident academically	-.21***	-.21**	-.23**	-.07	-.06	-.08	-.14**	-.15*	-.15*
5. Self-sufficient	-.20***	-.21**	-.20**	-.14**	-.14*	-.14*	-.05	-.06	-.05
6. Likes school	-.27***	-.24**	-.31***	-.13**	-.09	-.17**	-.14**	-.13	-.15*
7. Ambitious	-.26***	-.25***	-.27***	-.09*	-.08	-.11	-.16***	-.17**	-.15*
8. Feels valued and accepted	-.28***	-.30***	-.26***	-.10*	-.11	-.09	-.18***	-.21**	-.16*

Note. For sample size, see Tables 4-3, 4-4, and 4-5.
[a]Initiated use in 9th grade or earlier.
[b]Initiated use in 10th grade or later.
*p = .05.
**p = .01.
***p = .001.

105

TABLE 4-2 Point Biserial Correlations between Peer Rating Personality Variables Measured in Grades Seven and Eight and Drug Status Measured 2–4 Years Later

Variable	Nonusers versus early users[a]			Nonusers versus late users[b]			Late users versus early users		
	Total	Males	Females	Total	Males	Females	Total	Males	Females
Socialization variables with positive factor loadings									
1. Orderly	-.31***	-.37***	-.26***	-.09*	-.15*	-.04	-.21***	-.21**	-.21***
2. Curious, interested	-.36***	-.41***	-.31***	-.08	-.13*	-.04	-.23***	-.22***	-.25***
4. Tender	-.39***	-.50***	-.37***	-.13**	-.22***	-.09	-.24***	-.27***	-.25***
6. Determined, persistent	-.32***	-.35***	-.28***	-.10*	-.16**	-.04	-.18***	-.16*	-.21***
9. Obedient	-.45***	-.53***	-.37***	-.24***	-.29***	-.21***	-.21***	-.25***	-.16*
11. Likes hard thinking	-.36***	-.40***	-.32***	-.11*	-.12*	-.11	-.22***	-.25***	-.19**
13. Tries hard to achieve	-.34***	-.43***	-.26***	-.13*	-.16*	-.10	-.18***	-.21**	-.14*
16. Feels in control	-.23***	-.27***	-.19**	-.05	-.12	+.03	-.15**	-.11	-.21***
18. Works hard	-.35***	-.44***	-.26***	-.14***	-.21***	-.07	-.19***	-.20**	-.18**
Socialization variables with negative factor loadings									
3. Does not concentrate	+.36***	+.43***	+.30***	+.14**	+.19**	+.10	+.21***	+.23***	+.18**
7. Immature interests	+.24***	+.33***	+.13	+.06	+.10	+.02	+.16***	+.21***	+.10
8. Slow worker	+.29***	+.38***	+.19**	+.08	+.16*	-.01	+.19***	+.20**	+.18**
12. Cannot always be trusted	+.38***	+.46***	+.30***	+.17***	+.24***	+.10	+.19***	+.21***	+.17*
14. Dependent	+.25***	+.28***	+.22***	+.14**	+.19**	+.10	+.09	+.07	+.10
15. Impulsive	+.41***	+.48***	+.36***	+.20***	+.26***	+.14*	+.20***	+.22***	+.18**
17. Not responsible	+.34***	+.45***	+.21**	+.13*	+.22***	+.03	+.18***	+.19***	+.17**
19. Pessimistic	+.27***	+.33***	+.21**	+.06	+.12	-.01	+.19***	+.19***	+.19**
20. Not considerate	+.37***	+.45***	+.30***	+.13***	+.21***	+.06	+.21***	+.23***	+.21***
Nonsocialization variables									
5. Emotional	+.15**	+.21**	+.10	+.02	+.04	+.00	+.12*	+.14*	+.09
10. Sociable, talkative, outgoing	+.29***	+.29***	+.29***	+.21***	+.19**	+.22***	+.06	+.07	+.05

Note. For sample size, see Tables 4-3, 4-4, and 4-5.
[a]Initiated use in 9th grade or earlier.
[b]Initiated use in 10th grade or later.
*p = .05.
**p = .01.
***p = .001.

Late users tend to score lower than early users on sociability, but the relationship is not statistically significant.

The point biserial results for the seven measures of attitudes toward cigarette smoking are not tabulated in this report; but all 63 had negative signs, and 56 were statistically significant. Thus, nonusers had the most unfavorable attitudes toward cigarette smoking; early users had the most favorable attitudes; and late users were intermediate.

Tables 4-3, 4-4, and 4-5 report means and standard deviations for each of the three drug-use groups on each of 12 predictor variables and evaluate the differences among those means, using analysis of variance. The results in Table 4-3 are for the total sample of 651.[1] Table 4-4 shows results for the 303 males; Table 4-5 gives results for the 348 females. The 12 variables in Tables 4-3 through 4-5 were selected from the larger battery of 37 on the basis of multivariate analyses not reported here. Of the 12, 3 are self-report personality variables; 4 are peer variables; 3 are measures of smoking attitudes; and the remaining 2 are cigarette smoking and grade-point average.

Examination of Tables 4-3 through 4-5 reveals that each of the 12 variables differentiates significantly among the three groups, both when the sexes are combined and when they are treated separately. Note also that the group means vary monotonically in all 36 analyses. This monotonicity of means and the consistent statistical significance reflect the same underlying uniformity of results seen for the correlation coefficients in Tables 4-1 and 4-2.

As expected, males and females differ on grade-point average and on certain personality characteristics when drug-use status is controlled. Although such differences are important in other respects, they did not appreciably influence the construction of the multivariate discriminant models reported in Table 4-6, and they therefore will not be considered further.

A three-group multiple discriminant analysis was performed for males alone; another was performed for females alone; and a third was performed for the total sample. In each analysis, the predictor battery contained the 12 variables listed in Tables 4-3 through 4-5. The first discriminant function was highly significant in all three analyses. The second was not significant in either of the single-sex analyses. It was significant for the total sample; but even there, it did not contribute substantially to increased accuracy of group classification. Since most of the discriminative information is summarized by the first discriminant function, we used it to define a composite variable for further analysis.

In developing the multivariate predictive models, we included only those variables that contributed significantly ($p = .05$) to the first discriminant function. Table 4-6 lists those significant contributors for each analysis (males, females, and both sexes) and gives their standardized discriminant function coefficients. Because the multivariate models were highly similar for the two sexes, the model derived from the total sample was used to produce a composite score for further analysis. As seen in Table 4-6, the model assigns negative coefficients to the self-report and the peer measure of obedience and also to two measures of unfavorability of

---

[1] All 651 subjects had scores for drug status, self-report personality, and grade-point average. Incomplete records on one or more of the remaining predictor scores occurred for 16 nonusers, 30 late users, and 6 early users. In those instances, the mean score of a subject's drug-status group was substituted for the missing value.

TABLE 4-3 Comparison of Nonusers, Late Users, and Early Users by Analysis of Variance: Total Sample ($N = 651$)

| | Means | | | Standard deviations | | | | |
Variable	Nonusers ($N = 206$)	Late users ($N = 317$)	Early users ($N = 128$)	Nonusers ($N = 206$)	Late users ($N = 317$)	Early users ($N = 128$)	F value	Probability
Self-report personality:								
Obedient, law-abiding	3.16	2.89	2.58	.45	.52	.57	52.84	.001
Confident academically	2.69	2.62	2.48	.50	.49	.48	7.89	.001
Likes school	2.84	2.70	2.65	.44	.49	.48	7.87	.001
Peer personality:								
Tender	+3.07	+1.60	−1.26	5.57	7.20	6.83	16.81	.001
Obedient	+4.07	+1.37	−1.53	5.77	5.81	7.02	34.44	.001
Impulsive	−1.98	+0.13	+1.97	4.04	5.14	5.64	26.44	.001
Sociable	−1.03	+1.62	+2.05	4.66	5.17	4.24	23.53	.001
Cigarette attitudes:								
Views smokers negatively	2.74	2.56	2.39	.52	.53	.52	18.58	.001
Views smoking as hazardous	3.22	2.96	2.76	.45	.48	.60	36.58	.001
Finds smokers unattractive	3.50	3.11	2.62	.53	.74	.85	63.23	.001
Cigarette smoking	.41	1.06	1.58	.67	1.27	1.60	39.97	.001
Grade-point average	+.38	+.19	−.21	.90	.95	.96	15.58	.001

TABLE 4-4 Comparison of Nonusers, Late Users, and Early Users by Analysis of Variance: Male Sample (N = 303)

Variable	Means			Standard deviations			F value	Probability
	Nonusers (N = 96)	Late users (N = 146)	Early users (N = 61)	Nonusers (N = 96)	Late users (N = 146)	Early users (N = 61)		
Self-report personality:								
Obedient, law-abiding	3.07	2.80	2.52	.42	.52	.50	24.63	.001
Confident academically	2.83	2.78	2.64	.48	.43	.42	3.92	.05
Likes school	2.93	2.80	2.74	.40	.45	.47	4.11	.05
Peer personality:								
Tender	+0.71	−2.16	−4.74	3.29	5.53	7.23	20.04	.001
Obedient	+3.41	−0.47	−4.08	5.66	5.68	7.92	28.25	.001
Impulsive	−1.33	+2.04	+3.87	4.17	5.65	6.71	19.16	.001
Sociable	−0.31	+2.05	+2.18	3.96	5.11	4.08	9.05	.001
Cigarette attitudes:								
Views smokers negatively	2.73	2.59	2.47	.52	.52	.48	5.19	.001
Views smoking as hazardous	3.22	3.00	2.74	.47	.47	.58	17.57	.001
Finds smokers unattractive	3.50	3.20	2.70	.46	.66	.74	30.89	.001
Cigarette smoking:	.44	1.04	1.80	.58	1.34	1.66	22.73	.001
Grade-point average:	+.21	−.02	−.36	1.00	1.04	.95	6.09	.01

TABLE 4-5 Comparison of Nonusers, Late Users, and Early Users by Analysis of Variance: Female Sample (N = 348)

Variable	Means			Standard deviations			F value	Probability
	Nonusers (N = 110)	Late users (N = 171)	Early users (N = 67)	Nonusers (N = 110)	Late users (N = 171)	Early users (N = 67)		
Self-report personality:								
Obedient, law-abiding	3.23	2.97	2.63	.45	.50	.63	29.25	.001
Confident academically	2.57	2.49	2.33	.48	.50	.49	5.10	.01
Likes school	2.76	2.62	2.57	.47	.51	.48	4.26	.05
Peer personality:								
Tender	+5.14	+4.81	+1.91	6.30	6.91	4.56	6.27	.01
Obedient	+4.65	+2.94	+0.79	5.82	5.47	5.12	10.23	.001
Impulsive	−2.54	−1.51	+0.24	3.86	4.00	3.74	10.50	.001
Sociable	−1.66	+1.25	+1.94	5.14	5.22	4.41	14.73	.001
Cigarette attitudes:								
Views smokers negatively	2.75	2.54	2.32	.52	.53	.55	14.35	.001
Views smoking as hazardous	3.23	2.93	2.78	.44	.48	.62	19.70	.001
Finds smokers unattractive	3.50	3.03	2.54	.59	.79	.94	34.05	.001
Cigarette smoking	.39	1.08	1.37	.75	1.20	1.52	18.60	.001
Grade-point average	+ .52	+ .36	− .07	.78	.83	.95	10.47	.001

TABLE 4-6 Variables Contributing Significantly to the First Discriminant Function

Variable	Standardized discriminant function coefficients		
	Total (N = 651)	Males (N = 303)	Females (N = 348)
Obedient, law-abiding (self-report)	−.30	−.33	−.32
Obedient (peer)	−.27	−.40	
Sociable (peer)	+.27	+.18	+.32
Views smokers negatively	−.20		−.31
Finds smokers unattractive	−.44	−.42	−.46

attitudes toward cigarette smoking. It assigns a positive coefficient to the peer measure of sociability.

The composite variable was computed by applying to all raw scores the unstandardized coefficients for the first discriminant function in the analysis of the total sample. The resultant composite scores were then used to determine the degree and significance of separation among the three groups and to evaluate the accuracy of classification obtained when any two of the three groups were compared. As is shown in Table 4-7, the mean composite scores increase from nonusers to late users to early users. Both pairs of adjacent groups are separated by approximately two-thirds of a standard deviation; and in both instances, the difference between adjacent groups is highly statistically significant. The means for nonusers and early users are separated by more than a full standard deviation.

The percentage accuracy of classification for each two-group comparison was determined by plotting the composite scores and using the mean of the two distributions as the discriminant line. This procedure avoids spurious inflation of classification accuracy that might otherwise result from differences in the size of the two samples. The accuracy of classification of adjacent groups was 66% in both cases. This is consistent with the fact that the mean composite score for the late users is approximately equidistant from that of the nonusers and the early users. The accuracy for classifying nonusers and early users was 80%. In considering the level of accuracy achieved in those comparisons, it is important to recall that the

TABLE 4-7 Comparison of Nonusers, Late Users, and Early Users by Composite Scores Derived from Multiple Discriminant Analysis

	Mean	Standard deviation	Total N
Nonusers	−.61	.76	206
Late users	+.09	.89	317
Early users	+.75	1.01	128

	t test	Probability	Percentage accuracy of classification
Nonusers versus late users	−6.39	.001	66
Late users versus early users	−4.63	.001	66
Nonusers versus early users	−10.21	.001	80

classifications are made from information collected when all subjects, early users and late users as well as nonusers, were nonusers of marihuana.

SUMMARY OF FINDINGS AND CONCLUDING COMMENTS

Whether evaluated by self-report or by peer rating procedures, the variables in the present study that were designed to measure traits of personal competence and social responsibility (such as obedience, diligent work and study habits, self-confidence, determination and persistence, consideration for others, self-control, and orientation toward achievement) showed that nonusers scored highest, early users scored lowest, and late users were intermediate. The pattern of intermediate placement of late users held for all 37 pre-use predictor variables studied, although the mean of the late users was closer to that of the nonusers on peer ratings of emotionality and was closer to that of early users on peer ratings of sociability. On cigarette smoking and on favorability of attitudes toward cigarette smoking, early users scored highest and nonusers scored lowest. On grade point average, nonusers scored highest and early users scored lowest. A composite variable (derived from scores on self-report and peer ratings of obedience, peer ratings of sociability, and two measures of attitudes toward cigarette smoking) placed the mean for late users approximately equidistant between the mean for nonusers and the mean for early users. Accuracy of status assignment achieved by using that composite variable was 66% in the case of nonusers versus late users; for late users versus early users, it was also 66%; and for nonusers versus early users, it was 80%.

In a concurrently published analysis of data collected from 2,249 high school and junior high school students (Smith & Fogg, in press), we showed that rebelliousness, poor academic performance, cigarette smoking, and favorable attitudes toward cigarette smoking are associated with increased likelihood of subsequent use of illicit drugs and that these variables also predict subsequent *levels* of illicit drug use. The present analysis demonstrates that those same variables (and other related variables as well) distinguish among (1) nonusers who are destined to begin marihuana use before entering high school, (2) nonusers who will begin use after entering high school, and (3) students who will remain nonusers. In instances where similar predictor variables are used, the results of the present analysis concur with those of a previous analysis by Jessor and his collaborators (1973) that also examined antecedents of early and late marihuana use.

Four conclusions are drawn regarding predominantly white, middle-class, suburban seventh and eighth graders who have not yet begun using marihuana:

1. Precocity of marihuana use can be predicted with statistically significant accuracy from psychosocial variables that are quite similar to those that predict degree of subsequent drug involvement.
2. Earliest use is associated with low scores on pre-use measures of personal competence, social responsibility, and academic performance, and it is associated with high scores on pre-use measures of emotionality, cigarette smoking, and favorable attitudes toward cigarette smoking.
3. On most of the psychosocial variables we evaluated, the mean score for nonusers who will begin using in high school is approximately midway between the mean for nonusers who will begin using in junior high school and the mean for those who will remain nonusers.

4. The level of predictive accuracy found in the analyses reported here is sufficient to warrant further investigation of the theoretical and practical implications of these and related longitudinal relationships.

REFERENCES

Block, J. R., Goodman, N., Ambellan, F., & Reverson, J. *A self-administered high school study of drugs.* Hempstead, N.Y.: Institute for Research and Evaluation, 1973.

Gergen, M. K., Gergen, K. J., & Morse, S. J. Correlates of marihuana use among college students. *Journal of Applied Social Psychology,* 1972, *2,* 1–16.

Goode, E. *Drugs in American society.* New York: Knopf, 1972.

Groves, W. E. Patterns of student drug use and lifestyles. In E. Josephson & E. E. Carroll (Eds.), *Drug use: Epidemiological and sociological approaches.* Washington: Hemisphere, 1974.

Hogan, R., Mankin, D., Conway, J., & Fox, S. Personality correlates of undergraduate marihuana use. *Journal of Consulting and Clinical Psychology,* 1970, *35,* 58–63.

Jessor, R., Jessor, S. L., & Finney, J. A social psychology of marihuana use: Longitudinal studies of high school and college youth. *Journal of Personality and Social Psychology,* 1973, *26,* 1–15.

Johnson, B. D. *Social determinants of the use of "dangerous drugs" by college students.* Doctoral dissertation, Columbia University, privately published by the author, June 1971.

Johnston, L. D. *Drugs and American youth.* Ann Arbor: Institute for Social Research, 1973.

Josephson, E., Haberman, P. W., Zanes, A., & Elinson, J. Adolescent marihuana use: Report on a national survey. In S. Einstein & S. Allen (Eds.), *Proceedings of the First International Conference on Student Drug Surveys.* Farmingdale, N.Y.: Baywood, 1972.

Kandel, D. B. Stages in adolescent involvement in drug use. *Science,* 1975, *190,* 912–914.

McGlothlin, W. H., Jamison, K., & Rosenblatt, S. Marihuana and the use of other drugs. *Nature,* 1970, *228,* 1227–1229.

Mellinger, G. D., Somers, R. H., & Manheimer, D. I. Drug use research items pertaining to personality and interpersonal relations: A working paper for research investigators. In D. J. Lettieri (Ed.), *Predicting adolescent drug abuse: A review of issues, methods and correlates* (National Institute on Drug Abuse). Washington: U.S. Government Printing Office, 1975.

Naditch, M. P. Ego mechanisms and marihuana usage. In D. J. Lettieri (Ed.), *Predicting adolescent drug abuse: A review of issues, methods and correlates* (National Institute on Drug Abuse). Washington: U.S. Government Printing Office, 1975.

Robins, L. N., Darvish, H. S., & Murphy, G. E. The long-term outcome for adolescent drug users: A follow-up study of 76 users and 146 nonusers. In J. Zubin & A. M. Freedman (Eds.), *The psychopathology of adolescence.* New York: Grune & Stratton, 1970.

Sadava, S. W. *Becoming a marihuana user: A longitudinal social learning study.* Paper presented at the annual meeting of the Canadian Psychological Association, Montreal, 1972.

Segal, B. Drug use and fantasy process: Criterion for prediction of potential users. *International Journal of the Addictions,* 1974, *9,* 475–480.

Smart, R. G., Fejer, D., and White, J. The extent of drug use in metropolitan Toronto schools: A study of changes from 1968 to 1970. Toronto: Addiction Research Foundation, 1970.

Smith, G. M. Personality correlates of cigarette smoking in students of college age. *Annals of the New York Academy of Sciences,* 1967, *142,* 308–321. (a)

Smith, G. M. Usefulness of peer ratings of personality in educational research. *Educational and Psychological Measurements,* 1967, *27,* 967–984. (b)

Smith, G. M. Relations between personality and smoking behavior in pre-adult subjects. *Journal of Consulting Psychology,* 1969, *33,* 710–715.

Smith, G. M. Antecedents of teenage drug use. *Proceedings of the Committee on Problems of Drug Dependence.* Washington: National Academy of Sciences–National Research Council, 1973, pp. 312–317.

Smith, G. M., & Fogg, C. P. Teenage drug use: A search for causes and consequences. In D. J. Lettieri (Ed.), *Predicting adolescent drug abuse: A review of issues, methods and correlates.* Washington: U.S. Government Printing Office, 1975.

Smith, G. M., & Fogg, C. P. Psychological antecedents of teenage drug use. In R. Simmons (Ed.), *Research in community and mental health: An annual compilation of research* (Vol. 1). Greenwich, Conn.: JAI, in press.

Whitehead, P. C., Smart, R. G., & Laforest, L. Multiple drug use among marihuana smokers in eastern Canada. *International Journal of the Addictions,* 1972, *7,* 179–190.

5

Panel Loss in a High School Drug Study

Eric Josephson
Matthew A. Rosen
*Center for Socio-Cultural Research
on Drug Use, Columbia University*

The only correct method of handling persons
lost to follow-up is not to have any.

H. F. Dorn

THE PROBLEM

One of the major problems in prospective longitudinal research is the loss of cases in the sample. Unless attrition is extremely small or randomly distributed in the designated sample or original population studied, generalizations about the representativeness of the panel at Time 1, or about changes in attitudes and behavior that take place afterwards, may be compromised. This is especially true when research concerns the deviant behavior involved in illicit drug use. In addition, because longitudinal studies of drug use have tended to focus on young people of high school and college age, attrition is a problem because such individuals are so mobile.

This chapter is based on data from a two-wave combination trend-and-longitudinal study, conducted in 1971 and in 1973, of self-reported drug behavior among nearly 60,000 students in 18 selected U.S. junior and senior high school systems.[1] Of approximately 18,000 students grade eligible for follow up at Time 1 (1971), some 10,000 were lost to the study by Time 2 (1973).

Attrition in this study was fairly high (55%). What were the factors contributing to the panel loss? How did the cases lost to the panel after Time 1 compare on selected personal characteristics and the reported use of drugs, particularly marihuana, with those remaining? At Time 2, how did reported drug use by students in the panel compare with reports by students not in the panel, that is, those new to the study but of the same grade? These are among the questions addressed here.

[1] Columbia University School of Public Health, Division of Sociomedical Sciences, "A Study of Teen-Age Drug Behavior," supported by research grant DA-00043 from the National Institute on Drug Abuse; principal investigator, Jack Elinson; coinvestigator, Eric Josephson; coinvestigator and project director, Anne Zanes. Appreciation is expressed to Paul W. Haberman and Anne Zanes for helpful suggestions regarding this chapter.

Although the study was unique in many respects, our findings do have general implications for longitudinal research on drug use.

EXPERIENCES OF OTHER INVESTIGATORS

Before describing methods of data collection and presenting findings from this study, it is appropriate to review briefly the experiences of other researchers who have undertaken prospective longitudinal studies of drug use. The problem of panel loss is dealt with in a number of standard works on survey research (Kish, 1965; Zeisel, 1957), on epidemiology (MacMahon & Pugh, 1970), and on the life cycle (Nesselroade & Reese, 1973; Riley, Johnson, & Foner, 1972). This review is limited to prospective longitudinal studies of drug behavior in populations of the sort represented in this volume. Not included are retrospective studies or panel studies of drug users in treatment, comparison among these studies being difficult because they vary widely in the definitions of the original study population (sometimes an originally designated sample, other times, all those participating at Time 1), in methods of data collection, in the time elapsing between data collections, in the number of follow-ups attempted, and in the ways in which attrition is defined and reported. Not surprisingly, the attrition rates reported by these studies also vary widely. Table 5-1 presents the panel-retention rates from seven longitudinal studies of drug use, all except one included in this volume.

A look at the field procedures of these studies facilitates the understanding of these varying retention rates. Robins has conducted two follow-ups in samples of Army veterans who returned to the United States from Vietnam in September 1971. In the first follow-up, in 1972, 8–12 months after the men had returned from Vietnam, Robins drew two random samples from lists provided by the Veterans Administration. One was a general sample of 470 Vietnam war veterans, and the other was a drug-positive sample of 495 men who had shown urines positive for narcotics when they left Vietnam. Personal interviews were completed with 97% of the surviving members of the general sample and 95% of the drug-positive sample. In one case, 11 visits were made in order to obtain an interview (Robins, 1973, 1974; Robins, Davis, & Goodwin, 1974; Robins, Davis, & Nurco, 1974). Robins (Robins, Davis, & Nurco, 1974) notes that "since over 90 percent of every subgroup defined by race, age, rank, or type of discharge yielded interviews, unbiased estimates of responses by both drug free and drug using veterans were virtually insured" (p. 39).

In a second follow-up, conducted in 1974, more than 2 years after the veterans had returned from Vietnam, and based on a 25-state subsample of two-thirds of the men interviewed in the first wave of the study, Robins reinterviewed 94% of the eligible veterans interviewed the first time. (She also interviewed a control group of nonveterans.) Once again, the cases lost to the study were representative of the original sample on reported levels of drug use (Robins, 1975). The low panel-attrition rates reported by Robins are unmatched, not only by any other longitudinal study of drug behavior we have reviewed, but also by most panel studies, whatever the subject.

Experiences of a different order are reported in several longitudinal surveys of drug use among college students. Rossi and Groves (Groves, 1974) mailed questionnaires in 1970 to more than 10,000 randomly selected freshmen and juniors in a stratified sample of 48 colleges in the United States. Nearly 8,000 students, or

TABLE 5-1 Panel-retention Rates in Seven Studies of Drug Use

Investigators	Population	Designated sample (N)	Time 1 study population (N)	Number of data collections	Interval between data collections (years)	Retained panel[a] (N)	Percentage of Time 1 study population retained
Robins (1974, 1975)	Vietnam veterans	965	898	2	1	571	94[b]
Groves (1974)	College students	10,596	7,948	2	1	3,961	50
Mellinger, Somers, & Manheimer (1975)	College students	1,043 (est.)	960	2	$2\frac{1}{2}$	834	87
Johnston (1973, 1974)	High school students	2,277	2,213	5	1^{c}	1,599[c]	72
Jessor, Jessor, & Finney (1973)	College students	497	276	4	1	226	82
Jessor, Jessor, & Finney (1973)	Junior high and high school students	2,200	592	4	1	483[d]	82
Kandel, Single & Kessler (1976)	High school students		8,206	2	$\frac{1}{2}$	5,423	66
Elinson, Josephson, & Zanes (this chapter)	High school students		18,363	2	2	8,136	44

[a]In cases in which authors only report the percentage of the sample retained, we have estimated the N's. Our figures may not take rounding into account.

[b]The second follow-up was of veterans (N = 617) from the 25 most highly represented states in the first follow-up. Of these cases, six had died and six were stationed overseas. Of the effective target group, 94% (N = 605) were reinterviewed.

[c]There was a 4-year interval between Wave 4 and Wave 5. The total five-wave sample is 1,599. Drug-use data were collected at Wave 4 and Wave 5, with cumulative drug histories available for 1,265 students. The Time 5 sample represents 70% of the original designated population.

[d]The junior-senior high school panel (N = 483) contains cases not present for the four data collections. Those present all 4 years (N = 432) represent a retention of 73% of the Time 1 cohort.

75%, responded to the first wave. (Late respondents were more likely than early ones to report having used marihuana.) In a follow-up, conducted 1 year later, in 1971, addresses could only be obtained for 90% of the initial sample, and usable questionnaires were returned by less than 6,000 students—approximately 60% of those in the mailing and 54% of the originally designated sample. For matching purposes, respondents were asked in both mailings to produce a code number consisting of two 3-digit numbers, the first representing the months of the respondent's birthday and his or her mother's birthday; the other, the days of the month of the two respective birthdays. Fewer than 4,000 respondents could be matched—69% of the Time 1 respondents, but only 37% of the originally desig-nated sample of students who had been sent questionnaires in the first study year.

Comparing this matched subgroup with all respondents in 1970, Groves (1974) reports that the response rate was higher in the more selective colleges. The matched subgroup was slightly more likely to report experiences with socially acceptable drugs and slightly less likely to report use of illicit drugs. The panel of college students was more conventional than those lost to it, although "the differ-ences were not large and the relative proportions reporting usage of the different drug categories were similarly ordered" (Groves, 1974, p. 247) in the panel and among the lost cases.

A second longitudinal study of a college population has been conducted by Mellinger and his collaborators (see chap. 7) in a sample of men who enrolled as freshmen at the University of California at Berkeley in the fall of 1970. Time 1 data were obtained by a combination of personal interview and self-administered ques-tionnaire completed by 92% of the eligible sample. Time 2 data were collected $2\frac{1}{2}$ years later, in 1973, by a mail questionnaire completed by 87% of the Time 1 respondents, or 80% of the original eligible sample. Those who did not respond at Time 2 were more likely than those in the panel to report having used drugs other than marihuana at Time 1. Time 1 and Time 2 comparisons of drug use therefore tend to underrepresent the Time 1 users of drugs other than marihuana. Because of the high overall retention rate, however, the Time 2 respondents are distributed in terms of drug use in virtually the same proportions as the total Time 1 respondents (Davidson, Mellinger, & Manheimer, 1977).

Of several panel studies of high school students reviewed here, only one is national in scope—the University of Michigan Survey Research Center's project, "Youth in Transition," started in 1966. It has, over a period of 8 years, followed up an original national sample of more than 2,000 young men who had been high school sophomores in 1966 (Johnston, O'Malley, & Eveland, chap. 6). Four succes-sive annual personal interviews were conducted between 1966 and 1970, at which time (1 year after graduation from high school) respondents were first questioned about past as well as current drug use. By the fourth wave of interviews, 29% of the original sample had been lost. Johnston has compared those followed to 1970 with those in the original sample and reports that, with the exception of one group—high school dropouts—no subgroup in the panel was significantly underrepresented. In view of the probability that dropouts were more likely to be drug users than those who had completed high school, Johnston considered reweighting his estimates of reported drug use to correct for this loss but rejected the idea on the grounds that such weighting would not significantly alter his findings (Johnston, 1973).

In a more recent follow-up on his 1970 panel, conducted in 1974, Johnston (1974) reports a further attrition of approximately 13%. He also reports significantly more illicit drug use by the end of the 12th grade and in the year after high school among those in the 1970 sample who could not be recontacted in 1974.

Jessor and his collaborators have undertaken two separate, but parallel, panel studies, one of junior and senior high school students and the other of college students in a large university in the same community in one of the Rocky Mountain states (chap. 2). In the high school study, a random sample of 2,200 students, stratified by sex and grade level, was designated in three junior and three senior high schools. The entire designated sample was contacted individually by letter and asked to participate in a 4-year study of personality and social development in youth. Parents were also contacted by letter and asked to give signed permission for their child's participation in the study. Of the originally designated sample, 949 students (42%) agreed to participate in the first year of data collection in 1969. Of those who had not graduated in the interim, 81% were retained in Year 2, and of the latter, 82% were in turn retained in Year 3 and 82% were retained in Year 4. As Jessor (Jessor, Jessor, & Finney, 1973) notes,

> The fact that only 42 percent of the originally designated random sample of students ultimately participated in the research means that findings on the starting cohort cannot be generalized back with confidence as descriptive of the school population. While this limitation is unfortunate, it does not in any way preclude the testing of hypotheses nor does it diminish the significance of developmental analysis of the starting cohort itself. (p. 4)

The 483 students retained through the fourth year constituted Jessor's developmental cohort. Drawn from the seventh, eighth, and ninth grades, these students represented 82% of those questioned in the first year. Most of the analyses are based on 432 respondents for whom there was no missing year of data. Regarding the attrition, Jessor and Jessor (1975) report "only a few stable differences: the 'leavers' were significantly lower in grade point average than the 'stayers' of both sexes, and the same was true for expectations of achievement. The overwhelming impression from this attrition analysis, however, was of the sociopsychological similarity of 'stayers' and 'leavers' " (pp. 32–33).

Jessor's panel study of college students was started in 1970, a year after the high school study. A random sample of 497 students, stratified by sex, was drawn from the registration list of the freshman class. Of the designated sample, 276 freshmen, or 55%, agreed to participate. Of the initial cohort, 248, or 90%, were retained in Year 2, 83% in Year 3, and 82% in Year 4 (Jessor et al., 1973).

In the last of the projects reviewed here, Kandel has undertaken a panel study of drug use in a sample of New York State high school students, their best friends, and their parents (Kandel, Kessler, & Margulies, chap. 3). This was for most respondents a two-wave panel study carried out on a multiphasic random sample of the New York State secondary school population during 1 school year, that is, the first wave was conducted in the fall of 1971, the second in the spring of 1972, an interval of 5–6 months. Data were collected by self-administered questionnaires that students completed in their classrooms. Usable questionnaires were obtained from 8,206 students at Time 1, a response rate of 81%. Kandel attributes this attrition in part to a requirement that informed parental consent be obtained for each youngster invited to participate in the study. At Time 2, Kandel was able to administer questionnaires to 7,250 students in the same schools, a response rate of 76% of those in the first wave of the study. An additional requirement in this study was respondent anonymity. Therefore, to match students in the two waves, Kandel asked them to create a code number based on the middle letters of their names, their dates of birth, and the last 2 digits of their phone numbers, and, in five schools, to create a number also for their best friend. Based on these code numbers, 66% (5,468) of all students in the first wave of the study could be matched to themselves at Time 2. (In a third-wave follow-up of seniors only, conducted after graduation from high school, Kandel reports that 60% of the Time 2 respondents in this group could be matched to themselves.) Kandel (1975b) reports further that, "since unmatched cases contain a higher proportion of drug users than matched ones, the high school panel sample from time 1 to time 2 was weighted to reproduce the frequency of marihuana use observed at time 1 in the total cross-sectional sample" (p. 914).

Panel-retention rates are apparently highest when the investigator is able to identify respondents by name and when the time period between waves of data collection is relatively short. Thus those studies (for example, Robins) that have followed up on named cases and have conducted personal interviews have experienced the least attrition. On the other hand, those studies that have been required to preserve anonymity, to match by self-created code numbers, and to rely on self-administered questionnaires have experienced relatively high attrition (for example, Groves). The time between waves of data collection is obviously a factor, here, in attrition, but it does not explain it (Kandel). In some of the studies described above, panel attrition has meant the loss of drug users or those likely to become users. As Jessor suggests, however, even when attrition is high, plentiful opportunities remain for the analysis of the processes of change, as his own work and that of Kandel show.

THIS STUDY

The main study reported here had, as its primary objective, the measurement and analysis of patterns and trends in drug use between 1971 and 1973 among youngsters of junior and senior high school age in selected communities in scattered areas of the United States. The selection was based on certain a priori assumptions about differences in adolescent drug behavior on the two coasts compared with the Midwest and the Southeast, in small cities compared with large ones and their suburbs, and among different ethnic groups. The selection of schools was also determined in part by the willingness of their officials.

Participants were 18 school systems, including senior high schools as well as their feeder junior high schools, located in five metropolitan areas (one on the East Coast, two on the West Coast, one in the Midwest, and one in the Southeast) and in two small cities in the East and in the Midwest. Within the metropolitan areas, 3 schools were in upper-middle-class suburbs, 2 in lower-middle-class suburbs, and 11 in inner-city districts. Of the schools, 2, located in one midwestern city and in one southeastern city, were almost entirely black; 7 other schools had substantial percentages of black, Puerto Rican, or Chicano students enrolled. So far as can be determined, no important changes took place between 1971 and 1973 in the major socioeconomic and ethnic characteristics of the 18 school populations. Because the schools were selected rather than sampled randomly, findings reported here cannot be taken as representative of local or national trends in youthful drug behavior during the 2 years that elapsed between the two waves of data collection.

The schools also varied in size, grade structure, and attendance—each a factor in panel attrition. Two of the largest (an inner-city high school on the East Coast and a small-city high school in the Midwest) had more than 4,000 registered students. The smallest, an all-black high school in the Southeast, had a few more than 1,000 students registered. Grade structure also varied widely, with some school systems including 7th–12th graders and others only 10th–12th graders.

Attendance rates varied widely. At Time 1, attendance on the day of data collection ranged from less than 50% in one school (an ethnically mixed school on the West Coast) to a high of 96% in a school in a small Midwestern city. With the exception of two schools (one on the East Coast and the other on the West Coast, both registering increases in attendance rates by Time 2), there were no significant changes in attendance rates among the schools at the second wave of data collection in 1973.

Overall school participation rates (the ratio between enrollment and inclusion in the study) ranged in 1971 from a low of 46% to a high of 90%; in 1973, the range was from 50% to 86%. In all but three school systems, there were only minor shifts between 1971 and 1973 in the proportion of registered students who participated in the study. Two of the schools registered increases of more than 10% between Time 1 and Time 2; one recorded a drop of 10%. Differences in study participation rates were related closely to attendance rates on the day the survey was conducted; however, in one West Coast school system (consisting of a senior high school and two junior high schools), the participation rate was less than 50% in 1971 because students were required by school officials to obtain signed parental consent. Although few parents refused to give their permission, many students did not return signed consent forms before questionnaires were distributed. The resulting loss of study participants, and therefore of those eligible for the panel, was also experienced by Jessor and by Kandel. All of these factors—the socioeconomic characteristics of the populations served by the schools, their grade structure, and their attendance rates—figured significantly in panel-attrition rates among the schools.

The first wave of data collection was conducted between February 18 and June 4, 1971, with approximately 35,000 students providing usable questionnaires. More than half the students eligible for the panel were 7th–10th graders in 1971 (Time 1) who would presumably become ninth through twelfth graders in 1973 (Time 2). The remainder were eleventh and twelfth graders in 1971 who would presumably graduate by 1973, and who were therefore ineligible for the panel. The second wave of data collection was conducted between February 28 and May 3, 1973, with nearly 32,000 students returning usable questionnaires. Some of these students had entered the participating schools after the first wave of data collection and could not have been in the panel at Time 1; the remainder consisted of the panel and of those in the same grades as the panel who were not identified as participants in the first wave.[2] Just who among those eligible for the panel in this study did and did not remain in it is discussed later.

The questionnaire itself, procedures for its administration, and techniques for matching students for follow-up had been tested in a 1970 pilot study of nearly

---

[2] Two groups of students, the 11th and 12th graders at Time 1 and the 7th and 8th graders at Time 2, do not figure in this report. They will, however, figure in another report that will deal with overall school trends in drug use between the first and second waves.

1,000 students in two East Coast high schools (Haberman, Josephson, Zanes, & Elinson, 1972). To reach all students present in school and willing to participate in a single day of data collection, the questionnaire was administered in classes required of virtually all students in each school. The Time 1 questionnaire, which consisted of 75 items, was designed to be completed by student respondents of average reading ability in a class period of normal length, that is, 45 minutes. After the first wave of data collection in 1971, minor changes were made in the questionnaire used in Time 2 in 1973 to simplify its use.

Like school attendance and study participation rates, the proportions of students completing the entire questionnaire varied among the schools. In part, this reflected age differences within the schools (older students were generally better able to complete the questionnaire than younger ones), and in part, variation in reading levels and the length of the class period made available for questionnaire administration. A number of schools with the shortest class period available apparently also had students with the lowest level of reading ability. As a result, some students, particularly in the earlier grades, were unable to complete the entire series of questions on drug use, and even greater proportions failed to reach the items on socioeconomic characteristics. Items on drug use were in the middle of the instrument, and items on demographics were at the end. To illustrate, in one ethnically mixed high school on the East Coast in 1973, considerably more than half of 2,000 respondents failed to reach questions on their ethnic origin. In certain schools, as a result, demographic data are missing for substantial numbers of respondents. A usable questionnaire was therefore defined liberally to mean forms with matching information whether or not all the questions on drug use or on socioeconomic characteristics were answered.

Of 18,363 students eligible for the panel, that is, those in the 7th–10th grades in 1971, 44% were identified as members. In developing a procedure for matching eligible panel members, our assumption was that students promised anonymity would be more likely to respond honestly to questions on the use of illicit drugs. The matching technique involved asking all students in both waves of the study to create a 6-digit code number based on the second and third letters of their first and second names and on the date in the month of birth. This technique, which resembles the matching procedures used by Groves and by Kandel, had been tested in a 1970 pilot study conducted in two East Coast high schools. The results indicated that students are reasonably accurate in creating such code numbers and fairly reliable in reconstructing them on a second occasion (Haberman et al., 1972).[3] Perfect matching of these code numbers, that is, matching Time 1 with Time 2, accounted for approximately 90% of the panel. The remaining 10% consisted of hand-matched cases in which at least 4 of the 6 digits in the code were identical and in which there was correspondence in handwriting and in the

---

[3] These pilot studies also indicated no significant differences in the reporting of illicit drug use among matched groups of students who were either asked for no identifying information, asked to supply their names on detachable cards, or asked to construct code numbers. Further evidence that the reporting of drug use by adolescents may not require a promise of anonymity is provided by a special study, yet to be reported, that we conducted in 1973, of matched samples of high school students, half administered questionnaires in their classrooms and half at home. Because questionnaires were hand delivered to the home group, these respondents could assume they could be identified despite the assurance of anonymity, yet no significant differences in reported levels of illicit drug use in the two groups were found.

reporting of selected stable demographic characteristics. One of the major factors in attrition was the 2 years that elapsed between the two waves of data collection. Based on data obtained from 14 of the 18 high school systems, we estimate that at least 20% of the 18,000 originally eligible for the panel transferred or dropped out of the schools subsequent to the first wave of data collection. Not having been asked for their names and addresses, they could not be traced.

A second and related factor was the age distribution of eligibles for follow-up. The 18,000 eligible at Time 1 were not equally distributed among the four grades (7th–10th) eligible for follow-up. Indeed, more than 80% were in the 9th and 10th grades, youngsters who, by Time 2, were most likely to have dropped out of school. Table 5-2 shows the grade distribution of those eligible for the panel at Time 1, including those remaining and those lost. This table shows that, by Time 2, 47% of the 7th graders and 60% of the 10th graders had been lost to the panel.

A third factor was absenteeism at Time 2 among students who had completed questionnaires 2 years earlier. Although we have no way of calculating precisely how many were lost for this reason, school-wide attendance rates at Time 2 provide a clue. Among the 18 school systems, the absenteeism rate at Time 2 ranged from 5% to 50%; absentees averaged 15%. (The fact that the survey was conducted on only 1 day in each school meant that students grade eligible for the panel but absent from school at Time 1 also could not be matched; however, given the design of the study, they do not figure in panel loss.)

A fourth factor in panel loss was inability or unwillingness of students in the schools, both at Time 1 and at Time 2, to create a matching code number. Just how many were lost to the panel for this reason cannot be determined.

Panel attrition in the 18 school systems ranged from 40% in a middle-class suburban high school in the East to 86% in an ethnically mixed West Coast high school. This variation may in turn be attributed to the wide range among the schools in transfer and drop-out rates, grade distribution, attendance rates at Time 2, and the ability of students to create a matching code number.

Of the 18 school systems, 8 contributed 70% of the students retained by the panel; just 3 of the 18 contributed more than one-third. This was partly a reflection of school size, but also of school grade structure. Thus, only 4 of the 18 school systems included 7th graders, and 1 had none younger than 10th graders enrolled. Panel retention tended generally to be highest in upper-middle-class, white, suburban, and small-city schools; it was lowest in black or ethnically mixed large-city schools. Groves (1974) reports a range in response rate among participating colleges of 56 to 92%. He notes: "The more selective the school, the higher the response rate" (p. 245).

An additional 7,600 9th–12th graders, the so-called new cases in our study, were administered questionnaires at Time 2. They included students age eligible who had been absent from school at Time 1 or who, even if present, did not participate in the first wave. This group of new cases also included some students who had entered the schools between Time 1 and Time 2 and some who may have been present on both occasions of data collection but who could not or would not create matching code numbers. How many of the new cases fall into each of these categories cannot be determined. Although we deal, here, largely with a comparison of the Time 1 characteristics and self-reported drug behavior of panel and lost cases, we also compare self-reported drug use of panel members with the new cases in the study at Time 2.

TABLE 5-2 Grade Distribution of Panel and Lost Cases at Time 1 and of Panel and New Cases at Time 2 (in Percentages)

Grade	Time 1 (1971)				Time 2 (1973)		
	Eligible for panel[a] (N = 18,363)	Panel[b] (N = 8,136)	Lost cases[c] (N = 10,227)	Attrition rate	All 9th–12th graders (N = 15,736)	Panel[b] (N = 8,136)	New cases[d] (N = 7,600)
7	6	7	5	47			
8	9	11	8	49			
9	36	39	34	52	7	7	7
10	48	43	53	60	11	11	11
11					43	39	48
12					39	43	34

[a]All 7th–10th graders.
[b]Respondents matched at Time 1 and Time 2.
[c]Respondents only at Time 1.
[d]Respondents only at Time 2.

Selected Characteristics of Panel and Lost Cases at Time 1

As noted above, panel-retention rates were highest in upper-middle-class, white, suburban, and small-city high schools; lowest in black and ethnically mixed large-city schools. Unfortunately, we are unable to present more detailed demographic characteristics of these two groups because as many as 25% of the lost cases did not reach questionnaire items regarding ethnicity, religion, and parents' occupations, a proportion more than twice as high as in the panel. As also noted earlier, students' inability to reach such questionnaire items was concentrated particularly among schools in lower socioeconomic and ethnically mixed communities. If completion of such a questionnaire may be taken as a measure of reading ability, then panel members showed significantly greater reading ability than the lost cases.

This difference in reading or questionnaire-completion ability is worth noting because the panel was younger at Time 1 than the group of lost cases (see Table 5-2). Thus, although 43% of the panel were 10th graders (average age, 15 years) at Time 1, the corresponding proportion among the group of lost cases was 53%. Panel attrition for this study meant a significant loss of older high school students with presumably more involvement in illicit drugs.

Table 5-3 shows other significant differences between the panel and the lost cases at Time 1. The lost cases were significantly more nonconformist in educational aspirations and expectations, attitudes toward school, self-reported achievement, and self-reported absences from school during the preceding school term. Compared with panel members, significantly fewer of the lost cases aspired, expected, or were expected by their parents to complete college. The lost cases were more likely than panel members to have negative attitudes and behavior toward high school life and significantly lower grade averages, and they had nearly twice as many absences from school during the previous term as panel members. Lost cases were less likely to report absences because they were unable to reach the question. What is known about the relationship between absenteeism and drug use may help explain differences in reported drug use at Time 1 between those who stayed in and those who were lost to the panel by Time 2.[4] Cases lost to the panel were more pessimistic and fatalistic than those retained by it. Fewer expected to get ahead; more were disrespectful of the law; more were willing to endorse violence in order to effect social change; and fewer reported confidence in government. A reasonable assumption is that those most deviant in these respects were more likely to have had experiences with illicit drugs.

The cases lost to the panel at Time 1 were more likely than panel members to report either fair or poor health. They were more likely to report having used either pep pills or tranquilizers under prescription. The implication is that the most deviant students were more likely to have had experiences with illicit drugs. In addition, as Table 5-3 suggests, the lost cases were more likely to have positive attitudes toward marihuana and to report that most of their close friends were using marihuana, amphetamines, and barbiturates. Differences in patterns of drug use are discussed in the next section.

---

[4] A special study of chronic absentees, conducted in 1972, in 2 of the 18 school systems, shows twice as much reported illicit drug use among the absentees as among students in the 2 schools participating in the study at Time 1. Similar findings on drug use among absentees are reported by Kandel (1975a).

TABLE 5-3 Selected Characteristics of Panel and Lost Cases at Time 1 (in Percentages)

Item	Eligible for panel[a] (N = 18,363)	Panel[b] (N = 8,136)	Lost cases[c] (N = 10,227)
Questionnaire completion:			
Did not reach question on marihuana use	5	2	7
Did not reach question on father's occupation	19	11	26
School items:			
Want to finish 4-year college or more	54	62	48
Expect to finish 4-year college or more	43	51	37
Parents want me to finish 4-year college or more	61	66	56
Often feel I'm wasting my time in school	32	29	35
Think school rules and regulations are too strict	47	44	50
Have participated in school protest	43	38	48
Have B or better grade average[d]	56	63	51
Had 11 or more days of absences in preceding term[d]	16	10	20
Sociopolitical attitudes:			
Haven't much chance to be successful in life	13	9	16
When I try, something or somebody stops me	31	27	34
Think luck more important than hard work	16	12	19
Think laws should be obeyed even if you don't agree with them	75	79	72
Think it's OK to use violence to bring about needed changes	39	35	42
Have confidence in government to solve problems of the 1970s	59	64	55
Health items:			
Have fair or poor health	10	7	12
Have used pep pills by prescription	8	5	10
Have used tranquilizers by prescription	9	7	11
Drug-related items:			
Began to smoke cigarettes at age 14 or younger	42	36	47
Think it's OK to take a sleeping pill without a prescription	35	33	37
Think it's OK to smoke a little marihuana at parties	36	29	42
Think you can stop using grass anytime you want to	53	48	57
Think marihuana leads to stronger drugs	62	67	58
Report most close friends use marihuana[d]	16	10	21
Report most close friends use ups[d]	4	2	6
Report most close friends use downs[d]	4	2	6
Think marihuana should not be made legal[d]	58	63	53

[a]All 7th–10th graders.
[b]Respondents matched at Time 1 and Time 2.
[c]Respondents only at Time 1.
[d]More than 10% of the lost cases did not reach these questions.

Drug Use in the Panel and Among Lost Cases at Time 1

At Time 1, the cases subsequently lost to the panel were more likely than those retained to report more experiences with drugs (see Table 5-4). Grade-eligible students lost after Time 1 were more likely to report experiences with alcoholic beverages apart from the family and to be smoking cigarettes and were at least twice as likely as panel members to report use of illicit drugs. The proportion of lost cases reporting experiences with marihuana (ever, 60 or more times, or during the 2 previous months) was approximately twice as great as in the panel. So was the reported use of other drugs: amphetamines, barbiturates, cocaine, LSD, other psychedelics, and heroin. Panel attrition meant a significant loss of drinkers, smokers, and illicit drug users.

The different levels of drug use reported by panel members and lost cases at Time 1 can be attributed partly to variation among the 18 school systems in rates of panel attrition and of overall drug use. For example, in a West Coast school with

TABLE 5-4   Drug Use Reported by Panel and Lost Cases at Time 1 and by Panel and New Cases at Time 2 (in Percentages)

Drug	Time 1 (1971)			Time 2 (1973)		
	Eligible for panel[a]	Panel[b]	Lost cases[c]	All 9th–12th graders	Panel[b]	New cases[d]
Alcohol:						
Ever drunk apart from family	56	50	61	78	77	79
Drinks once a week or more apart from family	23	17	28	35	33	38
Cigarettes:						
Ever smoked	61	54	66	64	62	67
Smokes daily	24	16	31	29	29	38
Marihuana:						
Ever used	28	19	36	53	48	58
Used 60 or more times	6	3	9	20	16	24
Used in the last 2 months	20	13	26	39	36	44
Used 20 or more times in the last 2 months	4	2	6	12	10	15
Amphetamines: ever used	11	7	15	20	17	24
Barbiturates: ever used	13	8	18	22	18	27
Glue: ever used	10	7	13	11	9	14
Cocaine: ever used	4	2	7	10	8	13
LSD: ever used	6	3	9	12	9	15
Psychedelics other than LSD: ever used	8	4	11	14	12	17
Heroin: ever used	3	1	4	4	3	6

[a]All 7th–10th graders.
[b]Respondents matched at Time 1 and Time 2.
[c]Respondents only at Time 1.
[d]Respondents only at Time 2.

the highest panel-attrition rate (86%), 58% of all students in the first wave (which included ineligibles and 11th and 12th graders) reported experience with marihuana, the highest of all the schools. On the other hand, in an East Coast high school with the lowest panel-attrition rate (40%), only 36% reported marihuana experience.

The importance of interschool variation in panel-attrition rates is illustrated further by a comparison of two other schools, one with relatively low and the other with relatively high loss rates. In an East Coast, upper-middle-class, suburban high school with an attrition rate of 46%, the lost cases were twice as likely as the panel to report either any experiences with marihuana or its use during the past 2 months. At Time 1, 16% of the panel members and 34% of the lost cases in this school had used marihuana. Looked at another way, the panel in this school represented 54% of all grade eligibles but accounted for only 36% of marihuana users in those grades.

In a predominantly white, large high school in the Southeast with a panel-attrition rate of 78% the lost cases were three times as likely to report any experiences with marihuana and four times more likely to report use of the drug during the past 2 months. At Time 1, only 7% of the panel members, but 21% of the lost cases, in this school had used marihuana. The panel in this school included 22% of all grade eligibles but accounted for only 9% of marihuana users in those grades. The higher the attrition rate, the greater the loss of drug users to the panel.

Older age may also have bearing on the higher level of reported drug use among the lost cases at Time 1. As noted earlier, attrition was highest among the oldest students, that is, the 10th graders. Consequently, the panel was significantly younger than the lost group. Inasmuch as use of marihuana and other illicit drugs increases with age among high school students, greater use might be expected among lost cases.

When age, or more precisely grade, is controlled, however, differences in the proportions reporting marihuana use persist at every grade level. As Table 5-5 shows, the proportion of 7th graders in the panel reporting any experiences with

TABLE 5-5   Marihuana Use (Ever) Reported among Panel and Lost Cases at Time 1 and among Panel and New Cases at Time 2 by Grade in School (in Percentages)

	Time 1 (1971)			Time 2 (1973)		
Grade	Eligible for panel[a] (N = 18,363)	Panel[b] (N = 8,136)	Lost cases[c] (N = 10,227)	All 9th–12th graders (N = 15,736)	Panel[b] (N = 8,136)	New cases[d] (N = 7,600)
7	8	3	15			
8	14	8	20			
9	26	18	33	35	29	42
10	35	25	42	43	36	51
11				54	50	57
12				58	53	65
All grades	28	19	36	53	48	58

[a]All 7th–10th graders.
[b]Respondents matched at Time 1 and Time 2.
[c]Respondents only at Time 1.
[d]Respondents only at Time 2.

TABLE 5-6   Selected Characteristics of Panel Cases and Lost Cases Who Had Ever Used Marihuana at Time 1 (in Percentages)

Item	Eligible for panel[a] (N = 4,710)	Panel[b] (N = 1,486)	Lost cases[c] (N = 3,224)
Want to finish 4-year college or more	44	52	40*
Expect to finish 4-year college or more	33	41	30*
Think laws should be obeyed even if you don't agree with them	57	60	56
Have participated in school protest	65	63	65
Think it's OK to smoke a little marihuana at parties	87	87	87
Think you can stop using grass anytime you want to	85	85	84
Think marihuana leads to stronger drugs	26	25	26
Have used marihuana at age 14 or younger	63	64	62
Most close friends use marihuana[d]	50	43	53*
Have B or better grade average[d]	44	50	41*
Had 11 or more days of absences in preceding term[d]	28	20	32*

[a]All 7th–10th graders.
[b]Respondents matched at Time 1 and Time 2.
[c]Respondents only at Time 1.
[d]A high proportion (more than 13% of panel cases and 23% of lost cases) did not reach these questions.
*Significant at $p < .001$ (chi-square test).

marihuana was only 3% whereas, among the lost cases, it was 15%. Among panel 10th graders, 25% reported such experience; but among 10th graders lost to the panel, the proportion was more than two-fifths. These data suggest that the differences in rates of reported drug use between panel members and lost cases at Time 1 are independent of the age distributions in the two groups of students.

Although attrition meant a substantial loss of drug users to the panel after Time 1, not all drug users at Time 1 eligible for follow-up were lost. Did panel attrition also mean the loss of different types of drug users? In an attempt to explore this question, we have also looked at selected characteristics of marihuana users in and out of the panel at Time 1. These data appear in Table 5-6. The two groups of users did not differ significantly in participation in school protests, attitudes toward marihuana, or age at which they had started to use the drug, but marihuana users among the lost cases *were* more likely to report that most of their close friends also used the drug. They also reported significantly lower educational aspirations and expectations, lower school achievement, and significantly more absences from school during the preceding school term. The last of these items is particularly important because, as noted earlier, absenteeism on the part of those grade eligible for the panel at Time 2 was a major factor in panel attrition. It seems reasonable to assume that panel eligibles reporting a considerable number of absences prior to Time 1 were more likely to be missing at Time 2.

Comparison of panel and lost cases who had used marihuana 60 or more times yields a similar picture. These data appear in Table 5-7. Those lost to the panel reported lower educational aspirations and expectations as well as more absences from school. With the exception of these items, however, the heavier marihuana

TABLE 5-7   Selected Characteristics of Panel Cases and Lost Cases Who Had Used Marihuana 60 or More Times at Time 1 (in Percentages)

Item	Eligible for panel[a] (N = 1,016)	Panel[b] (N = 216)	Lost cases[c] (N = 800)
Want to finish 4-year college or more	40	52	37**
Expect to finish 4-year college or more	30	41	27**
Think laws should be obeyed even if you don't agree with them	42	44	41
Have participated in school protest	74	76	74
Think it's OK to smoke a little marihuana at parties	98	99	98
Think you can stop using grass anytime you want to	91	94	90
Think marihuana leads to stronger drugs	16	13	17
Have used marihuana at age 14 or younger	86	91	85*
Report most close friends use marihuana[d]	88	88	89
Have B or better grade average[d]	40	46	38
Had 11 or more days of absences in preceding term[d]	38	31	40*

[a]All 7th–10th graders.
[b]Respondents matched at Time 1 and Time 2.
[c]Respondents only at Time 1.
[d]More than 10% of both panel cases and lost cases did not reach these questions.
*$p < .05$ (chi-square test).
**$p < .001$ (chi-square test).

users in the panel closely resembled the heavier marihuana users among the lost cases.

Drug Use in the Panel at Time 2 Compared with New Cases

Our data on changing drug experiences among panel members between Time 1 and Time 2 allows us to compare drug use reported by the panel at Time 2 (1973) with drug use reported by other students in the same grades as the panel at Time 2, that is, the new cases who entered the study at Time 2. As noted earlier, these new cases included students who had been absent from the participating schools at Time 1, who had entered the schools between 1971 and 1973, or who may have been questioned at Times 1 and 2 but who were unable to create a matching code number.

With regard to age, or more properly school grade, the Time 1 panel was disproportionately younger than all those grade eligible for it. By Time 2, the panel was disproportionately older than those students in the new-cases group. Table 5-2 shows that, by Time 2, 39% of the panel and 48% of the new cases were in the 11th grade. At the same time, 43% of the surviving panel members were in the 12th grade but the corresponding proportion among the new cases was 34%. Panel members are probably a self-selected subsample who are less deviant and therefore less likely to drop out of school. The new cases represent a cross section of the student population, including that proportion most likely to leave school prior to the 12th grade.

Between Time 1 and Time 2, the proportion within the panel reporting experiences with various drugs increased dramatically (Table 5-4). Marihuana use in the panel increased from 19% at Time 1 to 48% at Time 2. With the exception of glue (more popular with younger students), there were increases of a similar magnitude in the panel's use of other illicit drugs. Many factors contribute here. The panel had aged 2 years in a time of increasing and earlier drug use by the generation of which it is part; trend data from this study show that by 1973 students were initiating marihuana use 1 year earlier, on the average, than in 1971. Also, the panel reported a relatively low level of drug use at Time 1; although some may have stopped using certain drugs by Time 2, the proportion who had ever used them could only increase. Given the influences operating, usage could not decline. Yet, with the exception of alcohol use and cigarette smoking, the panel had still failed to catch up with the new cases in other kinds of drug use. Controlling for grade, and with the exception of alcohol use, a higher proportion of new cases at each grade level reported drug experiences than did panel members (Table 5-5). This Time 2 gap was far narrower than the gap between the panel and the lost cases at Time 1, but the new cases at Time 2 consistently reported more experiences with drugs (alcohol excepted) than did the panel.

One plausible explanation of this difference is that the group of new cases at Time 2 included a number of students who had been absent from school at Time 1 who therefore could not be matched. We do not know how many there were, but data presented earlier showed considerably more drug use among those reporting frequent absences from school prior to the first wave of data collection.

The so-called new cases at Time 2 also included an unknown number of students who may have been present at both times of data collection but were unable or unwilling to create a matching code number. Time 1 grade averages of B or better were reported by 63% of panel members, by 51% of lost cases, and by 41% of lost cases who had ever used marihuana. This suggests an inverse relationship between academic performance and drug use.

The major problem in comparing drug use of the panel at Time 2 with the grade-matched new cases is our inability to differentiate those who had been absent at Time 1 either from those who were actually new to the schools or from those who could not produce a matching code number. The relative proportion of new cases participating in the study varied widely among the 18 school systems. For example, in a southeastern school where the panel-attrition rate had been 78%, the new cases at Time 2 amounted to 58% of all students in the same grades as the panel at that time. The new students accounted for 62% of all students in these grades with marihuana experience at Time 2. On the other hand, in an East Coast school where the panel-attrition rate had been 46%, new cases at Time 2 amounted to only 32% of all those grade matched to the panel then and accounted for 39% of all in these grades with marihuana experience.

Data from the two schools described above suggest that, whatever the proportion of new cases at Time 2, they contributed relatively little to the overall increase in reported levels of marihuana use in the schools by Time 2. The increase is accounted for by the panel's low levels of reported drug use at Time 1 and by the group absent at Time 1 but present at Time 2. This group is presumed to have had more drug experience.

ATTRITION AND IMPLICATIONS FOR FUTURE RESEARCH

The attrition rate of 55% in this study had three principal sources: (1) student transfers or dropouts after Time 1, (2) Time 2 absentees who had participated at

Time 1, and (3) failure of some students to produce matching code numbers. These cases were lost to follow-up in the main because of our guarantee of anonymity. Hence, lacking the names of students who had left schools, we could not easily locate them, and we deemed such effort impractical. Nor could we identify absentees, and in turn, their demographic characteristics, for the sake of correcting for panel loss and for weighting estimates of panel drug use.

Yet we found that panel members and the lost cases at Time 1 differed significantly in a number of characteristics: age, attitudes toward school, behavior in school, attitudes toward drugs, and, especially, reported use of drugs. Lost cases were also much more likely than panel members to report drug use. These and other differences between the two groups bar any generalizations from the panel to the schools on levels of drug use at Time 1 or on later trends in drug use.

The discussion so far of the attrition in this study indicates that the 2-year interval between data collections is, by itself, insufficient to explain the loss. On the one hand, for example, investigators like Mellinger and his collaborators (chap. 7) have conducted follow-up studies over equally long periods of time without experiencing high attrition rates. Kandel (chap. 3), on the other hand, lost one-third of her panel within 1 school year.

High rates of absenteeism pose a special problem for longitudinal research, especially in costs of follow-up. The desire to hold contamination effects to a minimum and to reduce disruption of school routines must be weighed against the students missed on 1-day data collection schedules.

It may be that panel losses will shrink naturally if and when illicit drug use comes to be seen as less deviant. Until that time, investigators may wish to consider reporting more fully and more uniformly than they have on the causes and magnitude of panel losses, with particular focus on the characteristics of lost cases and the drug users among them. This would seem essential for the comparability of findings and for the general improvement in quality of longitudinal research.

REFERENCES

Davidson, S. T., Mellinger, G. D., & Manheimer, D. I. Changing patterns of drug use among university men. *Addictive Diseases, 1977, 3,* 215–233.

Groves, W. E. Patterns of college student drug use and lifestyles. In E. Josephson & E. E. Carroll (Eds.), *Drug Use: Epidemiological and sociological approaches.* Washington: Hemisphere, 1974.

Haberman, P. W., Josephson, E., Zanes, A., & Elinson, J. High school drug behavior: A methodological report on pilot studies. In S. Einstein & S. Allen (Eds.), *Proceedings of the First International Conference on Student Drug Surveys.* Farmingdale, N.Y.: Baywood, 1972.

Jessor, R., & Jessor, S. L. Adolescent development and the onset of drinking: A longitudinal study. *Journal of Studies on Alcohol, 1975, 36,* 27–51.

Jessor, R., Jessor, S. L., & Finney, J. A social psychology of marihuana use: Longitudinal studies of high school and college youth. *Journal of Personality and Social Psychology, 1973, 26,* 1–15.

Johnston, L. D. *Drugs and American youth.* Ann Arbor: Institute for Social Research, 1973.

Johnston, L. D. *Some preliminary results from Drugs and American Youth II: A longitudinal resurvey.* Unpublished manuscript, 1974.

Kandel, D. B. Reaching the hard-to-reach: Illicit drug use among high school absentees. *Addictive Diseases, 1975, 1,* 465–480. (a)

Kandel, D. B. Stages in adolescent involvement in drug use. *Science, 1975, 190,* 912–914. (b)

Kandel, D. B., Single, E., & Kessler, R. C. The epidemiology of drug use among New York State high school students: Distribution, trends and change in rates of use. *American Journal of Public Health,* 1976, *66,* 43–53.

Kish, L. *Survey sampling.* New York: Wiley, 1965.

MacMahon, B., & Pugh, T. F. *Epidemiology: Principles and methods.* Boston: Little, Brown, 1970.

Mellinger, G. D., Somers, R. H., & Manheimer, D. I. Drug use research items pertaining to personality and interpersonal relations: A working paper for research investigators. In D. J. Lettieri (Ed.), *Predicting adolescent drug abuse: A review of issues, methods and correlates* (National Institute of Drug Abuse). Washington, D.C.: U.S. Government Printing Office, 1975.

Nesselroade, J. R., & Reese, H. W. (Eds.). *Life-span developmental psychology: Methodological issues.* New York: Academic, 1973.

Riley, M. W., Johnson, M. E., & Foner, A. *Aging and society,* vol. 3, *A sociology of age stratification.* New York: Russell Sage, 1972.

Robins, L. N. *A follow-up of Vietnam drug users* (Interim Final Report, Special Action Office Monograph, Series A, No. 1). Washington, D.C.: U.S. Government Printing Office.

Robins, L. N. *The Vietnam drug user returns* (Final Report, Special Action Office Monograph, Series A, No. 2). Washington, D.C.: U.S. Government Printing Office, 1974.

Robins, L. N. *Veterans' drug use three years after Vietnam.* Unpublished manuscript, 1975.

Robins, L. N., Davis, D. H., & Goodwin, D. W. Drug use by army enlisted men in Vietnam: A follow-up on their return home. *American Journal of Epidemiology,* 1974, *99,* 235–249.

Robins, L. N., Davis, D. H., & Nurco, D. N. How permanent was Vietnam drug addiction? *American Journal of Public Health,* 1974, *64* (Suppl.), 38–43.

Zeisel, H. *Say it with figures.* New York: Harper, 1957.

III

AFTER HIGH SCHOOL: COLLEGE STUDENTS AND ADULTS

6

Drugs and Delinquency:
A Search for Causal Connections

Lloyd D. Johnston
Patrick M. O'Malley
Leslie K. Eveland
Institute for Social Research,
The University of Michigan

Drug use and criminal behavior are generally thought to be related, the usual assumption being that drug use causes crime; but there has been a shortage of good data available with which to investigate the possible causal relationships between these two variables. The study under discussion here, "Youth in Transition," contains longitudinal measures of both drug use and delinquent behavior, and hence it provides an unusual opportunity to examine the cross-time relationships between these variables. Using data collected from this longitudinal study of a national sample of young men, we are attempting to address the following questions:

- How strong is the relationship between illicit drug use and other illegal activities?
- Is illicit drug use associated with specific kinds of crime?
- Does illicit drug use lead to an increase or decrease in subsequent delinquency?
- Does delinquency predict later drug use?

It should be noted that an important group of drug users—addicts (however defined)—is not sufficiently represented in this study for our findings to be generalizable to them. This study deals only with nonaddicted users of illicit drugs.

STUDY DESIGN

This longitudinal study of drug use, entitled "Drugs and American Youth," constituted a supplement to an ongoing survey that primarily concerned an assessment of the causes and effects of dropping out of high school. The parent project, "Youth in Transition," was begun in 1965 under the primary sponsorship of the U.S. Office of Education (Bachman, Kahn, Mednick, Davidson, & Johnston, 1967). The design called for a nationwide longitudinal study of young men in high school. The sample was exclusively male because the dynamics of dropping out were known to be somewhat different for boys than for girls.

Sample

The initial sample consisted of approximately 2,200 10th grade boys located in some 87 public schools across the United States. Through stratified random sampling, these boys were representative of all young men beginning 10th grade in public high school in the continental United States in the fall of 1966—a group that would eventually constitute the high school class of 1969 and many of whom would comprise the college class of 1973.

Field Procedures

The initial data collection, which lasted nearly 4 hours, was conducted in the schools. It included a personal interview, a group-administered paper-and-pencil questionnaire, and a series of ability tests. A very broad range of variables was covered, including background characteristics, affective states, delinquent and other behaviors, plans, attitudes, values, and cognitive abilities. Many of these variables were then remeasured on subsequent occasions to permit the assessment of change.

Over 97% of the initial sample of subjects agreed to participate and provided a full set of completed Time 1 instruments. This very high response rate provided a valuable set of initial data against which to calibrate the nature of eventual attrition from the longitudinal panel. Since the initial survey, four follow-up studies have been conducted. Individual interviews conducted at locations outside the schools were used to obtain data for the first three follow-up studies. These interviews were conducted in the spring of 1968, 1969, and 1970. Subjects were paid $2 for completing the first follow-up interview, $5 for the second, and $10 for the third. A self-administered questionnaire was used for the fourth follow-up survey. The questionnaires were mailed to respondents in the spring of 1974, 5 years after the majority of subjects had graduated from high school. Respondents were paid $10 for returning the completed questionnaire.

Retention Rates

The target sample for the fifth data collection in 1974, nearly 8 years after the initial data collection, consisted of the 1,994 members of the original panel who were still living and who had not explicitly refused to participate in the past. Full follow-up information was obtained from 73% of the original sample (1,608 out of the original 2,213 responded). The sample on which the analyses in this chapter are based represents a subset of the total sample obtained at Time 5. Because this chapter focuses on changes in delinquency across time, the most appropriate sample seemed to be one that contained only those subjects who responded at all five time points. This restriction reduced the sample to 1,365. The size of the longitudinal sample was further reduced in an effort to assure that varying amounts of missing data did not distort real cross-time differences on the delinquency indexes and items. Cases with missing data values for any of the five time points on a delinquency index measuring theft and vandalism were excluded from the analyses. While this procedure did not completely equalize the number of responses on delinquency items and indexes, it did reduce differences to an insignificant level. The final cross-time sample filtered for missing data on the index of theft and vandalism consisted of 1,260 cases.

In order to determine whether discrepancies existed between this longitudinal sample and the original sample contacted at Time 1, we compared the disaggregated composition of the two groups by region of the country, community size, socio-economic level, race, intactness of family, measured intelligence, and rate of delinquency in ninth grade (as reported in the first data collection). The longitudinal sample differed in composition from the original sample in several ways. There were: relatively fewer subjects from medium- or large-sized cities in the longitudinal sample (19% versus 24%); fewer respondents in the lowest socioeconomic category (17% versus 22%); more respondents from intact homes (85% versus 80%); more white respondents (93% versus 87%); fewer respondents in the highest delinquency category (21% versus 25%); and more in the higher intelligence categories (40% versus 35%). While differences of this magnitude, in the range of 4% to 6%, are not trivial, we think that they are not likely to alter seriously the results of the kinds of correlational analyses emphasized in this report.

Drug-use Questionnaires

Many of the variables discussed in this chapter were measured at all five administrations; however, the questions specifically dealing with drugs were included only in the fourth and fifth surveys, after the investigators decided that the drug phenomenon merited some focused consideration in the study. In the fourth data collection (spring 1970), approximately 1 year after most of the subjects had graduated from high school, the first set of drug-related questions was included in a confidential information questionnaire. Such a questionnaire had been administered during the first three data collections but had asked only about the respondents' involvement in various other delinquent behaviors. At Time 4 (1970), subjects were also asked about their personal use of each of seven drugs during two different time intervals.

The time interval covered by the first set of questions corresponded to the year after high school graduation, that is, spring 1969 to spring 1970. The second set of questions was identical to the first, except that it asked about the interval *prior* to graduation from high school. The latter questions were retrospective, which would normally make them suspect due to the potential for unreliable recall. Accurate recall on these activities, however, should have been enhanced immensely by the clear social and psychological significance of the activities under investigation as well as by the demarcation of the time interval by a major event—high school graduation.

Questions concerning drug use were also included in the fifth data collection. At this time, the subjects had reached an average age of 23 and had moved through a variety of environments, including college, military service, and civilian employment. Respondents once again were asked to report their drug usage for two time intervals. The first interval covered the most recent year (spring 1973 to spring 1974): "How often have you done this during part or all of the *last year* for other than medical reasons?" The second interval covered the full 4-year span between data collections. Respondents were asked to report their level of use during the 1 year between 1970 and 1974 in which they used each drug most often: "Think back over the last *4* years—that is, since we last talked to you in the spring of 1970. Now, for each drug, pick the 1 year since then in which you used it most often. *During that 1 year,* how often did you use that drug? (Do not include drug use for medical reasons.)" Two additional drugs, cocaine and methaqualone, were added to the list of seven drugs studied in 1970.

Thus, the study contains self-reports of drug use for four different time intervals: (1) pre-1969 (that is, before graduation for most), (2) spring 1969 to spring 1970, (3) spring 1970 to spring 1974, (4) spring 1973 to spring 1974. The pre-1969 measure of use probably provides a reasonable estimate of drug use during the senior year, although it does not ask about that specific period. Insofar as some subjects may have stopped using certain drugs before reaching their senior year, it may actually overstate the annual prevalence figures. Earlier analyses (Johnston, 1973, pp. 42-44) suggested, however, that very few users stopped using drugs in the year after graduating from high school, and it seems just as reasonable to conclude, at least for the high school class of 1969, that very few decreased their illicit drug use prior to graduation. The figures in this chapter referring to drug use in 1969 actually represent upper limits on annual usage for 1969, however.

One relevant assumption about drug use is worth noting. We assume that for this cohort of high school students (the class of 1969), illicit drug use was virtually negligible prior to our Time 1 measurement (fall 1966), when these students were beginning 10th grade. While such an assumption would not be reasonable for high school seniors today, illicit drug use in the mid sixties simply had not reached the vast majority of young people of junior high school age.

MEASUREMENT

Drug Measures

To examine relationships across time between a number of separate illicit drugs and two indexes of delinquency would quickly generate an unmanageable quantity of analyses. Instead, we built a single composite measure of illicit drug use. The concept of seriousness of involvement with illicit drugs underlies the series of categories we created. The categories were based on a combination of the judged or perceived seriousness of the drug (marihuana; any other illicit drug, except heroin; and heroin, in that order) and the degree of involvement with each (experimental use, that is, one-to-two times, versus more than experimental use).

Our first attempt resulted in a 10-category version. Further bracketing of this 10-category variable down to 7, 5, and finally 3 categories indicated that little information was lost in going to 5 categories. The product-moment intercorrelations among the 5-, 7-, and 10-category variables were all greater than .98. More than 96% of the variance in the 10-category version was explained by the 5-category version. Because so little information is lost, we concentrated on this 5-category version. The category definitions, percentage distributions, means, and standard deviations are given in Table 6-1.

There is a clear increase in use of illicit drugs for this cohort, from 21.0% using some illicit drug before 1969 to 52.6% in the year 1973-1974. Over half of the users during 1973-1974 used only marihuana (27.0%). Categories 3 and 4 distinguish between experimental users of one-to-three pills versus more than experimental use of one or two pills. For convenience, and in spite of the obvious inaccuracy, by *pills* we mean amphetamines, barbiturates, hallucinogens, and—when measured—cocaine or methaqualone. These categories contain 8.2% of the sample for pre-1969 and 19.6% of the sample in 1973-1974. The highest category of drug use, which includes all heroin users plus users of three pills more than experimentally, increases from 2.3% to 6.0%.

Heroin users were not separated out from the others because there were very few

TABLE 6-1 Percentage Distributions, Means, and Standard Deviations for Five-Category Index of Drug Use at Three Time Points

Index of drug use	1969	1970	1974
1. No use of illicit drugs	79.0%	63.8%	47.4%
2. Use of marihuana only	10.5%	19.5%	27.0%
3. Experimental use of one, two or three pills[a]	3.9%	5.8%	8.7%
4. More than experimental use of one or two pills[a]	4.3%	8.3%	10.9%
5. More than experimental use of three pills[a] or any use of heroin	2.3%	2.6%	6.0%
Mean	1.40	1.66	2.01
Standard deviation	.92	1.07	1.24

Note. These percentages are based on the unweighted analysis sample of 1,260.

[a]In 1974, *pill* is defined as "amphetamines, barbiturates, hallucinogens, cocaine, or methaqualone." Cocaine and methaqualone were not measured earlier and hence are not included in the 1969 and 1970 indexes. Inasmuch as the use of these drugs is believed to have been negligible in this cohort during 1969 and 1970, their exclusion from the earlier calculations should make virtually no difference in the classification of individuals.

in this study (1969, 1970, and 1974 frequencies are 14, 22, and 34). Furthermore, a seven-category version that does separate out heroin users correlates .98 with this five-category version. It should be noted that the composite drug-use scale has Guttman-like properties: A person exhibiting the behaviors required of each scale location has a very high probability of having exhibited the behaviors required of all lower scale locations.

In some later analyses, we used a trichotomous measure of illicit drug use that distinguishes among nonusers, users of marihuana only, and users of an illicit drug other than marihuana. This measure correlates .94 with the five-category version.

Delinquency Measures

Delinquency was measured at all five time points, from 1966 to 1974, using a self-report scale adapted from Gold (1966). The original set of 26 delinquency items asked in 1966 was reduced to 21 in 1970, and to 18 in 1974. Deletions were made because some of the early school-related items were no longer relevant and because, as the boys became older, some items were less suitable (such as, run away from home). The focus in this report is on two indexes of delinquency, based on a total of 15 items, all of which were asked at all five data collections.[1]

[1] There were several changes in the time interval for which retrospective reports of delinquent behaviors were obtained. The first data collection asked respondents to report on things done in the last 3 years. At Time 2, 18 months later, they were asked to report on things done in the last 18 months. At Time 3, 12 months later, this instruction was repeated, but through oversight, the time interval was not changed to 12 months. At Time 4 and Time 5, respondents were asked how often they had done each thing "during the past year." The use of several different time intervals for retrospective self-reports on delinquent behavior is an unfortunate flaw in our measurements. Because our primary focus is on relational analyses rather than overall shifts in delinquency rates, however, however, these problems do not seriously limit our ability to draw conclusions from the data.

The first index, theft and vandalism, is based on nine items that encompass a variety of illegal behaviors: (1) arson, (2) car theft, (3) theft of an expensive car part, (4) vandalism of school property, (5) theft of an inexpensive car part, (6) major theft, (7) trespassing, (8) shoplifting, and (9) minor theft (see Bachman et al., 1967, for specific text of items). Arson, vandalism, and trespassing are nonincome producing, whereas minor (less than $50) and major (more than $50) theft, theft of car parts, and shoplifting clearly produce monetary gain or material goods. Car theft is ambiguous in that it can be for joy riding or for permanent gain. The second index, interpersonal aggression, is based on six items, all involving striking someone or threatening someone with harm (Bachman et al., 1967).

In the early phases of the study, there was no grant from the U.S. Department of Justice to protect the confidentiality of the data. Consequently, in order to insure that no specific delinquent act could be linked to any respondent, all item-level data were discarded. As a result, for Times 1, 2, and 3 (1966, 1968, and 1969), only index-level data are available and therefore no changes in specific items across time can be linked to individuals. Correlational analyses across this time interval are restricted to the two delinquency indexes.

Neither can we perform other item-level analyses for the first three data collections. Such analyses were done, however, for the 1974 items. In general, there was a fairly high degree of intercorrelation among the items in each index. With the exception of arson, which did not correlate very well with the other theft-and-vandalism items, all the item-index correlations for both indexes were greater than .35.

Because each index is a simple unit-weighted mean of its ingredient items (with up to two missing data cases allowed), the items contribute differentially to the total index. The more frequent offenses of shoplifting and minor theft explain much of the variance in the theft-and-vandalism index (72.8%). Two items involving fighting account for over 70% of the variance in interpersonal aggression (75.5%).

Given the loss of item-level data for the first three time points, it is a moot point as to whether a unit-weighted index is optimal. It is worth noting, however, that a number of investigations have shown that, across a wide range of conditions, unit-weighting schemes are not greatly inferior to other, more optimal schemes (for example, Einhorn & Hogarth, 1975; Quinn & Mangione, 1973; Wainer, 1976). A related problem is that the index fails to account for the seriousness of the offenses. The same criticism has been directed at the Federal Bureau of Investigation index reported in the bureau's Uniform Crime Reports. But Blumstein (1974) demonstrated that an index derived from an elaborate procedure that weighted the crimes by their seriousness was almost perfectly linearly related to the simple unit-weighted FBI index. Blumstein concluded that the weighted index, though useful for certain purposes, contributed no significant information to a national crime index.

Validity

A basic question that must be faced in all survey work relying on self-report is that of the validity of the data. This question is particularly troublesome with questions dealing with illegal behaviors such as delinquency and drug use. Although we have no direct, objective validation of our measures, we think there is convincing inferential evidence indicating that they have considerable validity:

1. Well over 50% of the sample admit to some illegal behavior.
2. Although respondents were asked to leave the confidential items blank if they felt they could not answer them honestly, the percentage of missing data was essentially identical to that in the nonconfidential sections of the questionnaires.
3. There are consistent and reasonable relationships between the drug-use and delinquency items on the one hand, and other variables dealing with attitudes and behaviors on the other.
4. Some methodological studies (for example, Petzel, Johnson, & McKillip, 1973) have included fictitious drugs in the questionnaires. Invariably, these fictitious drugs show very low levels of reported use, indicating that intentional over-reporting is not a problem.
5. The longitudinal nature of the study precluded provision of anonymity to our respondents. This appears to make little difference for validity, however, inasmuch as a number of studies have found no difference in reported incidence of drug use among groups differing in anonymity (for example, Luetgert & Armstrong, 1973; Haberman, Josephson, Zanes, & Elinson, 1972).
6. Studies like the present one have shown similar prevalence rates of drug use for the same age group (Abelson & Atkinson, 1975; O'Donnell, Voss, Clayton, Slatin, & Room, 1976).
7. Gold (1970) used peer reports to establish that 77% of the boys age 13 to 16 in a study of delinquency were "truthtellers." Another 11% were questionable, while 12% appeared to be concealing at least one offense.
8. Finally, considerable effort went into convincing the boys in the interview situations that their data were completely confidential. By 1974, the young men had been confiding in us for 8 years. It is difficult to believe that we would have observed as much stability in our data if there had been a great deal of lying.

RESULTS AND DISCUSSION

Static Relationships between Drug Use and Delinquency

In exploring the relationships between drug use and the two indexes of delinquency, we began by looking at the static relationships observable at a given time point. We began here partly because it is this kind of information that is typically available from cross-sectional studies and partly because it provides a good starting point for getting into the more complex issues of cross-time relationships.

Figure 6-1 gives the mean value on each of two delinquency scales for the individuals in each drug-use category, during 1973-1974. It can be observed that the two delinquency indexes tend to have an ordinal relationship with the composite drug-use index: The higher the level of drug use, the higher the level of delinquency. Further, the relationships tend to be quite strong, though considerably more so for theft and vandalism than for interpersonal aggression. The product-moment correlations between the 1969-1970 drug-use index and the simultaneous measures of theft and vandalism and of interpersonal aggression are .319 and .201 respectively. The corresponding numbers for the 1973-1974 interval are .335 and .156. In other words, the kinds of illicit activities associated with drug use tend more to be crimes against property than against people.

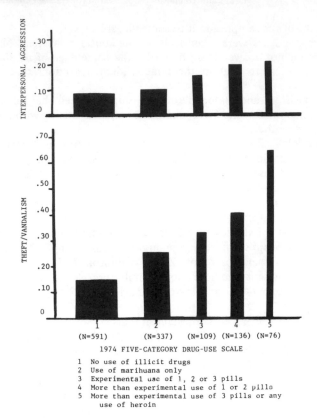

INTERPERSONAL AGGRESSION

THEFT/VANDALISM

1974 FIVE-CATEGORY DRUG-USE SCALE

1   No use of illicit drugs
2   Use of marihuana only
3   Experimental use of 1, 2 or 3 pills
4   More than experimental use of 1 or 2 pills
5   More than experimental use of 3 pills or any
     use of heroin

FIGURE 6-1   Indexes of interpersonal aggression and of
theft and vandalism by five-category drug-use index, 1974.

Analyses of Specific Delinquency Items

As a further check on both the ordinality and strength of the relationship between delinquency and our composite drug measure, we also examined the relationship of the latter with the 15 delinquency items that comprise the indexes. The predominant pattern was that of ordinality, although there were a few minor deviations from it. The data also showed that the items comprising each index vary greatly in the strength of their relationships with drug use. Of the theft-and-vandalism items, those most highly related to drug use (based on the eta value for each item) are shoplifting, minor theft (under $50), and trespassing. Of the interpersonal-aggression items, the one most strongly related to drug use is participating in gang fights.

It is worth noting in these item-level analyses that those using only marihuana in 1973–1974 are really quite close to the abstainers in their levels of interpersonal aggression, despite any public belief to the contrary. It is the offenses in the theft-and-vandalism category on which marihuana users are appreciably higher than the abstainers. Those who use illicit drugs other than marihuana, however, score substantially higher than the abstainers or marihuana-only users on both kinds of delinquency.

Drug-specific Analyses

It is worth considering whether any important relationships between the various kinds of delinquency and the use of *specific* drugs have been masked as a result of our utilizing a composite drug-use variable. To check, we examined the correlations between the individual drug-use measures for the seven illicit drugs included in the period 1973–1974 and the 15 individual delinquency items measured in the same period (see Table 6-2). In addition, we calculated a comparable set of regression coefficients predicting the score on each delinquency item from each drug item (Table 6-2, in italics). The resulting unstandardized regression coefficient constitutes a measure of the slope of the relationship. Unlike the correlation coefficient, such a slope measure is much less affected by the nature of the distribution on the items. As a result, a fairly rare behavior like heroin use turns out to have a

TABLE 6-2 Item-Level Correlation and Regression Coefficients for Delinquency by Drug Use, 1974

Items	Mari-huana	Amphet-amines	Hallu-cinogens	Cocaine	Barbitu-rates	Quaa-ludes	Heroin
Theft-and-vandalism							
1. Arson	.06	.06	.05	.01	.02	.04	.04
	.06	*.01*	*.01*	*.00*	*.00*	*.01*	*.02*
2. Car theft	.08	.12	.07	.09	.14	.07	.09
	.01	*.04*	*.03*	*.04*	*.06*	*.04*	*.07*
3. Theft: expensive	.09	.17	.12	.12	.19	.10	.13
car part	*.02*	*.07*	*.07*	*.07*	*.11*	*.07*	*.14*
4. School vandalism	.10	.14	.16	.11	.07	.02	−.01
	.02	*.06*	*.10*	*.07*	*.04*	*.01*	*−.01*
5. Theft: inexpensive	.11	.18	.11	.10	.17	.08	.13
car part	*.03*	*.09*	*.08*	*.08*	*.12*	*.07*	*.17*
6. Theft: over $50	.16	.16	.15	.19	.17	.15	.21
	.05	*.10*	*.14*	*.17*	*.15*	*.15*	*.34*
7. Trespassing	.17	.19	.21	.19	.22	.14	.10
	.10	*.24*	*.38*	*.34*	*.39*	*.28*	*.34*
8. Shoplifting	.30	.28	.29	.29	.28	.19	.16
	.18	*.36*	*.55*	*.55*	*.51*	*.41*	*.52*
9. Theft: under $50	.18	.19	.18	.14	.17	.12	.04
	.13	*.28*	*.40*	*.30*	*.36*	*.30*	*.16*
Interpersonal-aggression							
10. Hit instructor	.03	.05	.05	.02	.03	.04	.00
or supervisor	*.00*	*.01*	*.01*	*.00*	*.01*	*.01*	*.00*
11. Armed extortion	.05	.06	.08	.15	.08	.10	.09
	.01	*.02*	*.03*	*.06*	*.03*	*.05*	*.06*
12. Extortion	.06	.13	.09	.14	.13	.10	.06
	.02	*.08*	*.07*	*.12*	*.10*	*.10*	*.08*
13. Injurious assault	.07	.13	.12	.10	.15	.08	.09
	.02	*.08*	*.10*	*.08*	*.12*	*.07*	*.13*
14. Gang fight	.14	.18	.09	.13	.15	.04	.08
	.04	*.11*	*.08*	*.12*	*.13*	*.04*	*.14*
15. Fight at school	.03	.08	.02	.04	.03	−.01	.01
or work	*.01*	*.06*	*.02*	*.04*	*.03*	*−.01*	*.01*

Note. The product-moment correlation is given first in each case. The unstandardized regression coefficient predicting the delinquency item from the drug use item is given second, in italics.

strong relationship to a number of delinquency variables in the slope of the relationships, even though the corresponding correlation may be quite weak.

A quick scan of Table 6-2 shows that virtually all drug measures relate positively to all delinquency measures and that those delinquency items that were found to be related most strongly to the composite drug measure (that is, minor theft, shoplifting, and trespassing) are the three that also relate most strongly to all of the individual drug items (with the exception of heroin, which is much less predictive of minor theft and more so of major theft). Table 6-2 also demonstrates that all drugs are more predictive of theft-and-vandalism items than they are of interpersonal-aggression items; that the drugs most strongly predictive of interpersonal aggression are heroin, barbiturates, amphetamines, and cocaine; and that the drug least predictive of virtually all delinquency items is marihuana. In sum, whereas these drug-specific analyses yield some interesting distinctions, the basic similarity among these relationships with delinquency suggest that little is lost by using a composite variable. Further, the major distinction among them is the *degree* of their association with delinquency. The composite index places the drug that is least related (marihuana) in the lowest category of use and the drug that is most related (heroin) in the highest category, thus tending to maximize the ordinal quality of its relationships with delinquency.

Testing the Linearity Assumption

Because correlations were used in some of the dynamic analyses that follow, it is appropriate to test the assumption that the composite drug-use index has a linear relationship with the delinquency scales. We compared the product-moment correlation coefficients with the corresponding eta values derived from one-way analyses of variance. The latter procedure treats drug use as a categorical scale and does not assume interval properties on the independent variable, although the dependent variable is assumed to be intervally scaled. The square of the product-moment coefficient (r) is a measure of the proportion of variance in the dependent variable (delinquency) that can be "explained" by drug use, assuming a linear model with an interval scale on both the dependent and independent variables. Eta-squared is a measure of the proportion of variance that can be explained by a model that includes both linear and nonlinear effects, and therefore it is never less than r-squared. To the extent that a correlation coefficient approaches the value of the corresponding eta for the same pairwise relationship, a linear model captures most of the available variance.

Fortunately, we found a very high degree of similarity between the etas and the corresponding rs. Using the 1973–1974 index (five-category) to predict theft and vandalism, we obtained an eta of .341 and an r of .335. Substituting interpersonal aggression for theft and vandalism, we obtained values of .159 and .156. Thus, the linearity assumptions seem highly reasonable, which in turn make correlation coefficients appropriate statistics for use in analysis.

Dynamic Relationships between Drug Use and Delinquency

The static relationships just reviewed would be typical of what one might find in a cross-sectional study. Such a study would show that drug use relates positively and strongly to other forms of illegal behavior, particularly theft and vandalism. Use of heroin is more related to such behaviors than use of pills or of marihuana.

What is left unanswered, however, is whether (as many believe) drug use *causes* the criminal behavior either directly or indirectly or vice versa, or whether both are caused by other factors, which would account for their high level of association. The last explanation is consistent with an interpretation that illicit drug use and these other delinquent activities are all manifestations of a single construct, which might be labeled "deviance" or "antisocial behavior."

Short of experimental manipulation, the question of causality is best approached with data gathered over time on all variables of interest. Only then does it become possible to begin to disentangle the temporal sequence of events and to determine whether changes on one variable tend to precede or succeed changes on another. Unfortunately, a failure to find such temporal connections in a given study does not preclude the possibility of a causal connection, inasmuch as the time intervals between measurements could have been too long or too short; nor does the presence of an orderly temporal sequence necessarily indicate the existence of a causal connection, inasmuch as variables might have a common causal factor with differential time lags in its effects on each. Nevertheless, longitudinal data can do a great deal to illuminate the nature of a relationship and to address definitively at least some of the possible hypotheses.

For example, if we found that the various drug-using groups were fully as different in their rates of delinquency before they started using drugs as they were afterward, it would be hard (though not impossible) to argue that drug use caused delinquency. Conversely, if the drug-using and nonusing groups were all equally delinquent before drug use and subsequently became as different in their delinquency as we know them to be, then it would be hard to argue that these other, nondrug forms of delinquency caused drug use (unless the causal connections were quite short in their time lag).

Average Cross-time Delinquency Scores

The remainder of this chapter is devoted to our exploration of such issues. Because of the complexities of the problem, several different analytical approaches were used. The first, and probably most important, involved tracing the delinquency rates of the various user groups backward in time. We classified the sample into five categories based on their self-reported drug use in the year prior to the 1970 data collection. We then examined delinquency scores at all five time points for each of the five groups defined by this drug-use categorization. The results of these analyses can be found in Figure 6-2. The relationships turned out to be quite dramatic, and we think, quite important.

The figure shows that user groups were substantially more delinquent (on the interpersonal-aggression scale as well as on the theft-and-vandalism scale) *before* they ever used drugs and that the more "serious" their involvement with drugs in 1970, the more serious their prior delinquency. For example, those using heroin (or three-plus pills on a more than experimental basis) in 1969–1970 were more than one full standard deviation higher in their pre-1966 levels of interpersonal aggression than were drug abstainers (Figure 6-2). Other users of pills were more than one-half a standard deviation higher than abstainers, and those who used only marihuana were more than one-third of a standard deviation higher. The eta value, predicting interpersonal aggression from 1969–1970 drug use in a one-way analysis of variance, is fully as strong for pre-1966 interpersonal aggression (eta = .250) as for 1969–1970 interpersonal aggression (eta = .249). Classifying respondents

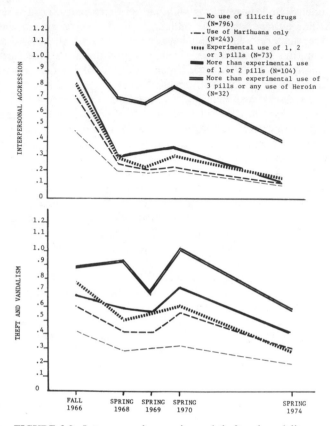

FIGURE 6-2 Interpersonal aggression and theft and vandalism across time by 1969–1970 drug use.

according to their 1973–1974 drug use (Figure 6-3) yields even more dramatic results of this kind. The value of eta derived from "predicting" pre-1966 interpersonal aggression is actually larger than it is with the simultaneous measure (eta = .238 and .162, respectively).

Turning to the theft-and-vandalism index (Figures 6-2 and 6-3), we find a similar picture, although the etas based on the simultaneous measures do turn out to be somewhat higher. For the 1973–1974 drug-usage index, the eta for the simultaneous measures of theft and vandalism is .341 versus .258 for the pre-1966 measures. On the 1969–1970 drug measure, the comparable figures are .323 versus .244. Because one would expect some enhancement of the relationships between simultaneously measured variables from method artifacts alone, these data are rather surprising: It is clear that the preponderance of the delinquency differences among the nonusers and various drug-user groups existed *before* drug usage and, therefore, can hardly be attributed to drug use.

Further, it should be noted that by age 23, the various user groups from 1969–1970 are beginning to converge with each other and with nonusers in their levels of interpersonal aggression (see Figure 6-2). Thus, any effects drug use may have had on interpersonal aggression (and the evidence is certainly not strong for its having *any* such effects) must be short-lived.

A similar case can be made for theft and vandalism, although the evidence is less dramatic (see Figure 6-2). The 1969-1970 user groups are tending to converge by 1973-1974 in that (1) the absolute differences among groups are less in 1974 than at any prior time point, and (2) the eta drops from .323 to .230 between 1970 and 1974. The groups are still some distance apart, however, even in 1974.

Inasmuch as we know that most of the differences in delinquency among the various drug-user groups predate the onset of drug use (and are, therefore, rather difficult to attribute to drug use), the question still remains whether becoming involved with drugs has some *incremental effects* on delinquency. In the kinds of figures just discussed, the most convincing evidence would be a divergence of the lines *after* the point of identified use, but not only is there no evidence of such divergence for the 1969-1970 user groups, there was actually a convergence over time. Perhaps the 4-year period between measurements was too long, however. If drug use had relatively short-lived effects on delinquency, the divergence would only be seen over a shorter period, or even *within* the same 1-year interval on which the drug categorization was based. If the latter were the case, we would expect a divergence of the lines at the time point labeled "spring 1970" in Figure 6-2, and at the time point labeled "spring 1974" in Figure 6-3. In fact, in three of the four

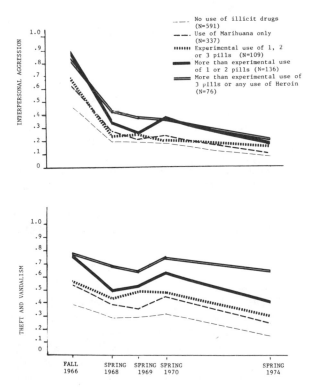

FIGURE 6-3 Interpersonal aggression and theft and vandalism across time by 1973-1974 drug use.

cases, we do observe such a divergence. The various user groups in 1969–1970 tend to increase on both kinds of delinquency during 1969–1970, whereas the nonuser group remains fairly steady. The eta values reflect that fact: Between spring 1969 and spring 1970, the eta rises from .209 to .323 for theft and vandalism and from .195 to .249 for interpersonal aggression. For the various user groups as of 1973–1974, the picture is more mixed. Between spring 1970 and spring 1974, the various user groups do *not* show any divergence in their absolute scores on the interpersonal aggression index because all groups decline about the same amount (the eta also remains steady at .160). On the theft-and-vandalism index, three of the four user groups show no divergence from abstainers with the exception of users of heroin, or three pills on a more than experimental basis. The eta value, however, does increase between 1970 and 1974 from .266 to .341. This is partly due to the heroin group diverging but perhaps even more to the sharp decrease in total variance between the two time points.

In sum, our analysis of the user groups defined at 1969–1970 shows some support for the notion that drug use and delinquency covary (inasmuch as the lines diverge during that time interval). The user groups defined at 1973–1974, which contain a number of people who were not users in 1969–1970, show less evidence of covariation. Such covariation might have several explanations, however, only one of which is that drug use increases short-term criminal behavior. Others are: (1) the association between the variables, when measured simultaneously, is enhanced by method artifacts such as carefulness, accuracy of recall, or tendency to conceal; (2) the overall increase in delinquency rates that occurred in the year after high school (1969–1970) enhanced the level of association between drug use and delinquency for reasons unrelated to the drug use per se (with the weakening of social controls in the year after high school, we would expect a greater increase in delinquency among users than abstainers, given the fact that proportionately far more "delinquency-prone" youth are found among users); (3) those who became more delinquent *subsequently* took up drug use within the same year; (4) drug use and delinquency covary in tandem, not sequentially, because of other common causative factors, or because they are really different manifestations of the same phenomenon.

Thus, we came away from these analyses with some evidence that *could* support the notion of drug use causing some modest incremental changes in delinquency in the short term, but the evidence also supports a number of plausible alternative explanations. The next task was to see if different analytic approaches offered anything more definitive about the existence of any incremental effects of drug use on delinquency.

Cross-lagged Panel Correlations

One analytic method available for addressing the sequential nature of relationships between variables is the cross-lagged panel correlation. This is a technique for assessing whether Variable A predicts Variable B at a later time point better than Variable B predicts Variable A at the same later point. The underlying assumption is that if Variable A has causal impact on Variable B, but Variable B does not have causal impact on Variable A, then the correlation between the early measure of A and the later measure of B will be greater than the correlation between the early Variable B and the later Variable A. As a technique to analyze causation, the method has a number of problems, and the literature concerning them continues to grow (for example, Kenny, 1975). Further, we do not think the method is the most powerful one for the particular data set under consideration here, because we are in the fortunate position of having measures of one of the variable classes (delinquency) at a time point *before* the behavior measured by the other variable (drug use) even *started*. Cross-lagged panel correlations are more appropriate for two variables both of which already have an ongoing rate of occurrence, and thus changes in those rates of occurrence is really what is being investigated.

Nevertheless, we find the diagrams of cross-lagged panel correlation useful heuristically and appropriate for examining change in drug use once drug use has already begun. Figure 6-4 shows the drug-use index related to the two delinquency indexes across a 4-year interval (1970–1974). The means and standard deviations are given for each variable at each time point, as well as all pairwise correlations.

A number of the points made earlier in this chapter are summarized in the figure: (1) Drug use increases substantially over the 4-year interval, as does the standard deviation in the drug-use measure. (2) Both kinds of delinquency decrease substantially over the interval, as do their standard deviations. (3) The static correlation between drug use and interpersonal aggression declines between the two time points, while that between drug use and theft and vandalism remains about the

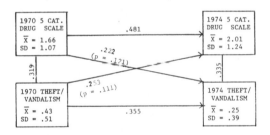

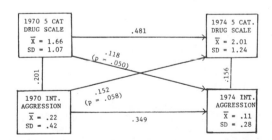

NOTE: The figures in parentheses are path coefficients (partial regression coefficients) in which each variable measured in 1974 is predicted from the two variables measured in 1970. The other figures adjacent to the connecting lines are product-moment correlations.

FIGURE 6-4 Cross-lagged panel correlations: index of theft and vandalism, index of interpersonal aggression, and five-category scale of drug use.

same. (4) Drug use and delinquency correlate with each other most strongly when measured at the same time points, rather than at succeeding or preceding time points. (5) Drug use shows a greater cross-time stability than either of the delinquency indexes. The information that is new to this discussion concerns the correlations and regression coefficients between one variable at the first time point and the other variable at a later time point, and the comparative size of these two correlations and coefficients.

If drug use caused an increase in delinquency, a cross-lagged regression coefficient between drug use and later delinquency would be higher than one between delinquency and later drug use (assuming that the time interval used captures the effect). In Figure 6-4 however, we do not find any significant difference in the cross-lagged coefficients. The coefficient linking 1970 drug use and 1974 theft and vandalism is .121; that between 1970 theft and vandalism and 1974 drug use is .111. The evidence does not support a hypothesis that one is more causative of the other. It suggests instead that there could be some small amount of mutual causation, or that some other factor or factors not included in the figures could account for the possibly spuriously nonzero coefficients.

For interpersonal aggression, there is even less difference between cross-lagged values, .050 versus .058, and neither is very different from zero. This suggests that drug use does not lead to an increase in interpersonal aggression. The 4-year time interval, however, would not have captured a limited, short-term effect. Of perhaps greater importance, the changes over time in the variance of all of the variables work in the direction of reducing the possible magnitude of one cross-lagged correlation (drug use predicting later delinquency) relative to the other (delinquency predicting later drug use). Thus while evidence against the hypothesis that drug use contributes to subsequent delinquency rates in the short term is not ironclad, it certainly provides no support for a hypothesis that drug use is predictive of any substantial increase in later delinquency.[2]

Our third and final analytic approach addressed the question of whether drug use has incremental effects on delinquency.

Delinquency Patterns for Beginners and Quitters

So far we have focused on drug-usage groups defined independently at two time points, and we have not at either point distinguished those who recently became users from the others. In our search for covariance between drugs and delinquency, it would seem that those individuals who shift position on the drug-use index would be most likely to show related changes in delinquency. Using a trichotomy, we distinguished among three groups of respondents: (1) those who

---

[2] In commenting on an earlier version of this chapter, Robert Hauser (1976) pointed out a logical inconsistency between the models implied in Figure 6-4: 1974 drug use depends specifically, in the one case, on earlier drug use and on theft and vandalism, and in the other case, on earlier drug use and on interpersonal aggression. Hauser also pointed out that some of the data are ignored (namely, the contemporaneous and cross-lagged correlations between the two delinquency measures). We chose not to present a model that would have dealt with these deficiencies because of the added complexities it would introduce. The results of the alternative analyses implied by Hauser do not conflict with any of the conclusions presented here. Interpersonal aggression and drug use show cross-lagged regression coefficients near zero (all less than .06); theft and vandalism shows a small impact on later drug use (less than .104); and drug use shows a small impact on later theft and vandalism (less than .127).

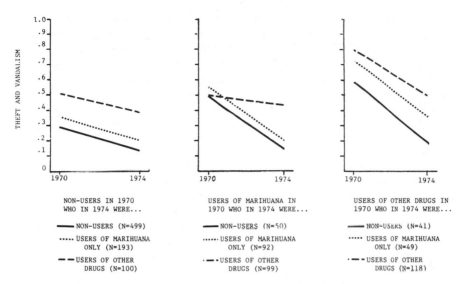

FIGURE 6-5　Theft and vandalism scores by patterns of cross-time drug use, 1970 to 1974.

use illicit drugs other than marihuana in 1969–1970, (2) those who use only marihuana in 1969–1970, and (3) those who use no illicit drug in 1969–1970. (This three-category drug-use variable was used instead of the five-category one to simplify analysis and descriptions.) Within each of these groups, we distinguished another three subgroups on the basis of the 1973–1974 trichotomy. Figures 6-5 and 6-6 show delinquency rates in 1969–1970 and 1973–1974 for the nine subgroups defined by all combinations of moves on the trichotomy across time.

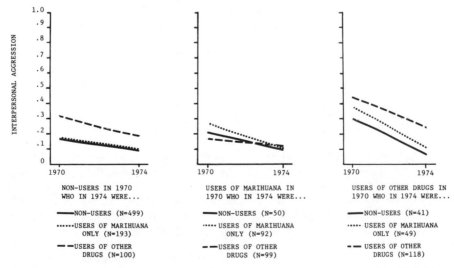

FIGURE 6 6　Interpersonal-aggression scores by patterns of cross-time drug use, 1970 to 1974.

The striking point of Figure 6-5 (left) is that, regardless of whether they became drug users by 1974, all three subgroups show a similar decrease in theft and vandalism between 1969–1970 and 1973–1974. In other words, in spite of the fact that one group of nonusers has begun to use marihuana, another has begun to use drugs other than marihuana, and a third group remains nonusers, there is no differential shift in delinquency rates. Figure 6-5 (right) also displays a remarkable parallelism, with only the middle panel departing from it. The subgroup that increases from marihuana use to other-than-marihuana use by 1973–1974 does not show the sharp decrease in theft and vandalism characteristic of the other two subgroups.[3]

The data for interpersonal aggression in Figure 6-6 are very similar to those in Figure 6-5. There is even more parallelism within panels, inasmuch as the single exception in the case of the marihuana to other-than-marihuana group is less pronounced.

It would appear that there is no differential change in delinquency rates associated with changes in drug use (with the one exception of the marihuana to other-than-marihuana users, $N = 99$). If drug use were causally linked to delinquency, then the groups that increase drug use (as indexed by the trichotomy) should show a relative increase in delinquency, and those who decrease in drug use should show a relative decrease in delinquency. The near-total absence of such findings argues against any causal relationship.

SUMMARY AND CONCLUSIONS

In this chapter, we have examined in detail the relationship between nonaddictive, illicit drug use and other forms of delinquent behavior in a national sample of young men. The age period encompassed in this longitudinal panel study was from approximately age 15 to age 23—the portion of the life cycle generally shown to have the highest incidence of both illicit drug use and other criminal behaviors. Of the cohort studied here—the high school class of 1969—over half had at least experimented with illicit drugs by the end of this period, and the vast majority of those also initiated their use within the same period (1966 to 1974).

The static analyses conducted on the data yielded a number of interesting findings:

1. Illicit drug use related positively and strongly to other forms of illegal behavior.
2. The greater the degree of an individual's involvement with drugs (as measured by his location on our composite drug-use index), the higher his expected level of delinquency.
3. Crimes against property (as measured by our theft-and-vandalism index) are considerably more related to illicit drug use than are crimes against people (as measured by our interpersonal-aggression index).
4. Of the specific crimes against property investigated here, those that tend to be most strongly related to illicit drug use are minor theft (under $50), shoplifting, and trespassing.
5. Heroin use is less related to the commission of minor theft (under $50) than is use of the various other illicit drugs, but it is more related to major theft (over $50) and to the theft of expensive and inexpensive car parts.

---

[3] This exception might suggest that involvement with the more serious drugs is critical to a relative increase in delinquency. If this were so, then the group that jumped from no drug use in 1969–1970 to the use of drugs other than marihuana in 1973–1974 should *also* show an absence of decline in theft and vandalism. In fact, however, this group shows a rate of decline in both forms of delinquency quite comparable to the rate of decline for continuing abstainers.

6. Young men who use only marihuana are lower than the other drug-using groups on both indexes of delinquency. In fact, their level of interpersonal aggression is quite close to that observed for abstainers.

Cross-time analyses were then used in an attempt to disentangle the temporal and causal connections between drug use and other forms of illegal behavior. By tracing the delinquency rates of the eventual drug-user groups back in time, we were able to show that the preponderance of the delinquency differences among the nonusers and various eventual drug-user groups existed *before* drug usage ever began and thus could hardly be attributed to drug use.

Given this central fact, the question became whether drug use may have incrementally affected the delinquency levels of the users. We used several different analytic techniques to address that question and reached the following conclusions.

There is no evidence of a lasting impact of drug use on delinquency levels. The various groups defined on the basis of drug use in 1969–1970 fail to show any divergence or even stable differences in their levels of delinquency between 1969–1970 and 1973–1974. Their annual rates of interpersonal aggression showed a strong tendency to converge with the levels of abstainers over the interval. There is also a tendency, though less marked, for their theft-and-vandalism rates to converge over the same time period. Cross-lagged panel correlations calculated across the same time interval also failed to show that earlier drug use had any causal effects on later levels of delinquency. Additional analyses of those who initiated or ceased use over that period also failed to indicate causal effects of drug use on delinquency levels.

We did not, however, assume the absence of evidence of longer term impact precluded the possibility of shorter term effects of drug use on delinquency; our conclusions here turned out to be more tentative. There was some evidence of modest covariance within the same 1-year interval for which drug use was measured. This in essence must be viewed as simultaneous covariation in the current research design because we do not have observations for time intervals of less than a year. If we did have shorter intervals, we *might* find that illicit drug use preceded an increase in delinquency; but, given what we know about the longer term relationships between these variables, the opposite sequence, or even simultaneous covariation, would seem more plausible. Further, it is quite conceivable that method artifacts accounted for some or all of that covariation. Some of the more plausible ones are discussed in the text.

We cannot conclude that drug use does *not* lead to crime, because one very important kind of user—the addict—is not sufficiently represented in this sample. Although our data would tend to suggest that the kind of person who progresses through drug use to heroin is likely to display substantially more criminal behavior than average, even before drug use, it seems quite likely to us that many addicts increase their levels of crime to support their habits. Neither would we suggest that alcohol, which was not investigated but which is certainly a drug, does *not* lead to criminal or violent behavior. Other investigators have developed evidence that suggests that alcohol may indeed be a contributing factor in assaultive crime (Tinklenberg, 1975).

What we *do* conclude from these explorations is that nonaddictive use of illicit drugs does not seem to play much of a role in leading users to become the more delinquent people we know them to be on the average. The reverse kind of causation seems considerably more plausible, that is, that delinquency leads to drug use. For example, we think it quite possible that delinquents who, because of their delinquency, became part of a deviant peer group are more likely to become drug users because drug use is likely to be an approved behavior in such a peer group. We also suspect that the correlation between delinquency and drug use stems not only from such environmental factors but also from individual differences in personality. Both delinquency and drug use are deviant behaviors, and therefore both are more likely to be adopted by individuals who are deviance prone. The fact that other forms of delinquency tended to precede drug use (at least in this cohort) may simply reflect the fact that proneness toward deviance is expressed through different behaviors at different ages. Further, for this cohort, the notion of using illicit drugs at all was just rising to consciousness among these young people as they passed through high school. Studies of a more recent class cohort would undoubtedly show less precedence of drug use by other forms of delinquency because the average age of first drug use has declined markedly.

So, while, we have relatively little direct evidence from this study to buttress these alternate hypotheses for explaining the connection between nonaddictive drug use and other forms of delinquency, we intuitively find them most convincing at present. Certainly the hypothesis that the association exists because such drug use somehow causes other kinds of delinquency has suffered a substantial, if not mortal, blow.

REFERENCES

Abelson, H. I., & Atkinson, R. B. *Public experience with psychoactive substances* (National Institute on Drug Abuse). Princeton: Response Analysis Corporation, 1975.

Bachman, J. G., Kahn, R. L., Mednick, M. T., Davidson, T. N., & Johnston, L. D. *Youth in transition*, Vol. 1: *Blueprint for a longitudinal study of adolescent boys.* Ann Arbor: Institute for Social Research, 1967.

Blumstein, A. Seriousness weights in an index of crime. *American Sociological Review,* 1974, *39,* 854–864.

Einhorn, H. J., & Hogarth, R. M. Unit weighting schemes for decision making. *Organizational Behavior and Human Performance,* 1975, *13,* 171–192.

Gold, M. Undetected delinquent behavior. *Journal of Research in Crime and Delinquency,* 1966, *3,* 27–46.

Gold, M. *Delinquent behavior in an American city.* Monterey, Calif.: Brooks/Cole, 1970.

Haberman, P. W., Josephson, E., Zanes, H., & Elinson, J. High school drug behavior: A methodological report on pilot studies. In S. Einstein & S. Allen (Eds.), *Proceedings of the First International Conference on Student Drug Surveys.* Farmingdale, N.Y.: Baywood, 1972.

Hauser, R. M. *Measurement and modelling in panel studies of drug use.* Comments prepared for the Conference on Strategies of Longitudinal Research on Drug Use, San Juan, April 1976.

Johnston, L. D. *Drugs and American youth.* Ann Arbor: Institute for Social Research, 1973.

Kenny, D. A. Cross-lagged panel correlation: A test for spuriousness. *Psychological Bulletin,* 1975, *82,* 887–903.

Luetgert, M. J., & Armstrong, A. H. Methodological issues in drug usage surveys: Anonymity, recency, and frequency. *International Journal of the Addictions,* 1973, *8,* 683–689.

O'Donnell, J. A., Voss, H. L., Clayton, R. R., Slatin, G. T., & Room, R. G. W. *Young men and drugs: A nationwide survey* (National Institute on Drug Abuse Research Monograph No. 5). Washington: U.S. Government Printing Office, 1976.

Petzel, T. P., Johnson, J. E., & McKillip, J. Response bias in drug surveys. *Journal of Consulting and Clinical Psychology,* 1973, *40,* 437–439.

Quinn, R. P., & Mangione, T. W. Evaluating weighted models of measuring job satisfaction: A Cinderella story. *Organizational Behavior and Human Performance,* 1973, *10,* 1–23.

Tinklenberg, J. Assessing the effects of drug use on antisocial behavior. *Annals of the American Academy of Political and Social Sciences,* 1975, *417,* 66–75.

Wainer, H. Estimating coefficients in linear models: It don't make no nevermind. *Psychological Bulletin,* 1976, *83,* 213–217.

7

Drug Use, Academic Performance, and Career Indecision: Longitudinal Data in Search of a Model

Glen D. Mellinger
Robert H. Somers
Susan Bazell
Dean I. Manheimer
Institute for Research in Social Behavior,
Berkeley, California

This chapter summarizes the major findings from a series of extensive analyses designed to identify possible adverse consequences of illicit drug use. The data come from a longitudinal study of 834 men, a probability sample of men who entered the University of California at Berkeley (UCB) as freshmen in fall 1970. We collected data from these men at two time points: Time 1, early in their freshman year, and Time 2, $2\frac{1}{2}$ years later in spring 1973. Although the majority (73%) of the men in the sample were still enrolled at UCB by Time 2, our sample also includes men who had transferred to another school or dropped out of school. This chapter is based on data from the freshman cohort.

Our search for adverse consequences has centered on three main outcome criteria at Time 2: (1) dropping out of school; (2) clarity of occupational goals; and (3) among men still enrolled at UCB by Time 2, academic performance as measured by grade point average recorded during the academic year 1972–1973. In the course of these analyses, we discovered that academic motivation and plans during the freshman year had an important conditioning effect on the relation of prior drug use to subsequent probability of dropping out of school (Mellinger, Somers, Davidson, & Manheimer, 1976, in press). For this reason, we added academic motivation at Time 1 to our list of criterion variables. Our findings on the relation of drug use to dropping out of school and to academic motivation have been reported elsewhere (Mellinger et al., 1976). In this chapter, we are focusing on academic performance and clarity of occupational goals.

Our interest in the various outcome criteria mentioned above is highlighted by widespread public and official concern about the possible amotivational effects of using marihuana as well as other drugs (Kolansky & Moore, 1972; Maugh, 1974a,

1974b). Underlying our analyses is the reasoning that an amotivational syndrome of apathy, mental confusion, and lack of goals is clearly inconsistent both with academic success in a competitive academic setting and with the process of finding a self-fulfilling and coherent sense of identity. Establishing clear occupational goals is an important part of this process (Erikson, 1959; Marcia, 1966). We have therefore been looking for evidence that drug use produces amotivational symptoms serious and long-lasting enough to be reflected in the academic and career progress of drug users compared with nonusers. Such evidence would be especially significant because respondents in this study represent a pool of exceptional talent for future leadership.

BACKGROUND

In his treatise on the uses of mathematics in sociology, James Coleman (1964) recognized how easy it is "to be intrigued by the rigor of formal techniques and led down the primrose path of too early formalization" (p. 7). Logically, he observed, the prior problem is to find the appropriate variables. Our primary goal in performing the analyses reported here was to locate the appropriate independent and intervening variables (drug use and other background and personal characteristics) that would be predictive of adverse outcomes. In this respect, our effort was prior to the task of formalization.

In searching for appropriate variables, we were able to capitalize on the fact that a great deal is known about the etiology of drug use in cross-sectional populations of young people. Increasingly, the data support the view that drug use can best be understood as a sociogenic, subcultural, or life-style phenomenon (Goode, 1972; Groves, 1974; Johnson, 1973; Johnston, 1974; Kandel, 1974). This view stresses the central importance of interpersonal influences and of participation in an adolescent subculture with a distinctive set of values at odds with the more conventional values of the adult or parent culture. Investigators generally find, as we have, that young marihuana and psychedelic drug users are more likely than nonusers to:

- Come from relatively affluent and educationally advantaged homes (Johnston, 1974; Josephson, 1974)
- Get high scores on intelligence tests (Johnston, 1974) but low high school grades (Jessor, Jessor, & Finney, 1973; Johnston, 1974)
- Espouse values that have been variously described as countercultural, alienated, and hang-loose (Groves, 1974; Johnson, 1973; Johnston, 1974; Suchman, 1968)

It is especially interesting that, in their longitudinal study of high school students, Jessor, Jessor, and Finney (1973) find that, even before they begin using drugs, drug users show higher levels of social criticism, alienation, and need for independence, lower need for achievement, and lower religiosity than nonusers.

In short, the available evidence indicates that drug users differ from nonusers in many important respects and that these differences are apparent as early as the high school years. Furthermore, it is reasonable to expect that differences in family background and values in particular are likely to be predictive of later differences in the academic performance and career aspirations of drug users compared with nonusers. The questions we pose are: (1) Does drug use show a relation to these Time 2 outcome criteria? and (2) To what extent is any observed relation independent of family background, of prior scholastic performance and aptitude, and of values espoused at Time 1?

Drug Use and Grades

It is generally recognized that high grades are not the sole (or perhaps even the best) criterion of success and motivation in college. Nevertheless, grade point average (GPA) continues to be the most widely accepted and objective way of determining the extent to which a student has both the motivation and aptitude to achieve the standards set by the academic community. College grades also have lasting consequences for subsequent job and educational opportunities.

Previous efforts to relate drug use to academic performance in college have not been entirely conclusive. Blum (1969) found no relation at all. Gergen, Gergen, and Morse (1972) reported that drug users get better grades than nonusers, whereas Johnson (1973) reported that drug users get worse grades, and Walters, Goethals, and Pope (1972) reported that differences between users and nonusers depend on year in school. Gergen, Gergen, and Morse explained their findings on the grounds that drug users were more intellectually curious and open to new experience, whereas Johnson stressed participation in a drug subculture that rejects conventional values of academic success.

The conflict among these results may exist because previous studies did not take into account several factors likely to influence the relation between drug use and academic achievement. These factors include scholastic aptitude and previous academic performance, which many studies have shown to be the major predictors of subsequent grades (Astin, 1971; Lavin, 1965), and also differential grading policies in various fields of study and possible bias in self-reported grades. Our study addresses each of these factors.

Drug Use and Career Indecisiveness

The choice of a career is an important decision for young people. It implies commitment to a set of tasks that will occupy most of one's waking hours, to a set of social relationships likely to generate many of one's friendships, and to a style of life likely to have significant effects on how one is seen by others and how one sees oneself. Marcia (1966), for example, has emphasized the importance of commitment to an occupation as a basic aspect of ego-identity. In short, it is a decision with a major bearing on how one will link one's energies to those of other people in the institutions of the wider society.

Although vocational theorists have given relatively little attention to career indecision as a variable, two contrasting viewpoints are evident in the literature. One view holds that indecisiveness about choosing a career originates in some kind of personality disturbance or general emotional instability (Baird, 1969). An amotivational syndrome of apathy, mental confusion, and lack of goals is certainly one kind of emotional disturbance that would lead to the expectation that drug users are less clear than nonusers about the kinds of careers they would like to pursue in later life.

Holland and Nichols (1964) take exception to the personality-disturbance theory and suggest that "in the past, we've been perhaps too ready to equate indecision with illness, confusion, and the need for counseling. For some people, the deferment of vocational choice may represent a slow and complex rate of personal development" (p. 33). In their study of National Merit Scholars these investigators found that boys with high indecision scores tended to have high verbal aptitude and good grades, to come from homes with more cultural and intellectual resources, to give themselves high ratings on independence of judgment, and to recognize the importance of contributing to human welfare as a life goal. Indecisive students were also less interested in religion. This cluster of traits, Holland and Nichols point out, is associated with potential for achievement and creative performance. Our study shows that these traits also tend to characterize college men who use drugs.

STUDY METHODS

Study Setting

Of our respondents, 99% were between the ages of 17 and 19 at the time of the first interview. They were predominantly Caucasian (82%); 12% were of Asian descent. Median parental income was between $15,000 and $19,999. Because this university has high standards for admission, most of these students had very good scholastic records in high school; 64% had high school GPAs of A— or better.

This university, along with other academically selective schools, was one of the centers of the newly emerging drug culture in the early 1960s. UCB has a relatively long tradition of drug use, and prevalence rates continued to be relatively high in the early 1970s (Davidson, Mellinger, & Manheimer, 1977). Statistically, drug use in this setting has become normal, rather than deviant, behavior—a situation that will prevail more widely if the young marihuana user of today continues to use marihuana in the future, or if use of this drug continues to diffuse through the general population.

Consequently, this university provided an unparalleled opportunity to study the personal and social implications of drug use among an academically select group of men. As Hollister (1971) has pointed out, "In view of the fact that many drug users are recruited from segments of our youth most favored with intelligence and opportunity, the future loss of a large number of these individuals from productive society could be of serious social consequence" (p. 26). Moreover, the drug user himself could suffer serious consequences if his drug use were to become a barrier to personal growth and self-fulfillment.

Sampling

Data from the freshman cohort were collected at two time points. Time 1 (fall 1970) data were obtained from 960 men early in their freshman year by personal interviews and self-administered forms. The completion rate, 92% of the originally designated sample, was exceptionally high (Manheimer, Mellinger, Somers, & Kleman, 1972). The same men were resurveyed at Time 2 (spring 1973) by self-administered mail questionnaires. We again achieved a very high completion rate, 87% of the Time 1 responders, or 80% of the originally designated sample. These response rates help greatly to reduce sampling biases that might be associated with nonparticipation (Davidson, Mellinger, & Manheimer, 1977).

Altogether, 834 students participated in both waves of the study, and all 834 are included in the analyses pertaining to career indecision. Not all were used in the GPA analyses, however, because these analyses required comparable data on grades both at Time 1 and at Time 2. Thus we excluded 117 men who had dropped out of school by Time 2 and 106 men who had transferred to another school, because, in many cases, these other schools have grading policies that are not comparable to those of UCB. Thus the analyses pertaining to GPA are based on the 611 men who participated in both waves of the study and who were still enrolled at UCB in spring 1973. Most of these men, of course, were in their junior year.

Data

Grades and SAT Scores

It is important to note that our data on university grades, high school grades, and SAT scores are largely free of any self-reporting bias that could be associated with these measures. For the most part, these data came from university records and high school transcripts that were obtained with the prior written permission of respondents.

University transcripts for the academic years 1970–1971 through 1972–1973 were obtained for 93% of the 611 men in this analysis. In 22 cases (3.6%), there was no information in the transcripts for the 1972–1973 year, and we used instead transcript information from the previous year (1971–1972) as an approximation of the Time 2 grades of these students. Another 22 men refused to give us permission to obtain their university transcripts but did report their GPAs in the questionnaire. We accepted these data as the basis for their freshman and junior grades. Self-reported grades are highly correlated (.86) with recorded grades.

Analysis of the relation between drugs and grades is complicated by the fact that grading policies differ in various fields of study, and as we have shown elsewhere, drug users tend to choose different fields of study than nonusers do (Somers, Mellinger, & Manheimer, 1974). By reputation, grading tends to be easier in the social sciences and the humanities than in other fields, especially engineering or the physical sciences; and our data show that men in the former fields did get higher grades than those in most other fields. For this reason we systematically included data on major field of study in our multivariate analyses of the relation between drug use and GPA.

We have taken respondents' scores on the SAT of mathematical and verbal aptitude as indicators of the level of aptitude they brought with them to college. These tests are required of all applicants to the university and are usually taken early in the senior year of high school.

High school GPA is a measure of academic performance prior to entering college that reflects level of aptitude as well as motivational and institutional factors. It is a crude measure of performance, partly because it was not possible to take into account differences in grading standards among the many different high schools from which these men came.

The average SAT math and SAT verbal scores of men in this sample were 635 and 570, corresponding approximately to scores in the upper 15th percentile for all college-bound high school juniors and seniors tested in the United States. The average GPA achieved by these men in high school was 3.54, further reflecting the high admission standards of this university.

Drug Use

In both waves of the study, drug-use data were obtained from a self-administered questionnaire. Questions about drug use were asked in an identical fashion at each time, although some additional questions were asked at Time 2. Our questions were restricted to use of illicit drugs and to illicit use of drugs that can be obtained legally. The drug classes about which we asked were: (1) marihuana, hashish, or both; (2) psychedelics; (3) cocaine; (4) heroin; (5) opium; (6) other opiates; (7) inhalants; (8) amphetamines and other stimulants; and (9) barbiturates and sedatives.[1] For the psychedelics, sedatives, other opiates, and inhalants, we supplied a short list of trade and street names of specific drugs to illustrate what was to be included in the class. It should be noted that only 2% of the men in this sample had ever used heroin by Time 2; but 14% had used opium, 19% had used cocaine, and 36% had used psychedelics (Davidson, Mellinger, & Manheimer, 1977).

Respondents were first asked to indicate whether they had ever used any drug in each of the classes and then asked about each of the classes they had used. Three of the additional questions provide the basis for this chapter: (1) How long ago did you first use it? (2) How long ago did you last use it? (3) How many days did you use it during the fall quarter [Time 1]? How many days in the past 2 months (60 days) [Time 2] did you use it? "Fall quarter" and "past 2 months" are essentially equivalent time periods inasmuch as we began interviewing in 1970 in the seventh week of the fall quarter, and 80% of the interviews were completed by the end of the fall quarter.

ANALYSIS STRATEGIES AND CLASSIFICATION

Because our methods of classifying drug users were contingent on the particular analytic strategies we used, we first describe the strategies, then return to the classification methods.

Which Comes First: Antecedents or Consequences?

As indicated earlier, this investigation was designed specifically to study the *consequences* of drug use rather than the *antecedents*. Our study population was one in which drug use was initiated, in the majority of cases, during high school, that is, prior to our first data collection. Because of the high prevalence of drug use at Time 1, we were in a good position to study what happens subsequently to men who are using (or have used) drugs. Some of the men in our sample did initiate drug use between Time 1 and Time 2, but for the most part, patterns of use among these late starters were relatively casual and experimental compared with men who began using drugs earlier (Davidson, Mellinger, & Manheimer, 1977).

---

[1] The drug variables used in this report do not include use of stimulants and sedatives because at Time 1 we unfortunately did not ask detailed questions about whether these drugs had been used for medical or recreational purposes. At Time 2, respondents indicated that, for the most part, these drugs were used infrequently and not to get high. Those men who did use these drugs to get high were, again for the most part, also using other drugs. Consequently, the number of possible misclassifications in the Time 1 data was presumably reduced by eliminating these drugs from consideration, and the Time 2 classifications were not materially affected by the omission. Use of inhalants is also excluded because there were very few men who reported using them.

In our view, previous research has focused attention prematurely on the antecedents of drug use. A fundamental premise of this study is that studies of the consequences of drug use have important implications for studies of antecedents, and can help give direction to them. If it can be established that certain patterns of use are essentially benign for most users, then the search for antecedents narrows to those that help to explain why specific patterns of use appear to have adverse consequences among people with specific characteristics, making them more vulnerable than others to the pharmacological effects of drugs or to the social (including legal) consequences of using drugs. This issue is obviously analogous to drinking behavior. Most people who drink do so without suffering any serious and lasting adverse consequences, whereas for others drinking either generates new problems or impairs their capacity to cope with already existing problems. In this sense, identifying the consequences of drug use should have priority over identifying antecedents.

Strategies for Studying Consequences of Use

A general conclusion emerging from all the analyses we have done to date is that, for most men in our sample, drug use was a relatively innocuous concomitant of life-styles prevalent in this kind of environment. Only in isolated instances did we find any evidence suggesting that drug use might have "caused" something. One such instance comes from our data on dropouts. One small cell of 19 cases accounted for virtually all of the observed relation between drug use and dropping out of school. These men had the following combinations of characteristics: (1) They had initiated multiple-drug use in high school and were still multiple-drug users at Time 1. (2) Unlike the majority of early multiple-drug users, they came from families in which neither parent had a college degree. (3) Early in the freshman year they expressed little interest in maintaining good grades and some doubt about staying in school. The drop-out rate (58%) in this small group was strikingly higher than the overall rate of 7% in the sample as a whole. This rate was also higher than would have been expected, even given the particular combination of characteristics of men in the group. On these grounds we cannot rule out the possibility that drug use had some kind of causal influence for this group.

In general, our data suggested that drug use per se does not have any consistent adverse consequences for most users. As is clear later, this conclusion is qualified by the fact that certain groups of drug users appeared to be doing *better* than the nonusers with respect to certain Time 2 outcome criteria but appeared to be doing *less* well with respect to others. In most cases, as shown below, these differences are reduced to insignificance in multiple regression analyses that include as predictor variables family background, scholastic aptitude (as measured in high school), and/ or values and interests that these men brought with them to college or acquired early in the freshman year. The analyses presented here employ two relatively simple strategies and conventional statistical procedures.

Strategy I asks the questions: To what extent does drug-use status at Time 1 predict each of the Time 2 outcome criteria, that is (1) mean grade point average (GPA 2) during the academic year 1972–1973, and (2) career indecision (the percentage either not very clear or not at all clear about their occupational goals) in spring 1973? Do men who had used particular drugs early in their university career, or in the previous year, differ $2\frac{1}{2}$ years later from men who never used drugs? If they *do* differ, can the differences be explained in terms of other characteristics that distinguish the drug users and the nonusers? If they do *not* differ, are their characteristics suppressing differences that are not apparent in simple bivariate comparisons?

For each criterion (GPA at Time 2 and career indecision at Time 2), we present two regression analyses. In one analysis, we contrasted men who never used drugs by Time 1 with those who had used only marihuana during the fall quarter of their freshman year, the previous year, or both. In the other analysis, we contrasted the same group of men who had never used drugs by Time 1 with those who were multiple-drug users during the fall quarter, the previous year, or both. The other predictors we used in these analyses are described below.

Strategy II also involves four regression analyses using the same two outcome criteria, but two different drug predictors. In these analyses, we combined information about drug use during the fall quarter of 1970 and the previous year with information about drug use in spring 1973 in order to identify two groups of continuing drug users (see the following section for definitions and rationale). In these regression analyses, we compared each group separately with men who had never used drugs as of spring 1973. We used the same set of nondrug predictors we used in Strategy I, but this strategy addresses a slightly different issue: Can observed differences between continuing (or long-term) drug users and nonusers at Time 2 be explained in terms of background or Time 1 characteristics, and so on.

In the final step in the analyses, we combined the two strategies. In earlier analyses, using the automatic interaction detector (AID) procedure developed by Sonquist and Morgan (1964), we often discovered strong statistical-interaction effects. For example, among men whose career goals were clear at Time 1, the multiple-drug users were less likely than the nonusers to be clear at Time 2 (a negative correlation); but among those whose goals were *not* clear at Time 1, the multiple-drug users were *more* likely than the nonusers to be clear at Time 2 (a positive correlation). For this reason, we included in each of the regression analyses a dummy variable that was coded as an interaction term, employing a coding procedure described by Kerlinger and Pedhazur (1973, pp. 154-197). The procedure specifies (1) the interaction of drug use and Time 1 GPA in relation to Time 2 GPA, and (2) the interaction of drug use and career indecision at Time 1 in relation to career indecision at Time 2.

In some of the analyses, the correlation of the interaction term with the Time 2 outcome was statistically significant and remained so after controlling for the effects of the other predictors. Thus, even if the partial correlation of drug use and the Time 2 outcome is not significant for the group as a whole, it could be that drug users compare unfavorably with nonusers given one of the two conditions at Time 1. In such cases, we did additional regression analyses separately for specific subgroups: men with high grades at Time 1 and those with low grades (in the GPA analyses), and men who were undecided about a career at Time 1 and those whose aspirations were at least fairly clear (in the career-indecision analyses).

Classifications of Drug Users

Our major goal in classification of drug users has been to identify characteristics or patterns of use most likely to produce amotivational symptoms. Some investigators have reported that such symptoms are associated with long-term use, use at high dosage levels, or both (Maugh, 1974b), but there is reason to believe that occasional use of the mild forms of marihuana generally available is unlikely to produce lasting symptoms associated with the amotivational syndrome (Hollister, 1971; Maugh, 1974a, 1974b). The question is whether the patterns of use that *actually occur* in a population of "normal" subjects are of sufficient duration or frequency to be detectable.

In earlier analyses, we used two main criteria for classifying drug users: (1) whether or not the respondent had used other drugs (psychedelics, cocaine, opiates) in addition to marihuana, and (2) the frequency of use during the fall quarter of the freshman year (Time 1) or during a comparable time period at Time 2. Throughout those analyses, the more useful distinction was consistently between multiple-drug users and men who used only marihuana. One reason is that the multiple-drug users as a group appeared to be substantially more involved in drug use and in the drug subculture than were men who used only marihuana. Compared with the latter, the multiple-drug users tended to use marihuana more frequently and were more likely to have many friends who used drugs and to say they identified with drug users.

Accordingly, in these analyses, we distinguished multiple-drug users (MDU) from men who used only marihuana (MAR). Our drug variables contrast each group separately with men who never used drugs (NEV) so that in each case the drug variable is coded as a dichotomy, for example, NEV (= 0) versus MDU (= 1), and NEV (= 0) versus MAR (= 1). This procedure has the distinct advantage of identifying specific patterns of use rather than simply assuming ordinality among the various patterns.

We further distinguished two kinds of drug variables: *drug-use status* at Time 1 and *continuing drug use* by Time 2. Drug-use status differs from other variables we used in earlier analyses in that it classifies users according to what drug they *had used* (during the fall quarter of the freshman year, previously, or both) and not necessarily according to what they *were* using most recently. Of the 188 men classified as MDU, 17% (32 cases) had not used any drugs during the fall quarter and 30% (57 cases) had used only marihuana during that period. We shifted to this method of classification because our analyses demonstrated that the fact of having been a multiple-drug user at some time was generally a better predictor of Time 2 outcomes than recent use, although the differences in predictive power were usually slight. The drug-status variables address the question: What subsequently happens to men who had used particular drugs by Time 1, compared with men who had never used drugs by Time 1?

The available evidence discussed earlier strongly suggests, however, that status, level of drug use at one time point, or both is not sufficient to describe the conditions of use most likely to have adverse consequences. Temporal continuity is equally important if we are to specify the extent to which a person has (1) become involved in the drug subculture, and (2) been exposed to the pharmacological effects of the drug or drugs he has used. Early initiation of use could be especially important as a precursor of later difficulties.

Our measures of continuing drug use retained the distinction between use of marihuana (MAR) and other drugs (MDU) but incorporated information about drug use during the 6 months prior to Time 2 as well as information about use during the fall quarter (Time 1) and the year before entering college. A *continuing user* is defined as "one whose pattern of use (marihuana only or multiple drugs) was consistent during each of the three time periods" (this does not imply continuous use between Times 1 and 2). Although we excluded from the continuing MAR group those who had used marihuana only a few (one to three) times during the fall quarter, during the year before, or both, the classification was not based on *level* of use. Continuity of use is, however, correlated with level of use, and thus the continuing users also tended to be more frequent users.

Another reason for focusing on continuing use rather than on level of use was that drug use in this kind of population generally appears to be experimental and casual, recreational, or both. Substantial levels of use were rare even at one time point, and there were too few men who were using drugs frequently over the entire period to permit multivariate analysis.

Nevertheless, by identifying continuing users among the MAR and MDU groups, we also identified not only those who began using drugs earlier but those whose levels of use tended to be relatively high. For example, the percentages of men who began using drugs *more* than 1 year before entering college were 61 among the continuing MDU, 44 among all other MDU, 33 among the continuing MAR, and 8 among all other MAR. Similarly, the percentages of men using marihuana nine or more times during the fall quarter (about once a week or more) were 87 (continuing MDU), 59 (other MDU), 48 (continuing MAR), and 5 (other MAR).

Table 7-1 shows distributions of drug use during the year before entering college, during the fall quarter 1970 (Time 1), and during the past 2 months in spring 1973

TABLE 7-1   Drug-use Prevalence during Year before Entering UCB, Fall Quarter 1970 (Time 1), and Spring 1973 (Time 2) (Total Sample 834)

Year before entering UCB			Time 1					Time 2		
						Those who ever used				
Days used	%	N	Days used	%	N	%	N	Days used in past 2 months	%	N
Never used										
	46	381		41	344	41	344		22	187
Used only marihuana[a]										
$\leqslant 3$	11	90	0 past 6 mos.	3	26	36	302	0 past 6 mos.	12	103
$4-13^b$	13	105	0 fall qtr.	5	44			0 past 2 mos.	9	71
$14-26^b$	6	50	1–3	11	93			$1-3^b$	14	118
$27-52^b$	5	42	$4-8^b$	10	82			$4-8^b$	8	70
$\geqslant 53^b$	4	34	$9-17^b$	8	67			$9-17^b$	4	36
			$\geqslant 18^b$	6	47			$\geqslant 18^b$	6	48
Multiple-drug use										
$\leqslant 3^c$	5	45	0 past 6 mos.	1	6	23	188	0 past 6 mos.	4	37
$4-6^c$	3	26	0 fall qtr.	3	26			0 past 2 mos.	8	67
$\geqslant 7^c$	7	61	$1-2^c$	6	50			$1-2^c$	7	56
			3^c	5	40			3^c	3	21
			$\geqslant 4^c$	1	9			$\geqslant 4^c$	2	20

[a]Includes 57 men who were multiple drug users before entering UCB.
[b]Continuing marihuana-only users ($N = 73$) met one of these criteria at all three time points.
[c]Continuing multiple-drug users ($N = 46$) met one of these criteria at all three time points.

(Time 2). The "ever-used" column shows the distribution of Time 1 drug-use status—the basis for the drug variables used in the Strategy I analyses. For reasons mentioned earlier, 223 of the 834 cases were excluded from the analyses of grade point average. "Time 1 days used" describes use specifically during the fall quarter, so that some of the men classified as MDU in the drug-use status variable show up as having used only marihuana during the fall quarter. Also for the MDU group, the number of days used refers to use of drugs other than marihuana, that is, psychedelics, cocaine, and opiates.

It is evident from Table 7-1 that use of illicit drugs was widely prevalent in this population. By Time 2, 78% of these men had used drugs at least once; 22% had never used any. At Time 1, 55% had used drugs during the past 6 months; at Time 2, the figure was 61%. At each of the three time points, there were more men using only marihuana than there were using other drugs as well. By Time 2, however, 39% had used other drugs at some time or other, almost exactly as many as had ever used only marihuana (Davidson, Mellinger, & Manheimer, 1977).

It is evident that prevalence of illicit drug use on the Berkeley campus was very high, even in 1970. There is evidence, however, that these high prevalence rates were not atypical. Data from a national study of college students conducted a year earlier (Groves, 1974) indicate that usage rates in our freshman panel at Time 1 were not much higher than the average nationally at similar schools and were below the high usage rates at some other schools. More recent Gallup Opinion Index (1974) data also show that prevalence of drug use among college students generally was about on a par, by 1974, with the prevalence we found at UCB in 1970.

In Table 7-1, the criteria we used for selecting the continuing MAR are signified by (*a*), the criteria for MDU by (*b*). There were 73 men who satisfied the criteria for continuing MAR at all three time points and 46 who satisfied the criteria for continuing MDU. These two groups together comprise a relatively small percentage (14%) of the total sample.

RESULTS

Drug Use and Time 2 GPA

In addition to the interaction term discussed previously, each of these regression analyses included three kinds of predictors: (1) family background (race or ethnicity, parents' income, and family politics); (2) scholastic aptitude and prior academic performance (scores on the SAT verbal test, high school grades, and freshman grades); and (3) two variables indicating the respondent's major field of study and vocational orientation (that is, degree of interest in preparing for a specific occupation) at Time 1. Race or ethnicity and major field of study are dichotomous variables. The variable for race or ethnicity identifies students of Asian, Black, or Latin ancestry. *Major* identifies those in the social sciences or humanities. *Family politics* identifies students whose own political views range from liberal to left of liberal and neither of whose parents are conservative.

Table 7-2 summarizes results of the four regression analyses using GPA 2 as an outcome criterion. In three of the four analyses there is a low ($\leq .10$) positive zero-order correlation between drug use and Time 2 grades. In each of these three analyses, the effect of the other predictors is to reduce this correlation. The resulting regression coefficient is not statistically significant. In these cases, therefore, the

TABLE 7-2   Regression Analyses of Relation of GPA 2 to Drug-use Status at Time 1 and to Continuing Drug Use by Time 2

Predictor	N	Zero-order correlation (r)	Standardized partial regression coefficient (beta)	F
		Drug-use status at Time 1		
IA-1. MAR: never used vs. used only marihuana	503	9	6	2.25[a]
IA-2. MDU: never used vs. multiple-drug use	382	8	−3	.424[a]
		Continuing drug use by Time 2		
IIA-1. CMAR: never used vs. used only marihuana	215	25	13	4.02
IIA-2. CMDU: never used vs. multiple-drug use	176	10	0	.00[a]

Note. Based on men (73% of total sample) still enrolled at UCB by Time 2. In addition to the pattern of drug use, the following eight variables were entered as predictors in each regression: parent income, race or ethnicity, family politics, high school GPA, SAT verbal scores, GPA 1, major, and degree of preparation for a specific occupation. For further details about the variables, see Appendix A.
[a]Not significant.
*$p < .05$.

somewhat higher grades of the drug users can be explained, statistically at least, by the fact that drug users had other prior characteristics that would lead one to expect that they would do well at a competitive and intellectually challenging university.

Analyses of continuing drug users show somewhat different results. In Analysis IIA-1, we find a moderate (.25) positive correlation between continuing use of only marihuana and Time 2 grades. Although this correlation is reduced substantially (to .13) in the regression analysis, it continues to be significant ($p < .05$). In this case, the other predictors do *not* succeed in explaining the fact that the continuing MAR group had *better* grades at Time 2 than the men who had never used drugs by Time 2. We return to this finding in the closing discussion.

Although space does not permit their presentation here, the four correlation matrices (available on request) on which the regression analyses were based provide an interesting picture of the ways in which drug users differ from nonusers. Careful examination of the tables reveals how these differences help to explain the *positive* bivariate correlations between drug use and grades. Although the details differ somewhat from one analysis to the next, the correlation matrices suggest that drug users were more likely than nonusers to:

1. Come from relatively well-to-do, liberal, and probably, intellectually oriented families
2. Go into the social sciences or humanities (but less likely to regard preparing for a specific career as an important reason for being in college)

3. Be white and non-Latin and (for the MDU but not the MAR) to get high scores on the SAT test of verbal aptitude
4. Have had *lower* grades in high school

The third and fourth findings suggest that the MDU, if not the MAR, tended to be underachievers in high school. We also return to these findings in the final discussion.

The final step in these analyses was to do eight additional regression analyses for subgroups defined in terms of Time 1 GPA, that is, for men with GPA 1 $\geq$ 3.0 and for those with GPA 1 $<$ 3.0 (data on request). These analyses produced one marginally significant ($p < .10$) partial correlation of $+.19$ between continuing MAR and Time 2 grades among men whose Time 1 grades were below 3.0. In this subgroup, as in the group as a whole, our background and other predictors did not account for the fact that the continuing MAR had better grades at Time 2 than did men who had never used drugs.

It may also be noted that we found a *negative* partial correlation ($-.16$) in the comparison of continuing MDU with nonusers among men whose Time 1 GPA was 3.0 or higher. Based on only 12 cases, this partial correlation was not significant. Further, even though these men had grades that were somewhat lower than the nonusers (controlling for other factors), the average GPA 2 for these 12 men was 3.11, indicating that as a group they were by no means in trouble academically.

Drug Use and Career Indecision at Time 2

Prior inspection of the large pool of available items indicated that background variables (for example, race or ethnicity and parents' income) would be less useful in the analysis of career indecision than they were in the analysis of drug use and grades. For the most part, the predictors that met our selection criteria for the career-indecision analyses reflect the values and interests that respondents brought with them to college or acquired early in the freshman year.

Some of these values have to do rather directly with vocational decisions: the extent to which respondents regarded preparing for a specific occupation as an important reason for being in college, how much thought they had given to choosing a career, and their choice of the social sciences or humanities as a major field of study. Other predictors reflecting personality and broader social values were current religious affiliation (Protestant or Catholic), "openness" (based on the self-descriptions, curious and questioning, creative and imaginative, and individualistic), and a measure that suggests a countercultural, hang-loose, present-oriented approach to life. One other important measure in the analysis is based on the respondent's report at Time 1 regarding the closeness of his relationships with his parents during high school. Career indecision at Time 1 was also included as a predictor in these regression analyses.

Table 7-3 shows the first clear instance so far in which a group of drug users (the continuing MDU in Analysis IIB-2) appeared to be doing less well than the non-users, that is, men who had never used drugs by Time 2. The positive correlation of .23 indicates that this group of drug users were significantly more likely than the nonusers to be undecided about their occupational goals at Time 2. In the regression analysis, however, virtually all of the difference is accounted for by the other predictors in the equation; the correlation is reduced to a nonsignificant coefficient of .03.

Put another way, as early as the first quarter in college (if not earlier), this group

TABLE 7-3 Regression Analyses of Relation of Career Indecision at Time 2 to Drug-use Status at Time 1 and to Continuing Drug Use by Time 2

Predictor	N	Zero-order correlation (r)	Standardized partial regression coefficient (beta)	F
Drug-use status at Time 1				
IB-1. MAR: never used vs. used only marihuana	646	2	−9	4.88[*]
IB-2. MDU: never used vs. multiple-drug use	532	7	−8	2.16[a]
Continuing drug use by Time 2				
IIB-1. CMAR: never used vs. used only marihuana	260	2	−13	4.08[*]
IIB-2. CMDU: never used vs. multiple-drug use	233	23	3	.192[a]

Note. In addition to the pattern of drug use, the following eight variables were entered as predictors in each regression: career indecision at Time 1, thought about occupation, degree of preparation for a specific occupation, major, closeness to family, current religion, living for now, and openness. For further details about the variables, see Appendix B.
[a]Not significant.
[*]$p < .05$.

of continuing MDU differed from men who had never used drugs in ways that would lead one to expect them subsequently to be undecided about their occupational aspirations. Data not shown (available on request) indicate that, as freshmen, the continuing MDU clearly were less vocationally oriented than the nonusers. They had given less thought to choosing a career, were less inclined to view college as instrumental to preparing for a career, and were more apt to be enrolled in the social sciences and humanities—fields that lead less directly than others to specific occupational choices.

These differences between the continuing MDU and men who had never used drugs were related, in turn, to other values that emphasize the conventionality of the nonusers (as reflected in their current religious identifications), as distinguished from the countercultural orientation of the continuing MDU. Most interesting of all, the conflict between the subcultural orientation of the drug users and acceptance of the conventional parental culture by the nonusers is highlighted by the fact that closeness to family is negatively correlated with drug use (−.21) and with career indecision (−.20) and is positively correlated with current religion (.31) and with the vocational variables (.15 and .27). These data lend strong support, it seems to us, to the subcultural theory of drug use discussed earlier.

Although a subcultural theory of drug use adequately explains the zero-order correlation between career indecision and continuing multiple-drug use shown in Table 7-3 (Analysis IIB-2), it appears to be less adequate in explaining the other outcomes in that table. In each of the other three analyses, there was a low, nonsignificant, and positive zero-order correlation between drug use and career indecision at Time 2. In the regression analyses, however, the partial correlations are negative and, in the two cases involving the marihuana-only users, these low partial correlations are statistically significant. The data thus suggest that men in the Time 1 MAR group and those in the continuing MAR group are somewhat *more* likely to be clear about their occupational goals than one would expect, given the fact that they were relatively less career oriented and more unconventional initially. We return to this point, also, in the discussion section.

Thus far, then, we can conclude that the apparently "adverse outcome" associated with continuing multiple drug use can be adequately explained, for the group as a *whole*, in terms of prior differences between these users and the nonusers with respect to career orientation and social values. There remains the possibility that these values do not completely explain adverse outcomes in smaller subgroups of users. For this reason, we again did eight additional regression analyses within subgroups defined in terms of Time 1 career indecision (available on request).

Three of the analyses involving men whose career goals were clear at Time 1 produced nonsignificant partial regression coefficients ranging from −.01 to +.06, indicating essentially no difference between users and nonusers after controlling for subcultural factors. In three other analyses involving men who were unclear about their goals at Time 1, the zero-order correlations were significant (though low) and negative, indicating that the various groups of users (MAR, MDU, and continuing MAR) were *less* likely to be undecided at Time 2 than were the nonusers. Further, the regression analyses produced partial correlations that were even more negative, ranging from −.18 to −.27, and all of which were statistically significant. Once again, cultural differences between users and nonusers appear inadequate to explain *favorable* outcomes associated with drug use.

The two remaining analyses, however, identified situations in which, at the bivariate level, the continuing MDU were *more* likely to be undecided than the nonusers and, in one analysis, the difference was not completely explained by introducing the other predictors. The basic relation is shown in Table 7-4.

Two groups are shown in Table 7-4: those whose career goals were clear at Time 1 and those whose goals were not clear. In both groups, the continuing MDU were more likely than the nonusers to be undecided at Time 2, although the correlation reflecting the difference was not significant in one case. Table 7-4 also shows that

TABLE 7-4   Relation of Career Indecision at Time 2 to Continuing Drug-use Status by Time 2 among Men Clear or not Clear about Occupational Plans at Time 1

| | Drug use status | | | | | | |
| | Never used | | Multiple drug use | | Regression analyses | | |
Status of career plans at Time 1	%	N	%	N	r	Beta	F
Very or fairly clear	16	122	45	22	.26**	.16	2.76*
Not very or not at all clear	48	65	63	24	.13	−.12	.82[a]

Note. In addition to the pattern of drug use, the following eight variables were entered as predictors in each regression: career indecision at Time 1, thought about occupation, degree of preparation for a specific occupation, major, closeness to family, current religion, living for now, and openness. For further details about the variables, see Appendix B.
[a]Not significant.
*$p < .1$.
**$p = .01$.

the regression analysis for men who were not clear at Time 1 reduces the correlation between drug use and career indecision at Time 2 (from $+.13$ to $-.12$), but neither is statistically significant.

The interesting case, however, occurs among men whose occupational goals were clear at Time 1. In this analysis, the other predictors (career values, social values, and closeness to parents) reduce the correlation from $+.26$ ($p < .01$) to $+.13$ ($p < .10$) but do not eliminate it entirely. Thus this small group of 22 continuing MDU appears somewhat more likely than the nonusers to be undecided about their career goals, even after controlling for other variables in the analysis. Although the difference is of marginal significance (partly because of the small number of cases), drug use retains a slight independent effect. We therefore cannot rule out the possibility that drug use contributed in some causal fashion to the difference in career indecision.

DISCUSSION

We have reported results from an extensive search for evidence that drug use has negative consequences for academic performance and for progress toward acquiring clear occupational goals. Perhaps the simplest way to summarize our findings is to say that they are comparable to the findings one would expect from a similar search for adverse effects of alcohol: For most users, there was no evidence that the generally moderate patterns of drug use prevailing in this kind of setting have any negative consequences that are independent of other prior characteristics of users compared with nonusers. Among two small subgroups of continuing MDU, however, we did find some evidence of adverse outcomes that could not be explained in terms of other prior characteristics. The possibility that drug use had some causal influence on these outcomes could not be ruled out.

In the eight analyses involving the four groups of drug users as a whole, we found only one outcome (career indecision at Time 2) with respect to which drug users (continuing MDU) compared unfavorably with nonusers. In this instance, the difference between users and nonusers was reduced to a statistically insignificant level in the regression analysis. The analysis demonstrated that these continuing MDU had the kinds of interests and values upon entering college that would lead one to expect them to make slower progress toward establishing specific career goals. In many respects these users were not unlike the vocationally indecisive men studied by Holland and Nichols (1964). Like those men, the continuing MDU as a group may have high potential for creative achievement and, for that very reason, may find it more difficult than others to evolve satisfying career goals.

As with alcohol, however, it would not be surprising to find smaller subgroups of users who are less able to cope with drug use and for whom drug use either creates new problems or impairs capacity to cope with preexisting problems. We did find some evidence that this may have been the case for one subgroup of continuing MDU. Among the 22 continuing MDU whose career goals were clear as freshmen, we found somewhat more (10 cases) who had become undecided by Time 2 than would be expected given their prior characteristics. Although we cannot clearly implicate drug use as a causal factor in this outcome, neither can we rule it out. Similarly, we found an even smaller subgroup ($N = 12$) of continuing MDU whose Time 2 grades were slightly (although not significantly from a statistical standpoint) lower than one would expect on the basis of their prior characteristics.

Thus our general conclusion with respect to the main goal of these analyses is that drug use may have had adverse consequences, of the kind considered here, in some small percentage of cases. For most users, however, no such adverse consequences could be demonstrated. Further, there was no clear, statistically convincing evidence, either in these analyses or in others we have reported elsewhere (Mellinger et al., in press), that using only marihuana has any adverse consequences. It was specifically among the MDU that the possibility of adverse consequences could not be ruled out, and this possibility occurred only in a small subgroup of users whose career goals were clear at Time 1. If drug use did play a causal role in these outcomes, it would be difficult to ascertain whether it was the use of other drugs (psychedelics, cocaine, or opiates), the relatively heavier use of marihuana, or a greater involvement in the drug subculture that contributed to the outcome.

Throughout the report, we have referred to the sociogenic or subcultural theory of drug use advanced by Goode (1972), Johnson (1973), Kandel (1974), and others. We find that theory to be consistent with much of our data. Variables reflecting the theory worked very well to explain the apparently adverse outcome involving the total group of continuing MDU. The theory is consistent with a restatement of one of our major conclusions: For most users in this setting, drug use (like drinking) is a social rather than pathological phenomenon.

It should not be overlooked, however, that the same set of variables did not adequately explain the possibly adverse outcomes (career indecision and GPA at Time 2) among the smaller groups of continuing MDU. It may be, of course, that we did not include all of the "right" questions pertaining to background and subcultural values; but it also may be that however useful sociogenic theory is for explaining drug use in the whole population of users, it is less adequate for explaining those isolated instances in which drug use is a concomitant or precursor of pathology.

Interestingly, our social–cultural variables also did not explain several of the cases in which drug use was associated with *favorable* outcomes, even after controlling for these other variables. Again this may be due to shortcomings in our data, our methods of analysis, or both. Nevertheless, there are other possibilities worth considering. One is that drugs, when used in moderation at least, can have the kinds of beneficial effects that drug users often ascribe to them (Goldstein, 1975). As our inquiry was not designed to investigate that possibility, we can neither support nor refute it.

Some of our findings call attention to a possibly neglected aspect of the theory of drug subcultures. A major goal of our study was to understand and explain drug use. Many of the questions derived specifically from what we knew about drug users. By focusing attention on drug users, however, we may have overlooked important characteristics of *nonusers* in a social setting where they represent, in several respects (including their nonuse of drugs), a deviant subculture. One intriguing finding, for example, is that the nonusers whose career goals were clear at Time 1 were more likely to remain clear; and nonusers whose career goals were *not* clear at Time 1 were more likely to remain unclear. In both cases, nonusers were less likely to change than the users were.

This finding suggests two further possibilities. One is that users and nonusers may differ with respect to *personality characteristics* (e.g., rigidity) not included in these analyses or in the data we collected. There is also the possibility that nonusers are out of step at a large, selective, and competitive liberal arts university where the prevailing academic atmosphere tends to be liberal and intellectually challenging, and where drug use is an integral part of the prevailing life-style. As we have seen, nonusers tended to come from less affluent and less liberal families, and their parents were less likely to have an educational background that is conducive to academic success at a school such as Berkeley (see Feldman, 1969). The nonusers also tended to lack the verbal skills necessary to take full advantage of the kind of intellectual stimulation Berkeley has to offer. Far from finding UCB a stimulating atmosphere in which to acquire occupational goals, or to question the goals they brought with them to college, the nonusers may have been turned off (or never turned on) by an academic environment that did not fit their particular needs. This line of reasoning, by the way, suggests that our findings might have been different if our study had been done at a small vocational or denominational school.

Although we have not been able to support these speculations with the data we have available, we believe they have some merit. We suggest that any comprehensive model of drug use should give more attention than we did to characteristics that make nonusers unique in a setting where they are in the minority.

In closing, we should call attention once again to the select nature of this population. These students were sufficiently talented and motivated to attain admission to a university with high academic standards. The majority of drug users had initiated drug use during high school but nonetheless maintained the levels of academic motivation and performance required to seek and gain admission. Early initiators who may have been more vulnerable to the effects of drug use (or to the effects of participating in the drug subculture) would not have been included in our study.

The results of the study cannot be lightly dismissed on these grounds, however. Alarmed public and official reactions to student drug use during the 1960s originated in reports of widespread drug use among college students at Berkeley and elsewhere. The evidence reported here, based on a rigorous attempt to identify adverse outcomes associated with drug use, suggests that public and official reactions to drug use at Berkeley were unduly alarmist. In retrospect, it would have been wiser to have raised earlier the difficult but essential question: Which patterns of use are associated with adverse outcomes among what kinds of individuals in what social settings?

APPENDIX A: TIME 1 PREDICTORS USED IN FOUR MULTIPLE REGRESSION ANALYSES WITH TIME 2 GPA AS THE OUTCOME CRITERION

Predictor	Question or item (response categories)
Parents' income	"What was your parents' income last year before taxes?" (0. Less than $10,000; 1. $10,000–15,000; 2. $15,000–20,000; 3. $20,000–30,000; 4. $30,000 or more)
Race or ethnicity	(1. Asian, black, or Latin American; 0. all others)
Family politics	Based on a typology of three items asking respondent to rate himself, his father and his mother on an 11-point scale of political views ranging from left of radical to right of very conservative. (−1. all three moderate or conservative; 1. all three left of liberal or liberal to moderate; 0. all others)

Predictor	Question or item (response categories)
High school[a]	
SAT verbal[a]	
GPA 1	Freshman grade-point average[b] (1. $\geq$ 3.00; 0. < 3.00)
Major	"Have you decided yet on a major; if so, what have you decided on?" (1. social sciences, humanities; 0. all others: engineering, physical sciences, life sciences, applied/ interdisciplinary, no major)
Degree of preparation for a specific occupation	"Students attend college for a variety of reasons. How important is each of the following reasons for you personally?" . . . "Preparing for a specific job or occupation." (1. not at all, not very important; 2. fairly important; 3. very important)

Note. Time 2 GPAs obtained directly from university transcripts with prior written permission of respondent.

[a]Obtained from university admissions records with prior written permission of respondent.
[b]Obtained directly from university transcripts with prior written permission of respondent.

APPENDIX B: TIME 1 PREDICTORS USED IN FOUR MULTIPLE REGRESSION ANALYSES WITH CAREER INDECISION AT TIME 2 AS THE OUTCOME CRITERION

Predictor	Question or item (response categories)
Career indecision at Time 1	Based on responses to the question: "How clear an idea do you have of which occupation you will choose?" (1. not very or not at all clear; 0. fairly or very clear)
Thought about occupation	"How much have you thought about what career or occupation you might choose after you finish your formal education?" (0. not at all or only a little; 1. some; 2. a lot)
Degree of preparation for a specific occupation	"Students attend college for a variety of reasons. How important is each of the following reasons for you personally?" . . . "Preparing for a specific job or occupation." (0. not at all important; 1. not very important; 2. fairly important; 3. very important)
Major	"Have you decided yet on a major; if so, what have you decided on? (1. social sciences, humanities; 0. all others: engineering, physical sciences, life sciences, applied/ interdisciplinary, no major)
Closeness of family	Index with scores ranging from 5 to 21 constructed from six items. A high score on this index indicates a person who:

> Identified and felt a sense of solidarity with his family
> Felt close to his mother when he was in high school (scored from 3 = very close to 1 = not close at all or not very close)
> Felt close to his father when he was in high school (scored from 3 = very close to 1 = not close at all or not very close)

Predictors	Question or item (response categories)
	Felt his mother approved of his general way of life and the way he spent his time (scored from 5 = approve strongly to 1 = disapprove strongly)
	Felt his father approved of his general way of life and the way he spent his time (scored from 5 = approve strongly to 1 = disapprove strongly)
	Would like his life to be similar to his father's (scored from 4 = similar in most respects to 1 = similar in few or no ways)
Current religion	"Which of the following best describes your present religious beliefs?" (1. Protestant or Catholic; 0. Jewish, Eastern religion or philosophy; agnostic, atheist, no religious beliefs, other)
Living for now	Index with scores ranging from 3 to 15 constructed from three items. A high score on this index indicates a person who:
	Described himself as being someone who doesn't take life too seriously, greatly values pleasure, has a lot of fun (scored from 5 = describes me very well to 1 = describes me not at all)
	Described himself as being someone who believes in living life to the fullest, experiencing as many new things as possible (scored from 5 = describes me very well to 1 = describes me not at all)
	Agreed with the statement that the future is so uncertain that we might as well live mostly for the present (scored from 5 = strongly agree to 1 = strongly disagree)
Openness	Index with scores ranging from 3 to 15 constructed from three items. A high score on this index indicates a person who described himself on an adjective checklist as:
	Individualistic (scored from 5 = describes me very well to 1 = describes me not at all)
	Curious, questioning (scored from 5 = describes me very well to 1 = describes me not at all)
	Creative, imaginative (scored from 5 = describes me very well to 1 = describes me not at all)

Note. Career indecision at Time 2 based on responses to the question: "How clear an idea do you have of which occupation you will choose?" (1. not very or not at all clear; 0. fairly or very clear)

REFERENCES

Astin, A. W. *Predicting performance in college: Selectivity data for 2300 American colleges.* New York: Free Press, 1971.

Baird, L. The undecided student: How different is he? *Personnel and Guidance Journal,* 1969, *47,* 429–434.

Blum, R. H. *Students and drugs* (Vol. 2). San Francisco: Jossey-Bass, 1969.

Coleman, J. S. *Introduction to mathematical sociology.* New York: Free Press, 1964.

Davidson, S. T., Mellinger, G. D., & Manheimer, D. I. Changing patterns of drug use among university men. *Addictive Diseases,* 1977, *3,* 215–233.

Erikson, E. H. The problem of ego identity. *Psychological Issues,* 1959, *1*(1), 101–171.

Feldman, K. A., & Newcomb, T. M. *The impact of college on students.* San Francisco: Jossey-Bass, 1969.

Gallup Opinion Index, July 1974, *109*, 14–30.

Gergen, M. K., Gergen, K. J., & Morse, S. J. Correlates of marijuana use among college students. *Journal of Applied Social Psychology,* 1972, *2*, 1–16.

Goldstein, J. W. Students' evaluations of their psychoactive drug use. *Journal of Counseling Psychology,* 1975, *22*, 333–339.

Goode, E. *Drugs in American society.* New York: Knopf, 1972.

Groves, W. E. Patterns of college student drug use and lifestyles. In E. Josephson & E. E. Carroll (Eds.), *Drug use: Epidemiological and sociological approaches.* Washington: Hemisphere, 1974.

Holland, J. L., & Nichols, R. C. The development and validation of an indecision scale: The natural history of a problem in basic research. *Journal of Counseling Psychology,* 1964, *11*, 27–34.

Hollister, L. E. Marihuana in man: Three years later. *Science,* 1971, *172*, 21–29.

Jessor, R., Jessor, S. L., & Finney, J. A. Social psychology of marijuana use: Longitudinal studies of high school and college youth. *Journal of Personality and Social Psychology,* 1973, *26*, 1–15.

Johnson, B. D. *Marihuana users and drug subcultures.* New York: Wiley, 1973.

Johnston, L. D. Drug use during and after high school: Results of a national longitudinal study. *American Journal of Public Health,* 1974, *64*(Suppl.), 29–37.

Josephson, E. Adolescent marijuana use, 1971–72: Findings from two national surveys. *Addictive Diseases,* 1974, *1*, 55–72.

Kandel, D. B. Interpersonal influences on adolescent illegal drug use. In E. Josephson & E. E. Carroll (Eds.), *Drug use: Epidemiological and sociological approaches.* Washington: Hemisphere, 1974.

Kerlinger, F. N., & Pedhazur, E. J. *Multiple regression in behavior research.* New York: Holt, 1973.

Kolansky, H., & Moore, W. T. Toxic effects of chronic marijuana use. *Journal of the American Medical Association,* 1972, *222*, 35–41.

Lavin, D. E. *The prediction of academic performance.* New York: Russell Sage, 1965.

Manheimer, D. I., Mellinger, G. D., Somers, R. H., & Kleman, M. T. Technical and ethical considerations in data collection. In S. Einstein & S. Allen (Eds.), *Proceedings of the First International Conference on Student Drug Surveys.* Farmingdale, N.Y.: Baywood, 1972.

Marcia, J. E. Development and validation of ego-identity status. *Journal of Personality and Social Psychology,* 1966, *3*, 551–558.

Maugh, T. H. Marihuana: The grass may no longer be greener. *Science,* 1974, *185*, 683–685. (a)

Maugh, T. H. Marihuana (II): Does it damage the brain? *Science,* 1974, *185*, 775–776. (b)

Mellinger, G. D., Somers, R. H., Davidson, S. T., & Manheimer, D. I. The amotivational syndrome and the college student. *Annals of the New York Academy of Sciences,* 1976, *282*, 37–55.

Mellinger, G. D., Somers, R. H., Davidson, S. T., & Manheimer, D. I. Drug use and academic attrition among university men. *Proceedings of the Conference on the Social Psychology of Drug and Alcohol Abuse.* In press.

Somers, R. H., Mellinger, G. D., & Manheimer, D. I. *Drug use and academic decisions: A longitudinal analysis of the freshman panel.* Unpublished manuscript, 1974.

Sonquist, J. A., & Morgan, J. N. *The detection of interaction effects.* Ann Arbor: Institute for Social Research, 1964.

Suchman, E. A. The hang-loose ethic and the spirit of drug use. *Journal of Health and Social Behavior,* 1968, *9*, 146–155.

Walters, P. A., Goethals, G. W., & Pope, H. G. Drug use and life-style among 500 college undergraduates. *Archives of General Psychiatry,* 1972, *26*, 92–96.

8

The Interaction of Setting and Predisposition in Explaining Novel Behavior: Drug Initiations before, in, and after Vietnam

Lee N. Robins
Department of Psychiatry,
Washington University School of Medicine

One of the most intriguing and important problems in social research is understanding the interaction between the immediate setting and the predispositions actors bring with them to that setting in determining what action will take place. In the term *predisposition*, I include every characteristic of actors that affects their readiness to show some behavior, whether a characteristic was acquired at birth, by socialization, or by past experience of others' reactions to their behavior, or demographic characteristics.

Recent controversy in the sociological literature pits the impact of the setting against the impact of the actors' sets of predispositions, but this is no either-or problem. Choosing sides between the system and the actors as *the* cause is as dated and inappropriate as choosing between nature and nurture to explain in turn the actors' predispositions. Geneticists and social scientists seem ready to agree that people inherit various genetic patterns, which are differentially expressed depending on such variables as prenatal experiences, socialization, and environmental stresses. (The analogy has been made that choosing nature *or* nurture is like choosing width *or* length as the more important determinant of the area of a rectangle.) Clearly, the rate of appearance of deviant behavior must similarly be a function of both the predispositions of the actors and the facilitating or inhibiting contexts in which they act.

To recognize that both context and individual predisposition contribute to action is a first step forward, but recognition alone is of no help in predicting changes in rates of behavior, given changes either in the population exposed or in the setting to which the population is exposed. This point is not novel. It was trenchantly stated by Walter Mischel (1969)

Supported by U.S. Public Health Service grants DA 01120, MH 18864, DA 4RG008 and Research Scientist Awards MH 36598 and DA 00013.

A tribute to the interaction of person and environment is usually offered at the front of every elementary textbook in the form of Kurt Lewin's famous equation: Behavior is a function of person and environment. In spite of such lip service to the stimulus, most of our personality theories and methods still take no serious account of conditions in the regulation of behavior. Literally thousands of tests exist to measure dispositions, and virtually none is available to measure the psychological environment in which development and change occurs. (p. 1014)

One would like to be able to estimate the size of the contribution of the setting for particular populations and to know whether a change to a more or less facilitating setting is likely to augment or decrease the contribution of the actors' predispositions. One would also like to be able to distinguish situational effects that merely delay or speed up the appearance of deviance from those that change final rates.

There has been little research that has satisfactorily estimated the effect of the setting as distinct from the effect of the predisposition of the actors. There are many difficulties in doing so. The first requirement is to identify a clear change in the setting so that a temporal association between a change in setting and the onset of a behavior can be established. One solution has been to study consequences of dramatic and datable life events. A problem that has plagued research on consequences of life events, however, is that predispositions of the actors strongly influence to what life events they will be exposed. Actors can influence their settings either by choosing the settings or by evoking responses from those around them, who then change the settings for them. For example, antisocial children have a high rate of separation from parents. In part, this is because they run away from home or are placed in detention. In such cases, it would be hard to decide how much of their later misbehavior to attribute to separation from the parents, inasmuch as the separation was brought about by their own behavior, which itself indicates a propensity to later behavior of the same kind.

Even when we consider settings over which actors have had no influence, there are problems in attributing effects to the settings when those who are responsible for creating actors' predispositions may also have contributed to creating the situations. For example, the experience of a parental death is one that children ordinarily have had no part in causing. Early death is, however, associated with characteristics in the parents that influence the children. Alcoholic parents, for example, not only die early, but may contribute a genetic predisposition to alcoholism and are also likely to have brought up their children in atypical ways. It becomes difficult in such cases to say whether the children's behavior can best be explained by the genetic contribution of their parents, the unusual way in which they were raised, or their experience of a critical life event, the death of a parent.

To demonstrate the effects of the setting as distinct from the effects of predispositions, then, requires being able to show a temporal association between the exposure to a new setting and a consequent change in behavior. The change in setting must be independent of influences either by actors themselves or by those who have influenced their sets of predispositions. There are not many opportunities to show such setting effects outside the laboratory, and laboratory experiments have their own serious drawbacks. The changes one can ethically produce in a laboratory are usually relatively unimportant and of brief duration. One alternative is to seek natural experiments that affect broad segments of the population both impartially (so that individual predispositions and family backgrounds have little to do with exposure to the setting), and dramatically (so that there is clear discontinuity with the previous setting).

In this chapter, I report on a study of the effects one approximation to a natural experiment in changing social settings had on the occurrence of a limited number of new behaviors—the initiation of use of four classes of illicit drugs. The "natural experiment" was the exposure of American soldiers in 1970 and 1971 to Vietnam. Of course, exposure to the Vietnam setting was not entirely uninfluenced by the predispositions of the soldiers. Those with prior histories of severe criminality, psychosis, mental retardation, or poor health were excluded by their draft boards. Those with money to hire good lawyers and those who had good grades in school often engineered their own exclusion from the draft. Those drafted with special skills were probably often able to arrange to serve out their terms elsewhere. Yet, however imperfect the natural experiment was, there seems little doubt that the Vietnam war exposed a large number of young men to opportunities to use hard drugs who would not otherwise have had that opportunity.

One can look at the Vietnam experience as a time of the coincidence of important factors facilitating drug use: (1) a great availability of drugs; (2) a desire to seek relief from the awareness of danger, the hardships of battle, and the regimentation of military life; and (3) a lack of constraints against use as a result both of separation from family and of the soldiers' definition of their enlistment period as distinct from "real life." One can contrast veterans' susceptibility to beginning drug use in Vietnam with their susceptibility before service, on first entering the military, and after service. One can further explore how the level of deviance of the soldier before he entered service and his demographic characteristics interacted with the change in his setting to predict drug initiation.

To measure the impact of a change in setting on drug-use initiations, one must be able to estimate how many initiations could have been expected in the same time interval if the exposure to the new setting had not taken place. Making an estimate for how many Vietnam veterans would have initiated drug use if they had not gone to Vietnam is no simple task. For instance, there is the issue of expected changes in risk with aging. The usual age at entering military service is 18 or 19, when young American men are also entering the period of highest risk of trying drugs. It would therefore be a mistake to assume that all increases in rates during the service period can be attributed to the change in setting that military service provided. Further, during the years 1969 to 1971, the period of their military service, drugs were becoming increasingly acceptable to young men in the United States. Men in service shared the changes in attitudes toward drugs that were characterizing their age group in the country as a whole. Thus to estimate the effect of the Vietnam experience, one needs to subtract increases in initiations that are a consequence of aging and of historical changes in attitudes toward drugs.

In our study, we resolved this problem as best we could by selecting a group of young men who, so far as we could tell, were equally eligible for military service but did not serve because they were not called up, due to high draft numbers in the lottery, or through other chance occurrences. This control group allowed us to estimate what the drug histories of the veterans might have been if they had not entered the military.

The study of drug initiations in successive periods carries with it another difficulty. The population at risk of initiating a particular drug is constantly diminishing. In our first period, that is, before entering service, the whole sample is at risk of initiating all drugs. By the time of entering the military, only those remain at risk who had not yet used a drug as civilians. By the time of arrival in Vietnam, the sample at risk has shrunk still further. This progressive reduction in the sample at risk means that statistical techniques ordinarily used to compare panels at different time points are inappropriate because they assume a constant sample size. Instead (to use the language of Bishop, Fienberg, & Holland, 1975), we have block, triangular tables resulting from many cells with structural zeros.

Not only is there a constantly declining sample at risk, but its characteristics change. Those with the highest liability to use tend to use early in the sequence of settings, leaving a sample at risk that is more and more biased toward the non-deviant and not demographically predisposed. To maximize the ability to perceive effects of predispositions on behavior, one ordinarily chooses predisposition scale categories so that they contain roughly equal numbers of individuals. The disproportionate loss of cases at the high end of predisposition scales over time means that in each successive period the scale categories become less well balanced. This in turn weakens the power of the statistical tests of the effect of predispositions at the same time their power is further reduced by the decreasing number of cases. Thus, the exhaustion of potential initiators over time is particularly critical among high-risk sample members.

THE VIETNAM PROJECT: PURPOSE AND METHODS

A follow-up of Vietnam veterans was undertaken at the request of the Special Action Office for Drug Abuse Prevention, an office that existed briefly within the Executive branch, in order to estimate treatment resources needed for Vietnam veterans who were addicted to narcotics as a result of exposure to heroin in Vietnam. A random sample was selected of all Army enlisted males who returned from Vietnam to the United States in September of 1971. In addition, a random sample was selected from the list of all men returning that month whose urine had been detected as positive for morphine (a metabolic product of heroin) just before departure. The first interview was carried out with 943 men. Approximately half came from each of the two samples, and there was an overlap of 22 men between the two samples. Interview rates were very high (95% of those surviving) and veracity seemed exceptionally high, with 97% of those known to be heroin users according to their military records admitting use in Vietnam (Robins, 1974).

When the men had been back 3 years, two-thirds of them were selected for reinterview. Those eliminated were men first inducted before 1969, because the previous study had shown these to be mostly career soldiers with very little experience with drugs either before, in, or after Vietnam, and men inducted from states that provided fewer than 10 men to the sample. The reduction in geographic distribution was decided on after it was found that there would have been virtually no change in estimates of drug use before, in, or after Vietnam in the first study had these less accessible cases been removed. Limitation of the sample to those inducted from the 25 more populous states reduced travel costs and thus freed funds for interviewing a control group of nonveterans. The control group was selected from Selective Service records, except for a few older men for whom no Selective Service records had been preserved. These few were obtained from schools in the towns from which the older veterans had been inducted. Nonveterans were required never to have been classified as ineligible to serve or exempt from the draft, that is, none had been classified as medically, mentally, or morally unsuitable (4-Y or 1-Y) nor as a conscientious objector; none was a minister or the only surviving son of a soldier killed in action. Each nonveteran was individually matched with a member of the general sample (that is, those from the random sample of all returnees) with respect to age, education, and location of residence as of the time the veteran was inducted.

The first veterans' interviews were carried out between May and September 1972. The second interviews were carried out between October 1974 and January 1975. Recovery rates for the second interview were again high, with 94% of the veterans and 91% of the nonveterans interviewed. Of the general-sample veterans interviewed, 91% had matched nonveterans also interviewed.

After each interview, urine samples were collected and analyzed to verify the honesty of the informant about his current drug behavior. In addition, military records and number of VA contacts were obtained for the veterans. In this chapter, all information other than age comes from interviews. Information about age comes from records for both samples, military records for the veterans, and the Selective Service or school records for the nonveterans.

To relate drug initiations to exposure to different settings, it was necessary for the respondents to assign their first drug use to the correct time period. This appeared to be easy for the veterans, who still at the time of the first interview could recall instantly their dates of induction, arrival in Vietnam, and return. They were doubtless also helped by the fact that the people providing the drug for that memorable first use were usually known in only one of the several settings experienced—either in the hometown, in basic training, or in Vietnam. In the second interview, the early periods were not reviewed; men were simply asked about use in the previous 2 years, in other words, the time since the first interview.

In order to get nonveterans to recall comparable time periods, each nonveteran was told that he had been matched to a specific veteran, and he was given that veteran's year and month of induction. He was asked a series of questions—about what he was doing that month (for example, in the fall of 1970, when he was 19 years old), where he was living, whether he was at school or at work, whether he was married or single—to help him fix the date firmly in mind. He was then asked about drug experience and other behavior with respect to their occurrence before or after that date.

We also asked nonveterans about drug experience in the previous 2 years. We did not attempt to divide the nonveteran's time period corresponding to the interval between the veteran's induction and 2 years before the second interview into the three subperiods corresponding to the veteran's basic training, time in Vietnam, and time between return from Vietnam and first interview. We felt it was impractical to ask the nonveteran to distinguish many intervals unmarked by the important transitions that made them memorable for the veterans. Therefore in comparisons between veterans and nonveterans, we are restricted to divisions into three time periods: before the date on which the veteran was inducted (Period 1), between that time and the date of the veteran's first interview (Period 2), and the last 2 years of the study (Period 3).

It is quite possible that this separation into time periods remained less clear for nonveterans than for veterans, despite our efforts. Not only did they lack equally dramatic changes in setting at the critical moments, but they covered all three periods in a single interview, whereas the veterans had been asked about earlier experiences 2 years before, at a time 2 years closer to that experience.

In presenting these data on drug use by veterans, I am using only those 571 men interviewed twice. We have weighted appropriately the sample members appearing on the surgeon general's list of men detected as drug positive at departure from Vietnam, so that our results can be generalized to all first-term Army enlisted men who left Vietnam for the United States in September 1971, without sacrificing the accuracy obtained by oversampling the part of that population who contributed the greater proportion of drug users. When we compared veterans with nonveterans, we restricted ourselves to the individually matched pairs. Because nonveteran matches were obtained only for the general random sample of veterans, these results are unweighted.

The soldiers I am describing spent a year in Vietnam at the height of a heroin epidemic. If we could not show an effect of a change in setting on drug initiations in this population, it would be hard to imagine one in which we could. Not only did almost all (85%) report having been offered heroin in Vietnam, but as first-term Army enlisted males, they represent the group believed by the U.S. Department of Defense to have the highest rate of narcotic use among all the service categories in Vietnam. Women, officers, Navy, and Air Force all had lower rates than these men. Because 95% were interviewed in the first round and, of those interviewed the first time, 94% were reinterviewed the second time, we have a reasonably representative sample of the population I am describing.

Most of the public concern about drug use in Vietnam centered on narcotic use. To cover narcotics broadly, we presented each subject with a list of commonly used narcotics, including heroin, opium, codeine and codeine cough syrups, morphine, Methadone, Dilaudid, Demerol, and paregoric. We asked which of these he had used in the relevant time period. The narcotic of initiation varied by time period. Those who began narcotic use before service usually began with codeine (74%). In service before Vietnam, the narcotic of initiation was usually opium (61%), with codeine second (37%). In Vietnam, the drugs of initiation were usually both heroin (78%) and opium (83%). The few men who began after Vietnam were equally likely to begin with codeine, morphine, heroin, or opium.

As a comparison, to test our ability to attribute initiation of drugs to a change in setting, we also included three other classes of drugs that both our veterans and nonveterans were asked about: marihuana, amphetamines, and barbiturates. Because the use of these drugs was not specially associated in the public mind with Vietnam, there was no reason to expect interviewers or respondents to be biased toward locating the veterans' first experience with those drugs in Vietnam.

The questions we attempted to answer are: (1) Was there an increase in drug initiations in Vietnam? (2) Was this a general increased liability to use drugs, or was it specific to certain classes of drugs? (3) Did the Vietnam exposure increase the number of men who would *ever* use illicit drugs, or did it only accelerate use in individuals who were likely to become users sooner or later anyway? and (4) Did the Vietnam exposure to drugs tend to equalize the drug experience of men with high and low predispositions to use?

Our measures of predisposition are divided into two types: demographic factors and preservice deviance. Our assumption is that demographic factors, that is, race, size of city of rearing, and age, have their primary importance in determining the degree of exposure to drug opportunities before service. The drug revolution has had a greater impact on the young than on older members of the population, and drug use has been found to be more common among blacks and among youths in the core city of large metropolitan areas. Analysis of our first interview with these veterans (Robins, 1974) confirmed these expected correlations between demographic variables and preservice drug use. Social class was not found to be a significant correlate. These results are consistent with Johnston's (1973) report for a national sample of young men of the same age, asked about the same period in their lives. We also found in that first interview that many forms of self-reported preservice deviance were associated with preservice drug use. School truancy, expulsion and dropping out, fighting before entering service, arrests before service, and early drunkenness were each independently related to liability to drug use before going to Vietnam. We combined these reports of demographic characteristics and preservice behaviors (other than drug use) into two measures that could be expected to indicate soldiers' predisposition to drug use.

We scored the demography scale as follows:

Black = 1
Other races = 0
Born:
    after 1950 = 2
    1949 to 1950 = 1
    before 1949 = 0
Teenage residence in:
    large city = 1
    suburb, small city, town or rural = 0

The sum was then coded as $0 = 1$, $1 = 2$, $2 = 3$, $3-4 = 4$. We scored the preservice deviance scale as follows:

Left high school because:
    expelled = 2
    dropped out = 1
    graduated = 0
Truanted:
    a lot = 2
    only in the final school year = 1
    rarely or not at all = 0
First drunk:
    before 15 = 2
    15-18 = 1
    19+ or never = 0
Arrested:
    three times or more = 2
    once or twice = 1
    never = 0
Fighting after 16:
    occasionally or often = 2
    once or twice = 1
    never = 0

The deviance scale used here is the sum of these scores, recoded as $0-1 = 1$, $2-3 = 2$, $4-5 = 3$, $6+ = 4$. The construction of these two scales, the correlations of items within and between them, and their correlations with narcotic use before Vietnam, in Vietnam, and after Vietnam are fully discussed in an earlier paper (Robins, Davis, & Wish, 1977).

To compare the impact of different settings on drug initiations, one needs to take into account differences in lengths of exposure to them by comparing annual rates rather than absolute differences. Calculating annual rates requires making assumptions about the duration of each interval of interest. The first period is the preservice period, ending with induction usually at age 19. Because other studies have shown that drug use commonly begins around 16, we assumed a 3-year period of being at risk of drug initiation for the preservice period. The middle period in comparisons between veterans and nonveterans dates from induction to 2 years before interview. It includes for the veterans about 1 year in the military before arrival in Vietnam, a 1 year tour of duty in Vietnam, and 8–12 months between return from Vietnam and the first interview. Therefore, we assumed that this middle interval also lasted about 3 years. The final period is the 2 years prior to the second interview. To calculate annual rates, we assumed that rates remained constant *within* each period. The formula is rate $(R) = (1 - \sqrt[n]{P_2/P_1})\ 100$, where n is the number of years in the period, P_2 is the number of people who still have never used the drug at the end of the period, and P_1 is the number of people who had not yet used the drug at the beginning of the period.

RESULTS

Figure 8-1 compares annual drug initiations in three periods for veterans and nonveterans. For veterans and nonveterans alike, the middle period, that is, the period between the date of induction for veterans and the 2 years before interview, showed the highest annual rates of drug initiations. The single exception was initiations to narcotics by nonveterans, which declined in both the middle and final periods. This rise in drug initiations in the middle period probably reflects the effects of both age and a historical period of increased drug use. It means that the

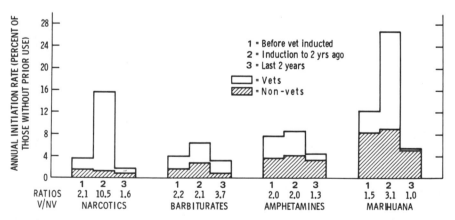

FIGURE 8-1   Annual drug-initiation rates in three time periods for veterans versus nonveterans.

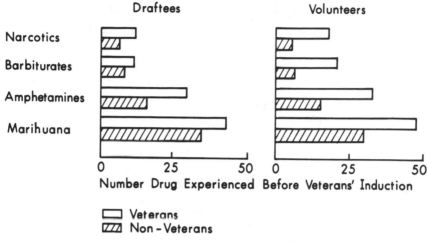

FIGURE 8-2 Preservice drug experience.

years that included the veteran's Vietnam experience might well have been their years of greatest liability for initiating drug use, even if they had not been sent to Vietnam.

We also noted that veterans had higher rates of drug initiations than nonveterans even *before* induction. This was the case for those drafted as well as for those who volunteered (Figure 8-2). Therefore, before attributing the higher rate of drug use among veterans after induction to their military experience, we had to take into account their initial higher likelihood of using drugs. This initial difference confirms the suspicion that the military draft did not select a completely unbiased sample of young draft-eligible men, despite the lottery system.

Figure 8-1 also shows that, for all drugs, the risk in the third period for both veterans and nonveterans was lower than the risk in Period 1. This means that in Period 3 there was no longer a sufficient increase due to aging and historical period to counterbalance the early selection of the more vulnerable members of the sample into the drug-experienced segment—which is a complicated if precise way of saying that by the end of the study, the period of risk for the appearance of new drug users was about over for these men, most of whom were then 24 or 25 years of age.

Comparing veterans and nonveterans shows that the veterans' excess initiations to narcotics and marihuana were much greater in Period 2 (which includes the Vietnam period) than in Period 1. The excess of veteran over nonveteran drug initiations in the middle period for barbiturates and amphetamines, in contrast, is of about the same magnitude as in Period 1.

For all drugs, veterans continued to surpass nonveterans in the final 2 years, although, except for barbiturates, the excess was smaller in the last 2 years of the study than it had been previously. For marihuana, the difference between veterans and nonveterans almost disappeared in the third period.

The convergence of veterans' and nonveterans' rates in Period 3 must in large part result from having used up that portion of the veteran population that was drug-use prone, by exposing them so thoroughly to opportunities to take drugs in Period 2, while in Vietnam. That is, having begun with a higher liability to drug use

TABLE 8-1 Proportions Still Inexperienced with Drugs: Actual Proportion Versus Expected
Proportion if Period 1 Rates of Initiations Had Persisted Throughout

	Still nonusers					
	Veterans			Nonveterans		
Drugs	Observed %	Expected based on Period 1[a] %	x^2	Observed %	Expected based on Period 1[a] %	x^2
Narcotics	52	75	18.1*	89	87	n.s.
Barbiturates	69	72	n.s.	85	86	n.s.
Amphetamines	54	52	n.s.	73	73	n.s.
Marihuana	22	35	13.8*	51	50	n.s.

$^a(1-R)^8$, where R = the annual rate in Period 1.
*$p < .001$.

than nonveterans, veterans could approach the level of nonveterans after Vietnam
only by having previously exhausted a larger proportion of their high-risk cases.
This implied that we should consider the possibility that the Vietnam experience
only *accelerated* the initiation of drugs by veterans due to become users anyhow,
rather than increasing the final number of users. To discover whether this was the
case, we needed to know whether there was a sufficient drop below the number of
initiations expected in the last 2 years to compensate for the excess new users in
Vietnam.

To learn whether the final number of users among veterans was any greater than
we should have expected based on their preservice rates, we projected the annual
rate of use in Period 1 for the full 8 years for which we have information, including
the 3 years after Vietnam. Table 8-1 presents the results. It compares the proportion never having used each drug as observed at the end of our 8 years of drug risk
with the proportion expected if the annual rate in the first period had persisted
throughout all three periods. We find that the early rates give very accurate estimates of observed rates of experience for all four drug classes for nonveterans. The
fact that the total period for nonveterans has been well predicted by their rates of
use in the first period shows that the slow rates of initiation before age 19 have
been balanced by decreasing risks in the last few years, as the vulnerable members
of the population were exhausted. [Tietze (1968) has a similar observation about
declining fertility risks in women discontinuing contraception as a function of the
number of years since discontinuation without becoming pregnant.]

While initial rates serve as excellent predictors of the final number of veterans
who used barbiturates and amphetamines, just as they did for nonveterans, many
more veterans became marihuana and narcotic users than we would have predicted
based on rates during the preservice period. Note, however, that even if the veterans
had never entered the military, we would have predicted that 25% of them would
have used narcotics by the time of their second interview, compared with only 13%
of the nonveterans, because they were clearly more vulnerable to begin with. In
fact, 48% of the veterans had tried narcotics—twice the expected rate. We would
have expected 65% of the veterans to have tried marihuana by the time of the
second interview, compared with half of the nonveterans, but actually, 78% of the

veterans had tried marihuana. If we are correct that the risk period for new drug use was near its end by the second interview, exposure to the Vietnam setting indeed markedly increased the proportion of veterans who would ever try narcotics and marihuana, but it had little or no effect on the number who would try barbiturates and amphetamines.

Effect of Military Induction and Return from Vietnam

Before dismissing the Vietnam experience as without effect on barbiturates and amphetamines, we needed to look at the course of drug initiation for veterans in a more detailed way. Exposure to Vietnam was only one of the changes in setting experienced by veterans during Period 2. That period includes not only the Vietnam experience but also a period in the military before going to Vietnam and a period of about 10 months after return from Vietnam.

It is possible that entry into the military may also have been a change in setting associated with a changed liability to drug use. To examine the role of entry into the military, we moved from our sample of veterans for whom nonveteran matches had been obtained to the whole veteran sample. Before doing so, we had to be certain that the vulnerability of those veterans who had been matched with non-veterans did not differ from that of the veteran sample as a whole.

The 259 matched veterans make up less than half of the total 571 veterans interviewed. The veterans interviewed include the matched veterans, members of the general sample for whom no nonveteran match was obtained, and those members of the drug-positive sample who are not also in the general sample and for whom no match was sought. To combine the general and drug-positive samples, the drug positives in the general sample and in the drug-positive sample are weighted to their proper proportion in the general sample. Because only 17 veterans in the general sample were not matched, and because the 287 drug positives *not* in the general sample were weighted down to the equivalent of only 20.6 persons, the move from the matched to the total sample involved adding new cases that are the statistical equivalent of only 15% of the matched sample. One would expect an expansion of this magnitude to make only a small difference. Table 8-2 shows that those veterans from the general sample who were matched with nonveterans are indeed an unbiased subsample of the total. Rates of drug use during the preinduction period are virtually identical, whether we look at the matched veterans or the weighted total sample.

TABLE 8-2 Comparison between Matched General Sample and Total Sample

	Incidence rates of drug use before induction (Period 1)	
Drugs	Matched general sample[a] %	Total weighted sample[b] %
Narcotics	10	10
Amphetamines	22	22
Barbiturates	12	11
Marihuana	32	33

[a] $N = 259$.
[b] $N = 571$.

TABLE 8-3 Veterans' Annual Rates of Initiation to Drugs during Parts of Period 2: Military Service before Vietnam, Military Service in Vietnam, and the First 8–12 Months after Vietnam

| Drugs | Period 1 Before induction (A) | | In service before Vietnam (B) | | | In Vietnam (C) | | | First 8–12 months back (D) | | |
| | | | | | | Period 2 | | | | | |
	N	%	N	%	B:A	N	%	C:A	N	%	D:A
Narcotics	571	3.3	476	2.3	.7	458	39.1	11.8	161	.0	.0
Barbiturates	571	3.8	464	2.7	.6	434	17.2	4.5	245	1.9	.5
Amphetamines	571	8.0	406	4.6	.7	368	15.2	1.9	260	6.6	.8
Marihuana	571	12.5	314	15.5	1.2	238	54.5	4.4	77	4.9	.4

Table 8-3 presents annual rates for the three subperiods of Period 2 (B, C, and D) and their ratios to Period 1 (A). Entry into the military was associated with a *decline* in the annual incidence of initiation of narcotics, amphetamines, and barbiturates. Only for marihuana was there a modest increase in incidence. It is conceivable that the decline in initiation rates at entry into service is only apparent. We have assumed a constant rate in Period 1. If it were actually declining, there might have been no sharp drop-off at entry into service. If we remember, however, that, among nonveterans, initiations to all drugs except narcotics rose in Period 2, a declining rate in Period 1 seems unlikely, particularly because it is well known from other studies that 1969 and immediately thereafter was a period of increasing drug use nationwide (Greene & DuPont, 1974). Therefore, it appears that entry into the military did temporarily depress the onset of drugs other than marihuana.

We have no direct evidence as to why entry into the military should have been associated with a decline in drug initiations. Perhaps it stemmed from a breaking up of peer networks through which drugs were available. We do know from other studies (Fisher, 1972) that rates did not remain low if soldiers were sent to duty stations other than Vietnam, but no other study has yet explored rates of initiation during basic training and immediately thereafter.

Use of all four drug classes rose markedly with arrival in Vietnam, with the largest increment in narcotics initiations. Barbiturates were as much affected as marihuana. Although amphetamines showed least effect, their level of initiations in Vietnam was almost double their rate before induction into the military.

On return to the United States, rates of initiations fell below preservice levels for all drugs. The decline was particularly striking for narcotics, with no new users at all in the first months after return, and for marihuana, for which the rate of initiation dropped to less than half the preservice rate.

We can conclude, then, that for *every* drug class, there was a high rate of initiations in the Vietnam setting. The failure to find an excess for amphetamines and barbiturates in Period 2 treated as a whole resulted from the depression of initiations on first entering the military and on returning from Vietnam.

Figure 8-3 plots the rates of initiations for veterans in the five periods we have studied: before induction (A), at entry into the military (B), in Vietnam (C), during the first 10 months home (D), and in the last 2 years (E). It also compares the observed curves of use with the curves we might have expected if these soldiers had not entered the military at all. Our estimate uses the veterans' level of initiation in the first period, when they were still civilians, as the starting point, and sketches the shape of the curve found for nonveterans as our guess of what would have happened thereafter if they had remained civilians.

Rates of initiation prior to induction were higher for marihuana and amphetamines than for the other drugs. Initiation of all drugs except marihuana rose markedly on arrival in Vietnam, and all fell below the preservice level after return from Vietnam. The drop in liability after return is much more striking for marihuana and narcotics initiations, which had risen most in Vietnam, than for amphetamine and barbiturate initiations. For marihuana and narcotics, but not for amphetamines and barbiturates, there has been some rebound in initiations in the last 2 years.

The decline in marihuana and narcotic initiations after Vietnam followed by a rebound suggests a temporary "immunity" following exposure to a high-risk situation. It would be interesting to explore whether such temporary periods of relative invulnerability can regularly be detected in those who have survived exposure to high-risk environments without succumbing. For instance, there has been a great interest in showing an increased risk of psychiatric symptoms after traumatic life events, but no exploration as to whether there may be a *reduced* risk in the posttrauma period among those who survived such events unscathed.

In Figure 8-3, the estimated net effect on drug experience attributable to having been sent to Vietnam is represented by the areas between the solid and dotted lines in the Vietnam period minus the areas between the dotted lines and the solid lines following induction and following return home. As we had found by our projection

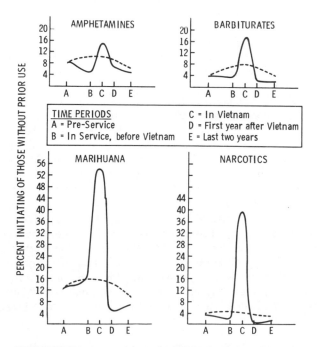

FIGURE 8-3 Veterans' annual initiation rates for each drug type in five time periods.

in Table 8-1, there has been no net increase attributable to the Vietnam experience for barbiturates and amphetamines, but there was a large net increase in the number of narcotic and marihuana users, even taking into account the drop in initiation rates on entering service and on returning from Vietnam. We conclude, then, that the effect of military service on amphetamine and barbiturate use was largely a change in the *timing* of initiations, whereas it produced a substantial net gain in the *number* of narcotic and marihuana users.

Role of Predisposition to Drug Initiation in High- and Low-risk Situations

The direction of causal associations between the demography scale and pre-service drug initiations would seem at first to be unambiguous. Age, residence, and race are not variables that change as a result of drug use. Although the causal direction *would* be unambiguous in a random sample of a total population, this is not true when a special sample is chosen, such as this sample of men who have been in the military. Being a *young* soldier means having enlisted before draft age, which in turn usually means having dropped out of school. If drug use led to dropping out of school, then, indirectly, drug use has "caused" being young! For the preservice deviance scale, it is obvious that any of its elements (dropping out, fighting, arrest, early drunkenness, truancy) could be caused by, as well as cause, preservice drug use. Ambiguity about the direction of cause–effect relationships between our two scales and drug initiations disappears, of course, when we look at associations after entry into service, because both scales describe the men before service and thus inevitably predate drug initiations after entering service.

The fact that preservice drug use can be a cause as well as an effect of high scores on the deviance and demography scales should tend to inflate correlations in the preservice period. Thus larger associations between the predisposition scales and preservice, as compared with later, initiations might occur even if the scales were not actually more potent predictors in the earlier period. Further reasons to expect a declining strength of association in later periods are (1) that the city-size element in the demography scale and the behaviors in the deviance scale are all more temporally proximal to the drug use in the preservice period than later, and (2) that the sample size at risk shrinks as men who use drugs in one period are no longer at risk of initiating them in later periods. This progessive reduction is particularly acute at the positive end of the scales, because the most predisposed use first, causing (3) a progressive imbalance in the distribution of the remaining sample at risk along the scale steps in later periods.

Weighing against these reasons for expecting an artifactual decrease in the statistical significance of relationships between our predisposition scales and the initiation of drug use in Vietnam as compared with preservice, is the consideration that the high rate of drug initiation in Vietnam makes the effect of predispositions easier to detect. Other things being equal, the closer the probability of an event approaches to .5, the more likely are correlations of predictor variables with that event to be found significant. Rates of initiation were closer to .5 in Vietnam than in any other time period.

Table 8-4 shows contingency coefficients as measures of the sensitivity of drug initiations to our predisposition scales in four time periods. The two periods after Vietnam have been combined because the number at risk at the high end of the

TABLE 8-4 Contingency Coefficients for the Relationship between Drug Initiations and Predisposition Scales in Four Time Periods

Period	Deviance				Demography			
	Nar-cotics	Barbi-turates	Amphet-amines	Mari-huana	Nar-cotics	Barbi-turates	Amphet-amines	Mari-huana
Before service (A)	.19	.23	.24	.27	.17	.23	.14	.20
In service (B)	.15	.24	.04	.14	.08	.13	$.11^a$	.13
In Vietnam (C)	.34	.25	.31	.21	.29	.24	$.20^a$	$.19^a$
After Vietnam (D)	$.13^a$	.20	.30	$.10^a$	$.14^a$	$.07^a$	$.18^a$	$.25^a$

^{a}All results except these come from 4 × 2 contingency tables. These results come from contingency tables that were collapsed to 3 × 2 because of small numbers in the highest category. For Ns see Table 8-3.

predisposition scales was near zero before the last time period began. Contingency coefficients are presented because they compensate for the decreasing number of people at risk in each successive period. (The upper limit for χ^2 is N. The contingency coefficient $= \sqrt{\chi^2/\chi^2 + N}$.) For narcotics and amphetamines, relationships between drug initiation and both predisposition scales were stronger in Vietnam than before service despite the facts that, in the preservice period, causal relationships could operate in both directions, the predictor variables were more temporally proximal to the drug use, and the categories of the predictor scales were more equal in size. Differences between the two periods were negligible for barbiturates. For marihuana, differences were negligible for demographic predictors, but the relationship with deviance was stronger before service than in Vietnam. For initiations to narcotics, the preservice predisposition scales had a greater effect in Vietnam than at any other period. Inasmuch as narcotics was also the drug category whose availability was most affected by the Vietnam setting, it would seem that preservice predispositions were considerably more important in determining who would begin drug use in high-availability, than in low-availability, conditions.

There still remains the possibility noted above that the strong relationships found in Vietnam are a spurious effect caused by the fact that the rate of initiations overall in Vietnam was closer to .5. But if this were the explanation, we would expect correlations between predispositions and marihuana initiation to be especially significant in Vietnam, because marihuana was the only drug begun in Vietnam by approximately half the men who had never used it before. Marihuana, however, is the exception to our finding that correlations between predispositions and drug initiations were greater in Vietnam than before service.

The fact that the measures of predisposition were even more strongly related to risk of drug initiations in Vietnam than before Vietnam meant that the Vietnam experience served to make the cumulative rate of narcotic and amphetamine experience increasingly reflect initial predisposition to use. This point is illustrated in Figure 8-4, which compares the cumulative use rates of veterans in the highest and lowest positions on the two predisposition scales. (Men at the middle levels of these scales are omitted for clarity's sake.) By the time they left Vietnam (point C on the graphs), veterans with high deviance scores differed considerably more from veterans with low deviance scores in the proportions who had ever tried narcotics and amphetamines than they had differed from them at the time they arrived in

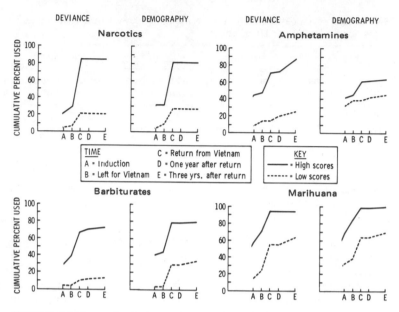

FIGURE 8-4 Preservice deviance, demography and drug initiation: cumulative percentage having used drugs at five time points.

Vietnam (point B). Similarly, though less dramatically, veterans with high demography scores increasingly differed from veterans with low demography scores for both drugs after Vietnam.

Only for marihuana did the Vietnam experience act as an equalizer of deviant and nondeviant soldiers and also of those high and low on demographic predisposition. These unique results for marihuana seem to be merely a ceiling effect. Almost all the highly predisposed men had already used marihuana before Vietnam. The remainder (with few exceptions) did begin in Vietnam. Indeed, every man in the high demography group (those black, young, and brought up in the inner city) had used marihuana by the end of the study. Only one of these men came back from Vietnam never having tried marihuana, and after his return, he did try it.

DISCUSSION

We have taken advantage of the natural (or better, unnatural) experiment of the Vietnam war to see how well it was possible to demonstrate the effect of a change in setting on the initiation of novel behaviors and to see whether exposure to a facilitating environment seemed to blur or sharpen the effects of underlying predispositions to behavior.

We restricted our study to the initiation of new behaviors because that is a far simpler problem than trying to show the effects of a change in setting on *rates* of behavior. Not only have we avoided the problem of quantifying the intensity and frequency of the behaviors of interest, but we have avoided the issue of the behavior's own natural history of rate change over time. Even in a constant setting, narcotic use, for instance, has a natural course characterized by moving from occasional to regular use, to daily compulsive use, to withdrawal and abstention, to the relapse that renews the cycle. It seemed an insuperable problem with our present techniques to show how a change in setting creates perturbations in this cycle, particularly inasmuch as the cycle's natural periodicity is still unknown.

We have also avoided an issue that would have been interesting to consider, but which we saw no easy way to cope with, that is, the relationships among our four dependent variables—the initiation of marihuana, amphetamine, barbiturate, and narcotic use. We have treated the four drug classes as though they were independent, despite the many studies showing that, among users of multiple classes of illicit drugs, marihuana is typically the first drug used.

The many newspaper stories about dogs trained to smell out marihuana in Vietnam and the scare headlines about the heroin epidemic among soliders in Vietnam both made it easy to believe that exposure to the Vietnam setting *had* increased the number of users of these drugs, but proving it was not so simple. At first blush, the obvious way to study the effect of a change in setting is to compare behaviors in that setting to the same behaviors during a previous baseline period, but when the probability of the behavior varies with age and historical period, one needs a control group going through the same aging and living through the same period. It was for this reason we selected a control group of nonveterans matched for age, education, location, and draft eligibility. They turned out, however, to differ from the experimental drug group in their baseline measures of drug use— variables we had no way of matching initially. Still, we were able to use the control group to predict the expected *shape* of the experimental group's curve of initiations over time, if not its level. We noted an echo of that shape in the experimental group for two of the drug classes studied—barbiturates and amphetamines—but a marked upward divergence for the other two—narcotics and marihuana—during the period that included Vietnam. Thus, we surmised that the Vietnam setting had indeed affected initiations of *these* two drugs.

A more detailed look at the veterans' initiations showed a temporary drop on return from Vietnam in initiations of the same two drugs—marihuana and narcotics—followed by a later rebound. This further supports the effect of the Vietnam setting on these drugs. Apparently the Vietnam setting was so great a facilitator of introductions to these drugs that almost all those predisposed to use in that time period had been sufficiently exposed, leaving a temporarily "immune" population. The fact that the Vietnam exposure showed a permanent effect on the number of users of narcotics and marihuana and a postsetting "immunity" for these two classes of drugs known to be remarkably available there, but not for amphetamines and barbiturates, gives us added confidence that we have found a setting effect and that our results are not merely the typical natural course in a group of men with a higher initial predisposition to drug use than our control group.

In addition to demonstrating that a change in setting has an effect on behavior, we explored how exposure to a facilitating setting affected the expression of the predispositions that the actors brought to the setting. We found that in a setting greatly facilitating narcotic use, preexisting differences in predispositions were more fully expressed than they had been in a more inhibiting environment, even against the odds of more temporal distance, smaller samples, and unbalanced samples. Rather than equalizing the drug experience of men from different social and behavioral backgrounds, easy access to narcotics in Vietnam seemed to increase their preexisting differences. We had not known whether to anticipate this finding or its opposite. Would black inner-city youths who did *not* use narcotics before service be more or less likely than rural whites to begin use in service? One could argue either way—that because narcotics use is common among their acquaintances, there are no serious taboos against use or fears of effects, and therefore they would be more likely to use, the more available the drugs became; or that if they had resisted use in the high-availability situation in which they grew up, they would also resist it in Vietnam. One could also have argued either way with respect to men with much preservice deviance. Those who did not use narcotics before service might merely have lacked opportunity, which certainly was not lacking in Vietnam. On the other hand, deviant youth who *had* the opportunity before service and chose not to use narcotics then might be expected to be especially invulnerable to their use, perhaps because they were satisfied with alcohol.

If the finding that a setting with greater opportunities to express deviant behavior *increases* the impact of prior predispositions to deviance is substantiated in studies of other forms of deviance, it will further underscore the fruitlessness of arguments about whether the situation or the predisposition to deviance is more important. If a setting favorable to deviance allows the fuller expression of underlying predispositions, whereas a setting unfavorable to deviance inhibits such expression, reducing levels of predisposition and reducing the facilitating nature of the setting should both be effective ways to reduce deviance. The issue, then, becomes simply the pragmatic one of which kind of change is easier to effect.

REFERENCES

Bishop, Y. M. M., Fienberg, S. E., & Holland, P. W. *Discrete multivariate analysis.* Cambridge: M.I.T. Press, 1975.

Fisher, A. H. *Preliminary findings from the 1971 DoD survey of drug use.* Alexandria, Va.: Human Resources Research Organization, 1972.

Greene, M. H., & DuPont, R. L. Heroin addiction trends. *American Journal of Psychiatry,* 1974, *131*, 545–550.

Johnston, L. D. *Drugs and American youth.* Ann Arbor: Institute for Social Research, 1973.

Mischel, W. Continuity and change in personality. *American Psychologist,* 1969, *24*, 1012–1018.

Robins, L. N. *The Vietnam drug user returns* (Final Report, Special Action Office Monograph, Series A, No. 2). Washington: U.S. Government Printing Office, 1974.

Robins, L. N., Davis, D. H., & Wish, E. Detecting predictors of rare events: Demographic, family, and personal deviance as predictors of stages in the progression toward narcotic addiction. In J. S. Strauss, H. Babigian, & M. A. Roff (Eds.), *The origins and course of psychopathology: Methods of longitudinal research.* New York: Plenum, 1977.

Tietze, C. Fertility after discontinuation of intrauterine and oral contraception. *International Journal of Fertility,* 1968, *13*, 385–399.

9

"Spontaneous Remission" among Untreated Problem Drinkers

Ron Roizen
Don Cahalan
Patricia Shanks
Social Research Group, School of Public Health,
University of California at Berkeley

Longitudinal data can be analyzed from a number of different perspectives. Different perspectives often imply both attention to different parts of the change tables and different techniques of analysis. Thus Lazarsfeld (1969) commenting on the differences in statistical techniques he and Campbell used, has noted the differences in research interests: "Campbell's approach deals with prediction, [whereas Lazarsfeld has emphasized] a structural analysis; the shift back and forth from consonant and dissonant positions" (pp. 11–12).

In this chapter, we take up an important substantive issue in alcohol research and attempt to tailor an analysis of longitudinal data to fit it. The issue, namely the existence, frequency, and character of "spontaneous remission" from alcohol problems, forces us to take some novel cuts at the data. In the first part of the chapter, we show the impact that varying the criteria of alcoholism and the definition of remission can have on the estimates of spontaneous-remission rates. In the second part of the chapter, we show how certain "background" features of spontaneous-remission research design (for example, choices about whether remission is scored in the "improvement" direction only or as a two-way change variable) can have important and often unnoticed consequences for the findings on spontaneous remission. This approach reflects our view that, in the varied and complex arena of longitudinal analysis, analytical strategies must be organized around and tailored to specific research questions. Equally important, the impact of such tailorings on the research's conclusions must be carefully assessed.

The authors wish to express their appreciation to the National Institute on Alcohol Abuse and Alcoholism, under whose auspices this research has been conducted (under grant AA 00275-6 and prior grants), and to Robin Room and Nicholas Robins for their assistance in this analysis.

VARYING CRITERIA FOR ALCOHOLISM
AND THE DEFINITION OF REMISSION

The concept of *spontaneous remission* is drawn from clinical language, in which it refers to improvement in a patient's condition in the absence of effective treatment. Estimating the rates of spontaneous remission for alcoholism or drinking problems is an important research problem on a number of counts. For example, without reliable knowledge about these rates, the effectiveness of alcoholism treatments cannot be established. By extension, treatment success rates cannot confidently be used as a test of their own conceptual foundations. Where alcoholism is regarded as a *progressive* and *irreversible* condition, spontaneous remission also indicates the degree to which either the *progressive characterization* or the *diagnostic criteria* for alcoholism require rethinking and revision.

In any case, knowledge of the predictors of remission would put estimates of the prognosis for alcoholism on a firmer footing. Even the hotly debated question of whether alcoholics can return to controlled drinking depends, in part, on the experiences of *untreated* alcoholics, if the influences of clinical ideologies about the matter are to be controlled for. Hence, the problem of spontaneous remission is nested in a variety of theoretical issues that bear on the definition of alcoholism, the validity of diagnostic criteria, rationales and impacts of differing treatments, factors in prognosis, and models of both the development and the abatement of problems associated with drinking.

The rate of spontaneous remission from alcoholism or problem drinking has been the subject of widely differing claims. Eysenck and Beech (1971), for example, have argued that "spontaneous remission is theoretically expected to be almost entirely absent, and clinical experience certainly suggests that lack of treatment would almost always mean absence of improvement" (p. 586). Drew (1968), on the other hand, has suggested that the age distribution of admissions for alcoholism implies that "alcoholism tends to disappear with increasing age" (p. 965), and though part of the apparent remission may be accounted for by differential morbidity and mortality, "a significant proportion of this disappearance is probably due to spontaneous recovery" (p. 965).

Current Knowledge

In spite of the significance of the issue, current knowledge about spontaneous remission of alcoholism is based on a weak and uneven collection of studies. Among them, one can find scraps of evidence to support expectations of very low or very high remission. From the clinical vantage point, these expectations have tended to dip toward the pessimistic end. Where alcoholism is regarded as both an intractable condition and one that is difficult to treat, even dimmer hopes are implied for the untreated cases. Every alcoholic in treatment was once an untreated alocholic, and, although the logic is fallacious, the modest expectations for enduring improvements among treated cases can easily be generalized to untreated counterparts.

Even a brief look at the literature on untreated alcoholics should give us a sense of how tentative and provisional our data have been in this area. One example is Lemere's (1953) study in which, over a period of 6 years, he asked psychiatric patients about "the incidence and details of serious alcoholism in their grandparents, parents, aunts, and uncles" (p. 674). Because these relatives lived during two preceding generations when formal treatment available was "very limited and seldom sought" (p. 674), he argued that they comprised a group of untreated cases. Among the 500 cases for which he collected data, one-third ultimately gave up drinking, but more than two-thirds of this abstinent group was described as quitting during a terminal illness. Another 10% moderated their drinking in time; and within this outcome group, which numbered 49 cases, 35 cases where characterized by "increasingly longer periods of sobriety, while in 14 the amount drunk and degree of intoxication abated to the point of normal drinking" (p. 674). An additional 29% of the full sample stayed the same in their drinking practices, and the remaining 28% became worse. Although for a time this study was the best available evidence on the subject, Lemere's data must be regarded as little more than speculative. As Kendell and Staton (1966) wrote,

> his information was derived solely from the patients' descendants, whose memory of events long past, which in many cases they would not even have witnessed themselves, cannot have been other than imperfect. It is difficult to believe that a reliable distinction between alcohol addicts and mere habitual excessive drinkers can be made on such a basis. It is also doubtful whether the assumption that these patients were necessarily untreated because no treatment was then available is really justified. (p. 31)

That Lemere's provisional report remains a useful resource in the literature probably tells us more about the low state of research than about the fates of untreated alcoholics.

In their own study, Kendell and Staton (1966) collected follow-up data on 57 diagnosed alcoholics who were refused, or themselves declined, treatment at the Maudsley Hospital in London between May 1950 and June 1961. The follow-up interviews were begun in 1963, both with the patient and with corroborating relatives or other sources where possible. The period of follow-up, therefore, varied from 2 to 13 years. About half of Kendell and Staton's cases had had previous treatments elsewhere before declining or being refused treatment at the Maudsley Hospital, and 40% of this sample obtained alcoholism treatment during the follow-up period. The overlap in these two groups was not reported, so we do not know how many of their cases were entirely free of formal treatment. Among those who received no treatment during the follow-up period (a total of 32 cases), only one became abstinent, two reverted to normal drinking (see Kendell, 1965), 13 continued drinking either continuously or intermittently but avoided serious disruption of their lives, 10 continued drinking but manifested serious disruption, and 6 died due to continued drinking (4 by suicide). A sample of treated alcoholics at Maudsley, followed up at 2 years by Davies, Shepherd, and Myers (1956) and at 4 years by Wing (1956) fared somewhat better, although Kendell and Staton noted that, except for the higher mortality rate in the untreated group, treated and untreated outcomes were more noteworthy for their similarities than for their differences. These data might be interpreted as reporting a 50% improvement rate and a 3% abstention rate among untreated cases, but of course these small numbers and the problem of prior treatment make these data difficult to generalize from.

Thorpe and Perret (1959) studied 278 cases referred for alcohol problems to the Medical Department of Esso Standard Oil Company in the period 1948 to 1956. In this group, 36 employees refused any formal treatment. When the data were collected, 2 were abstinent, 11 were drinking but rated "improved," and the remaining 23 were "unimproved." The authors pointed out that "every one of these people was subject to a variety of social pressures ... Reprimands, suspensions, demotions, and final warnings had beneficial effects in some cases" (p. 29). Hence, again, the "untreated" status of this group is at least arguable.

Very low remission was reported by Kissin, Rosenblatt, and Machover (1968) in a comparative test of three therapies, which included an untreated control group and in which 4% of the 50 control cases were judged improved. Although a randomizing scheme was employed in the distribution of cases to the experimental and control groups, this distribution was influenced to some extent by the patients' circumstances. Those who were assigned to the experimental group were advised that treatment was currently unavailable. Nonpatients whose requests for treatment persisted beyond 6 months were assigned to treatment and dropped from the control group. In addition, only about one-half of the total sample (experimentals and controls) contributed follow-up data, and all non-follow-up cases were classified as treatment failures. The attrition rate among untreated cases might well have been higher than among the experimentals. Because the attrition rates within groups are not reported, however, it is unknown how much of this 4% rate underreports remission in the total control group.

If 4% spontaneous remission seems too low, one can consult Goodwin, Crane, and Guze's (1971) study of alcoholics found in a sample of felons in which 40% were in remission at the time of follow-up 8 year later. This remission rate, as the authors noted, compares favorably with many, and perhaps even exceeds most, published accounts of improvement after clinical treatment. But, the authors also noted that, "rather than conclude that treatment has adverse effects on alcoholics, it is more likely that alcoholics who seek and receive treatment differ from untreated alcoholics in various characteristics influencing prognosis, although symptomatically the untreated alcoholism may be just as severe" (p. 144). Because most of these cases were apparently interviewed in prison, the diagnosis of alcoholism was, of course, based on retrospective accounts of drinking behaviors. It is difficult to gauge the biases in reporting that may have stemmed from conducting interviews in prison (see McCaghy, 1968). Robson, Paulus, and Clark (1965), Clancy (1961), and Clancy, Vornbrock, and Vanderhoof (1965) as well, have reported high improvement rates (37%, 40%, and 54%, respectively) among untreated cases.

One credible interpretation for these often widely varying estimates of spontaneous remission rates relies on the assumption that variations in alcoholics' (or groups of alcoholics') social characteristics influence their capabilities for improvement. Baekeland, Lundwall, and Kissin (1975) and others have argued that improvement rates among *treated* cases are strongly influenced by client characteristics such as social stability and social class, and we might assume that similar forces are at work among untreated cases. Of course, other sources of variation are also probable: Differences in diagnostic criteria and procedures, varieties of outcome measures, and differences in the follow-up interval (to name only some of the methodological variations in these studies) have long bedeviled clinical research in this area. These circumstances naturally suggest that we look for attempts to impose a common framework of measurement on the existing literature and, in addition, for studies using large and representative samples of alcoholics.

Emrick (1975) has recently published a comprehensive review of this literature, in which he found 24 studies of untreated or "minimally treated" samples, among which 7 were wholly untreated and 17 minimally treated. The data from 7 of these 24 studies met Emrick's quite lenient criteria of methodological sufficiency and could be combined in a common data pool. He found that roughly 15% of the combined untreated and minimally treated groups were abstinent at outcome and a little more than 40% could be counted as "improved." Even with rough controls for outcome measures, however, the range of remission rates among the studies was substantial. Among the studies in which abstinence was defined as at least 6 months of nondrinking prior to the follow-up point, the range of abstinence rates varied from virtually zero (Gibbins, 1954) to about one-third of the sample (Lemere, 1953); and among the studies that employed roughly comparable improvement measures, the range was from 37% (Thorpe & Perret, 1959) to 54% (Clancy, 1961). If these data are considered as one large sample, a base of 1,267 cases was available to a test by the abstinence criterion, and 634 were available for the "improved" criterion. But when used as an aggregate pool, the weakest studies (Lemere, 1953 and Gibbins, 1954), because of their large samples, tend to exert a numerical dominance over the rates produced. However tentative the summary calculations in Emrick's study must be, they are doubtless pretty close to the best estimate the literature can provide. Emrick, of course, was reporting on the relevant literature rather than on original data, and in a sense this fact makes his findings all the more noteworthy. In spite of a climate of opinion in which spontaneous improvements are often regarded as rare, what literature exists on the subject suggests that remission in the sense of 6 months of abstinence can be expected in 15% of the cases, and remission in the sense of some improvement in about 40%.

The need for larger and more representative samples of alcoholics has been partially satisfied by reports stemming from the data-gathering system surrounding treatment centers funded by the National Institute on Alcohol Abuse and Alcoholism (Armor, Polich, & Stambul, 1976; Ruggels, Armor, Polich, Mothershead, Stephen, with others, 1975). The first fruits from this system suggested spontaneous-remission rates even higher than those reported in Emrick's review. Ruggels and his associates (1975) found that, among untreated and minimally treated clients, 30% had been abstinent for 1 month whereas 66% either were abstinent, drinking less than 1 ounce of pure alcohol per day on the average, or scored low on a multi-item alcohol-impairment index at the point of follow-up 18 months after their contact with the treatment center. Unfortunately, intake or Time 1 data were not collected on the untreated group, so this picture of remission depends on the assumption that alcoholics who received treatment and those who did not were similar groups at Time 1.

Spontaneous Remission
in a General-population Sample

In light of the deficiencies of even the better studies of untreated alcoholics, we have conducted an analysis of remissions from alcohol-related problems in a panel sample of white, adult males living in San Francisco. We have focused this analysis on two questions: (1) What is the rate of spontaneous remission from alcohol-related problems in this general-population sample? and (2) What are the strengths of a variety of factors in the prediction of "spontaneous remission" in this group? We return to these questions after a brief account of the surveys themselves.

METHODS

The data for this analysis are drawn from a two-wave panel study of a probability sample of white, noninstitutionalized males aged 21 to 59 in San Francisco, California. The *R. L. Polk City Directory* of dwelling units was used as the primary sampling base, although the sample was supplemented and checked by area probability methods (see Cahalan & Room, 1974, pp. 236–239 for a fuller description of the field methods and sampling procedures).

The interview schedule employed in the first wave of the study was a lengthy and detailed instrument that inquired into respondents' drinking patterns and problems, psychological adjustment, life circumstances, and demographic characteristics. These interviews took place between September 1967 and May 1968. Of the first-wave sample, 80% were successfully interviewed. The follow-up wave of the study was completed approximately 4 years later in the early months of 1972. This time, a much shorter instrument was used that concentrated on respondents' drinking practices and problems at Time 2. The second wave used a self-administered questionnaire, which the respondents returned by mail. When the mail method did not generate a response, respondents were first telephoned and then visited by an interviewer, who either administered the questionnaire or waited while the respondent completed it. These methods in combination produced follow-up data on 78% of the first-wave sample, providing a total of 615 respondents about whom there were usable panel data.

This analysis is especially concerned with the outcomes among respondents both who report some drinking problems at the time of the first wave of interviewing, *and* who do not report having ever been exposed to alcoholism treatments of one sort or another. Therefore, for the purposes of this analysis, we initially excluded all respondents who either did not drink at the time of the first interview ($N = 39$) or reported, at the time of the second wave, having had contact at any time with a treatment agency or group concerning problems with alcohol ($N = 55$). This reduced the panel sample to 521 "untreated drinkers" about whom we have both Time 1 and Time 2 data.

Both instruments collected data on each respondent's drinking practices and on the problems he may have experienced in connection with his drinking. Scales for 11 drinking problems, each scale covering a different sort of problem associated with drinking, have been constructed from these data. Each scale was designed to tap both the *recency* and the *apparent severity* of a particular problem event or condition. In this analysis, problems reported by the respondent have been limited to those occurring within the 12 months prior to the interview (except in some instances where ordinary language required that questions simply be stated in the present tense). The severity of a problem was judged on (1) the face value of an item (for example, losing a friend qualified as a "high level" of severity, whereas a friend's expression of concern qualified as a "moderate level" of severity), and (2) the relative rarity of problem reports at that level on the scale (for example, "high level" = overall drinking volume in the top 5 percentiles of the sample; "moderate level" = drinking volume in the next 5 percentiles).

These problem scales cover alcohol-related problems in three more or less distinct domains: (1) problems associated with the *interpersonal consequences* of drinking; (2) problems suggested by the respondent's *intake of alcohol per se*; and (3) *subjective problems* (to be explained). Three corresponding summary scales were constructed from the 11 problem scales. The *interpersonal problem scale* is based on self-reports of negative sanctions over drinking. These include troubles with the police and strains or actual breaks in relationships (with spouse, other relatives, friends, co-workers, or job supervisors). The *problematic intake scale* is based on reported consumption practices that put the respondent at risk of intoxication on a fairly regular basis. This scale is made up of four subscales measuring (1) the frequency of drinking fairly large quantities at a sitting; (2) the occurrence of going on binges and drinking episodes longer than 1 day; (3) the usual quantity consumed per drinking occasion; and (4) the total volume consumed in a month. Finally, the *subjective problems scale* is based on feelings of loss of control over drinking, concern with reliance on alcohol to cope with stress, and acknowledgment of a number of alcoholism symptoms based on Jellinek's (1952) original symptomatology.

Finally, an overall problem scale, the sum of the respondent's scores on the three summary scales, was constructed. (See Appendix A for operational definitions of the individual drinking problem scales, the summary scales, and the overall problem scale.)

RATES OF SPONTANEOUS REMISSION

Ideally, the first order of analytical business would have been the selection of the "alcoholics" from our subset of untreated current drinkers. This could have been accomplished by applying a consensual set of diagnostic criteria to our problem scales. Unfortunately, such diagnostic expertise is nowhere to be found. Clinical conceptions of alcoholism, as Knupfer (1972) has pointed out, have tended to regard the condition as an all-or-nothing matter, like pregnancy; and this presumption has never fitted well the findings from general-population studies. Our samples have consistently revealed continua on these problem dimensions, so that no clearly discernable trough could be used to divide normals from alcoholics. In the absence of a clearly bimodal distribution on these problem scales, the next best alternative is probably that of matching respondent characteristics with a criterion group of labeled alcoholics. Comparable data on both clinical and nonclinical groups have not, as yet, provided a basis for better classification schemes, although Armor and colleagues (1976) have made some progress in this area, and Bruun (1963) apparently used this method some years ago in a study comparing Finnish alcoholics with a general-population sample. Conventional screening tests for alcoholism (for example, Selzer, 1971), and even ostensibly more exhaustive diagnostic inventories (for example, National Council on Alcoholism, 1972), tend to employ disjunctive sets of criteria that would yield positive diagnoses for an uncomfortably large sector of the male general population.

We have opted to consider the "alcoholism criteria" as a variable rather than as a fixed element in the remission picture. Table 9-1 shows the Time 1 frequency distributions for several different formulations of problem drinking or alcoholism (based on the 11 individual drinking problem scales, the three summary scales, and the overall problems scale). Also shown are the frequencies of drinking problems at differing severity levels. For example, if "problematic intake," is used as the criterion of problem drinking or alcoholism, then 8% of the sample qualifies for the label if the "high severity" cutoff point is used, whereas 15% reported "at least minimal" problems in this area.

TABLE 9-1 Time 1 Drinking Problems among Untreated Drinkers

	Severity level (%)		
Problem scales	No problems	At least minimal	High
Overall problem scale	61	39	17
Summary scales			
A. Problematic intake	85	15	8
B. Interpersonal problems	81	19	10
C. Subjective problems	74	26	5
Individual scales			
A1. Binge	97	a	3
A2. Heavy intake	90	10	3
A3. Overall volume	90	10	5
A4. Usual quantity	94	6	4
B1. Spouse problems	93	7	3
B2. Interpersonal problems	89	11	3
B3. Job problems	97	a	3
B4. Police problems	98	a	2
C1. Symptomatic behavior	91	9	2
C2. Psychological dependence	82	18	1
C3. Loss of control	90	10	2

Note. This table should be read as follows: The first row of figures shows that, at Time 1, 61% of the sample had no problems or scored 0 on the overall problem scale (OPS), 39% had at least one minimal level problem (score of 1 or higher on the OPS), and 17% had at least one higher level severity drinking problem (score of 5 or higher on the OPS). $N = 521$.
[a]No minimal level defined for these scales.

Table 9-2 shows the spontaneous remission rates associated with a variety of Time 1 criteria for problem drinking and Time 2 definitions of remission. Time 1 and Time 2 data are presented for both the overall problem scale and the three summary scores of drinking problems in the areas of problematic intake, interpersonal problems, and subjective problems. With respect to the overall problems score (OPS), outcome data are presented for four criteria: (1) R had no problem at Time 2; (2) R had no or minimal problems (OPS = 3 or lower) at Time 2; (3) R had no or minimal problems or his problem score showed a drop of 2 or more problem points at Time 2, and finally; (4) R had no or minimal problems or showed a drop of 1 or more problem points at Time 2.

Each of the summary scales is split into three severity categories at Time 1: (1) no problem; (2) at least one "minimal-level" problem (which is inclusive of higher level problems); and (3) at least one "high-level" problem. The Time 2 data have been coded to show respondents with no problem and respondents with a mild problem only. With respect to both the overall and the summary drinking problems scales, this mode of presentation allows us to assess the impact of varying definitions and cutting points on estimates of the apparent rate of spontaneous remission.

Because only one respondent with one or more current drinking problems at Time 1 turned up at Time 2 as abstinent during the preceding 12 months, an abstinence column in the outcomes was not needed. (We had initially intended to use the respondent's self-definition as an alcoholic or problem drinker as a criterion variable, but virtually all of the few respondents who reported that they "thought they might be an alcoholic" at Time 1 were excluded because they had received some form of treatment for alcoholism at some time in their lives.)

TABLE 9-2 Remission from Drinking Problems among Untreated Drinkers as Indicated by Various Time 1 Criteria of Problem Drinking and Various Time 2 Criteria of Remission

		Time 2 criteria of remission (%)									
		Time 2 overall problem scale				Time 2 summary scales					
						Problematic intake		Interpersonal problems		Subjective problems	
Time 1 criteria of problem drinking	N	No problems	No or minimal problems	No or minimal problems or a drop of 2+ points in problem score	No or minimal problems or a drop of 1+ points in problem score	No problems	No or minimal problems	No problems	No or minimal problems	No problems	No or minimal problems
Time 1 overall problem scale											
No problems	316	72	88	88	88	86	94	88	94	86	98
1+	205	30	55	60	63	61	77	65	75	48	79
2+	112	15	43	51	57	46	68	56	68	36	71
3+	89	18	38	48	56	47	64	54	66	37	71
5+	86	19	40	50	58	47	64	54	66	38	71
6+	59	14	32	48	59	36	58	46	61	29	64
7+	29	14	28	59	66	38	52	31	48	24	59
10+	27	11	26	59	67	37	52	30	48	22	59
11+	17	12	24	59	71	41	47	29	53	24	53
Total	521	56	75	77	78	76	87	79	87	71	90
Time 1 summary scales											
Problematic intake											
No problems	445	62	81	82	82	83	93	82	89	77	94
At least minimal problems	76	20	37	46	54	41	55	62	72	38	68
High problems	43	21	37	49	58	35	44	61	74	47	72
Interpersonal problems											
No problems	421	63	80	81	82	81	90	85	91	77	93
At least minimal problems	100	26	52	60	63	57	76	55	67	45	78
High problems	50	20	38	54	60	54	70	40	56	30	68
Subjective problems											
No problems	385	67	83	83	83	83	91	85	92	82	96
At least minimal problems	136	24	52	59	64	58	78	62	73	39	73
High problems	25	0	24	52	60	32	60	32	44	20	56

Implications

At Time 1, about 39% of the current drinkers reported at least one minimally severe drinking problem. Hence, the complete absence of a current problem characterizes only a little more than half the sample. Therefore, reporting one current problem should not be regarded as strongly implicative of deviant drinking. Equivalently, setting the "remission criterion" at "no current problems" at Time 2 is a stringent remission criterion.

Column 2 in Table 9-2 shows the proportion of respondents reporting zero current problems at Time 2. As would be expected, the Time 1 criterion groups defined by the lower problem scores are more likely than those groups defined by higher scores to cross over into the no problem group at Time 2. But the degree of variation in this transition probability does not appear to be strongly affected by varying the Time 1 criterion level. Respondents with one or more problems at Time 1 have a 30% chance of reporting no problem later on, whereas respondents at the highest end of the Time 1 distribution have about a 10% chance of reporting no problem later on. In part, this relatively small difference in transition probabilities results from the cumulative character of these cutting points: the group defined by 1+ (one or more) problems at Time 1 *includes* 2+, 3+, and so on, respondents as well. This cumulativeness was imposed on the table so that it would provide a closer parallel to a treatment center sample, in which anyone who meets certain criteria for alcoholism is admitted regardless of by how much the criteria are exceeded. Respondents with one *and only one* current problem at Time 1 had 48% probability of no problem at Time 2. (Noncumulative transition probabilities appear in Appendix D.) In the third column of Table 9-2, the remission criterion is relaxed to include respondents who reported only minimal problems at Time 2. The variation in remission rates shows roughly a 30-point spread (from 55% to 24%) across the range Time 1 of problem drinker criterion scores. The biggest single jump in remission rates is between the one-problem-plus group and the remission of the no problem group. The differences in remission rate between the second column (no problem) and third column (no or only minimal problems) are greatest at the low end of the Time 1 criterion scores and smallest at the high end. Relaxing the definitions of remission brings in an additional 25% of the sample (30% to 55% in this case) at the 1+ Time 1 criterion, but it brings in an additional 12% to the remitted group at the very highest end of the Time 1 scores. Both columns 2 and 3 reflect absolute standards of remission rather than measures of change, so that the distributions show a trend toward smaller remission as the initial status of the respondent involves a greater number of problems.

In column 4 of Table 9-2, the criterion of remission is relaxed again to include a 2-point or greater amount of decline in problem scores between the Time 1 and Time 2 surveys, as well as a decline in the absolute problem score to no or minimal problems. If this column had been defined solely in terms of decline, the trends in the second and third absolute columns would have been reversed, and remission rates (in the fourth column) would have increased as the Time 1 criterion rose. Although this sort of distribution would reflect accurately the probabilities of improvement in the sense of change for the better across the Time 1 criterion scores, it would omit from the remission picture the cases that at Time 1 are substantially problem free or minimally problematic but that showed no change. Therefore, we have conjoined the absolute criterion of no or minimal only problems with a measure of change so that respondents who qualified on either grounds would be counted among the remitted.

The group with 1+ problems now shows a 60% remission rate; the groups defined by 2+ through 6+ problems dip to roughly a 50% remission rate; and the groups with 7+ or higher Time 1 scores rise again to about a 60% rate. Notice that the impact of the relaxation in the remission criterion is more strongly felt at the high end of the Time 1 measures than at the low end. At the high end, remission rates in column 3 are more than doubled in column 4, but at the low end, switching the criterion does not result in as dramatic a change.

The fourth column's requirement that remitters drop at least 2 points on their overall problem scale provides something of a buffer against measurement error. This buffer is set aside in the fifth column of the table wherein any reduction in the respondent's problems is counted as remission (again, respondents with no or minimal only problems at Time 2 are included regardless of the amount of change). Once more, the remission rates show modest to modestly great increases emerging from 3 to 12 points higher than they were in column 4.

Table 9-2 also shows the remission patterns for the Time 2 summary scales. These are illustrative of the remission patterns that follow from rather different criteria of "alcoholism." We have cross-tabulated the Time 1 summary scales by both the Time 2 overall problem scale and the Time 2 summary scales to present all the bivariate dependencies among the summary and the overall scales.

We are not describing this part of the table in detail. The reader might notice, though, that the likelihood of losing higher level problematic intake, interpersonal problems, or subjective problems scores by Time 2 are respectively, 44%, 56%, and 56%. These rates of defection are in each instance higher than the defection rate from *any* problem by Time 2. For example, the probability that someone with high-severity interpersonal problems will diminish or lose them by Time 2 is .56, but the probability that this person will have *no* Time 2 high-severity problems is only .38. This patterning suggests a considerable amount of flow among the problem indicators. Having a particular problem at Time 1 carries a stronger implication for having *some* problem at Time 2 than for having the *same* problem at Time 2 (see Cahalan & Roizen, 1974, for similar findings in a national sample).

By now we may have at least a provisional answer to the question: What is the rate of spontaneous remission in a general population sample of adult males? If abstinence is the criterion, the rate is virtually zero. Taken together, different criteria of measurement would permit different researchers to claim *improvement* rates as low as 11% or as high as 71% with these same data, depending on the cutting points. It seems that the establishment of a single remission rate for this sample is not quite so pertinent as an appreciation of the sway on the remission rates that differing Time 1 and outcome measurement criteria imply.

RESEARCH DESIGN AND ANTICIPATING REMISSION

Diagnostic Versus Prognostic Approaches

One of the by-products of the fact that "remission" touches on different conceptual and practical issues in the field of alcohol problems is that there is no *single* remission research problem but a number of problems, each requiring somewhat different approaches. Consider two of these: Remission can be regarded—especially in the classical model of alcoholism as a disease—as a failure of *diagnostic criteria* to perform the task of keeping nonalcoholics out of that diagnostic group (the failure to identify false positives). Alternatively, remission can be regarded as a *prognostic problem.* In this case, the same outcome variance will be searched for prognostic factors that anticipate the future course of a patient's condition.

Several different research strategies divide these two approaches: First, diagnostic studies typically involve tests of criteria against both an alcoholic criterion group and a sample of supposed normals (for example, Selzer, 1971) in order to validate the discriminating abilities of the proposed criteria; the literature on prognosis, on the other hand, is universally confined to samples of alcoholics only. Second, the two sorts of studies also tend to differ in the independent variables they use. For instance, prognostic studies tend to focus on social stability and personality variables that would not be employed in a diagnostic analysis. In fact, the use of *social* (prognostic) *characteristics* in the *diagnosis* of alcoholism is regarded as a weakness or failing in diagnostic practice (see, for example, Blane, Overton, & Chafetz, 1963). Third, the two sorts of approaches also carry different implications about the way the dependent variable is conceptualized and scaled. Prognostic analyses, for example, sometimes view negative change as simply as "unimproved" case or a treatment "failure" but provide scale values for the degree of improvement that patients seem to have experienced (for example, Gillies, Laverty, Smart, & Aharan, 1974; Mindlin, 1959). Logically, diagnostic studies, on the other hand, should focus on identifying people who will turn up with *high problem scores* at Time 2. All the while, the diagnostic and prognostic questions address ostensibly the same problem: ways to anticipate the future course of a patient's condition based on limited (and, as we have seen, socially conditioned) sets of predictive information.

In considering these differential implications for the analysis of remission from drinking problems, we wish to stress that the choices mentioned above (which sample should be studied, which independent variables should be employed, which form of the dependent variable should be used) are not resolvable in a single, encompassing analytical solution. Consequently, as we have already done with regard to the description of remission, we have considered the alternatives mentioned as themselves variables in research on remission.

Three alternatives pertaining to the sample, the dependent variables, and the independent variables have been varied in the analysis:

1. *Sample: full sample versus "clinical" subgroup.* Respondents with at least one drinking-related problem at the higher level of severity and an additional problem at at least the minimal level of severity are treated as a surrogate for a clinic population sample. The choice of cutting points is arbitrary but poses no particular problem because our interest here is merely to examine the differences introduced in the analysis by focusing on either the full or the "clinical" samples.

2. *Dependent variables: Time 2 problem level versus improvement versus raw change.* The "Time 2 problem level" refers to a respondent's overall problem score at Time 2. Thus, it is not a change measure but an outcome score that defines the "remission variable." The dependent variable labeled "Improvement" is a scale of "changes for the better" in which decreases in the respondent's overall problem score are scored, but both worsening and unchanged scores are set to zero.

With this scoring method, the dependent variable corresponds to clinical studies in which worsening and unchanged cases are lumped together in an "unimproved" category. "Raw change" is simply the difference between the Time 1 and Time 2 overall problem scores, with both changes for the better and for the worse scored.

3. *Independent variables.* We have separately considered social and diagnostic variables. Measures of social stability were drawn from those common in the literature (see Appendix B). Time 1 problem scores have been used as stand-ins for diagnostic criteria (see Appendix A). Many of these problem scores were originally drawn from various conceptions or criteria for alcoholism (see Keller, 1960). In general, the array measure of social stability and drinking problems that are used might correspond well to the data routinely collected for diagnosis and prognosis in a clinical setting.

It is interesting to note, incidentally, that locating this analysis in the medical language of diagnosis and prognosis permits us to bypass the problem of multicollinearity in the interpretation of our findings. Both diagnostic and prognostic approaches to these data are primarily concerned with the discovery of signs or symptoms rather than with the etiological significance or the causal structure that they suggest. Hence, these studies tend to rely on the multicollinearity of the factors on which they collect information and do not necessarily regard the lack of independence as a problem.

The three analytical alternatives described above imply 12 different analyses covering (1) the full and the "clinical" samples; (2) the social stability and the problem scale predictors; and (3) alternative scoring procedures for the dependent variable, the Time 2 problem level, improvement, and two-way change. So that these analyses would reflect the medical goal of selecting the most parsimonious set of prognostic and diagnostic indicators, in each case a *stepwise* multiple regression was run. Each of the regressions was terminated when the next additional step failed to add at least .01 to the multiple correlation coefficient (see Table 9-4).

Table 9-3 shows the final multiple correlation coefficients in each of the 12 regression analyses. Some general observations are suggested by this table. First, the multiple *R*s vary over a substantial range of values, from a low of .183 (prognostic factors, full sample, raw change) to a high of .684 (diagnostic factors, full sample,

TABLE 9-3 Final Multiple Correlation Coefficients in 12 Stepwise Regressions

Sample	Prognostic factors	Diagnostic factors
Full ($N = 521$)		
Time 2 overall score	.260	.527
Improvement	.238	.684
Raw change	.183	.353
"Clinical" ($N = 59$)		
Time 2 overall score	.518	.579
Improvement	.556	.547
Raw change	.547	.486

Note. The final step was established for each regression when the subsequent step failed to add at least .01 to the multiple correlation coefficient.

improvement). This range of variation alone suggests that studies of remission among problem drinkers are strongly affected by the independent-variable domains, sample definitions, and dependent variables used in the research strategy.

Whereas *prognostic variables* account for a substantial amount of the improvement variance in the "clinical" sample for each of the three dependent variables, the multiple Rs for prognostic variables in the full sample are much lower. It seems that the predictive strengths of prognostic factors partly derive from the fact that they are universally employed in "clinical" samples. *Diagnostic factors,* on the other hand, achieve more *similar* multiple Rs in both the "clinical" and full samples.

This pattern of multiple Rs does not suggest a perfect fit with the classical model of alcoholism as a single disease entity. If a diagnosis of alcoholism implies, without appropriate treatment and abstinence, the worsening of alcohol-related problems, we should expect diagnostic factors to flag this likelihood: Diagnostic factors in the full sample should be strongly predictive of Time 2 problem scores, particularly because the classical model of disease alcoholism regards the condition as permanent once it is acquired. But in a group of already diagnosed alcoholics (that is, the "clinical" sample), the pragmatic implication of the diagnostic factors is simply that all the members of this group—by virtue of their common diagnoses— face a more or less common alcohol-problems fate. Accordingly, in an untreated sample of alcoholics, we should expect little outcome variance and little or no relationship between individual diagnostic criteria and what outcome variance there is.

Some alcoholics get better and others do not. If the concept of alcoholism referred to a common condition shared by all people with that diagnosis, then *prognostic factors*—those that concern the relevant features of the environment of the disease—should best account for the outcome variance in an already diagnosed sample. The finding from our "clinical" sample that diagnostic factors account for about as much outcome variance as prognostic factors suggests either that there is no common clinical disease entity or that this set of diagnostic factors includes signs or symptoms that are far from being equivalently diagnostic. Whichever is the case, a perfect fit between classical disease imagery and these data would have generated: (1) very low multiple Rs for (a) prognostic factors in the full sample, and (b) diagnostic factors in the "clinical" sample; and (2) on the other hand, high Rs for (a) diagnostic factors in the full sample and (b) prognostic factors in the "clinical" sample. Such a pattern did not fully show itself in our data.

The clinical literature on prognostic factors for alcoholism tends to follow an implicit bad-leads-to-bad model (Hirschi, 1973) in which patients with few social and psychological resources are rated the poorer treatment bets. This general trend is offset, somewhat, by the notion of "hitting bottom" in the standard Alcoholics Anonymous account for the path to recovery. Here, the theory seems to suggest that recovery follows the complete exhaustion of social and personal resources. The two perspectives can be brought into something of a synthesis by adjusting the point of hitting bottom for different alcoholics. For example, the bottom point for most middle-class alcoholics might be substantially above the bottom point for most skid row alcoholics. In terms of this synthesis, the positive associations between social and psychological resources and improvement in the patient's condition are compatible with both perspectives, although such a relationship certainly is not always confirmed in clinical studies (see, for example, Gillies et al., 1974).

Remission and Prognostic Variables

This analysis employs nine prognostic variables: family income, educational level, marital status, age, geographical mobility, whether there are children in the home, occupational level, employment status (working or not working), and an index of interpersonal isolation. In our surrogate for a clinical sample, the regression equation for Time 2 problem level by prognostic factors (see Table 9-4, unit A) exhausted nearly all of the explanatory potential after three steps. *Low* Time 2 scores were anticipated by *low* occupational level, *higher* educational level, and by being currently (at Time 1) employed rather than unemployed. Each of these variables is uncorrelated with Time 1 problem scores in the "clinical" sample. (See Appendix C for the zero-order correlation coefficients among all of the variables.) This implies that the association between occupational level, education, and work status and Time 2 problem scores is not a by-product of the relationship between these prognostic variables and *initial position* in the "clinical" group. In order to get a more concrete feeling for the predictive improvement won by this equation, the unstandardized regression coefficients were used to construct an index of the likelihood of remission. The "clinical" group consisted of respondents with a 6+ overall problem score at Time 1 ($N = 59$). By Time 2, 26 respondents, or 44%, reported problem scores less than 6, or became "subclinical." Among respondents whose occupational level, education, and work status suggested an upcoming remission (based on the regression equation), 70% did report subclinical scores at Time 2; and among those whose prognostic characteristics indicated less chance for remission, 23% reported subclinical scores. As calculated by Lambda, this equation netted a 35% improvement in the prediction of outcome when outcome is defined as either retaining or losing a problem score of 6 or more by Time 2.

The "clinical" sample imposes on the data a rough control for initial position. Most of the change in drinking problems in this group was in the downward direction. Consequently, in the "clinical" sample, the three alternative forms of the dependent variable (Time 2 problem level, improvement, and raw change) are highly intercorrelated. In the limiting case, in which all Time 1 problem scores are the same in the "clinical" group and all change is in the downward direction, respondents would score identically on all three forms of the dependent variable. Predicting who at Time 2 will be *low* in problems, who will show the most *decrease* in problems, and who will *change* most boils down to the same question. For the prognostic variables, the regression equations tend to show this pattern of rough equivalence across the forms of the dependent variable (see Table 9-4, units A, E, and I).

In the *full* sample, though, the correlations among the forms of the dependent variable are lower (see Appendix C). This circumstance implies that the regression equations for prognostic variables in the full sample may be substantially affected by the particular form of the dependent variable employed. When the Time-2 problem score is the remission criterion, *low* outcomes are predicted by *higher* education, being *older, having a job,* and *lower* occupational prestige (see Table 9-4, unit C); but when improvement is the criterion, *high* remission is predicted by being *younger,* by *lower* interpersonal isolation, and by *lower* occupational prestige (see unit G). Finally, when raw change is the criterion, change in the direction of improvement is predicted by *having a job*, by being *unmarried,* and by *lower* interpersonal isolation (see unit K).

The relationship between age and each of the outcome variables is particularly

TABLE 9-4 Twelve Stepwise Regressions for Remission, Varying (1) the Dependent Variables Scoring, (2) the Types of Independent Variables (Prognostic or Diagnostic), and (3) the Sample

Variable	Final-step beta	Variable	Final-step beta
	Predicting Time 2 overall problem score		
A. Clinical sample, prognostic ($N = 57, R = .518$)		B. Clinical sample, diagnostic ($N = 59, R = .579$)	
Occupational level	−.467	Job problems	.322
Educational level	.307	Symptomatic behavior	−.265
Employment status	.244	Binge problems	−.252
(high = employed)		Spouse problems	−.250
		Loss of control	−.170
C. Full sample, prognostic ($N = 504, R = .260$)		D. Full sample, diagnostic ($N = 520, R = .527$)	
Educational level	.236	Symptomatic behaviors	−.227
Age	.168	Spouse problems	−.169
Employment status	.126	Loss of control	−.155
(high = employed)		Overall volume	−.140
Occupational level	−.110	Interpersonal problems	−.130
		Usual quantity	−.121
	Predicting improvement		
E. Clinical sample, prognostic ($N = 57, R = .556$)		F. Clinical sample, diagnostic ($N = 59, R = .547$)	
Occupational level	−.537	Job problems	.440
Interpersonal isolation	−.347	Heavy intake	.289
(high = more isolated)		Police problems	.237
Educational level	.262	Interpersonal problems	.105
Children at home	.143		
(high = yes)			
G. Full sample, prognostic ($N = 504, R = .238$)		H. Full sample, diagnostic ($N = 520, R = .684$)	
Age	−.160	Job problems	.326
Interpersonal isolation	−.122	Heavy intake	.301
(high)		Police problems	.219
Occupational level	−.121	Interpersonal problems	.139
		Coping	.139
		Spouse problems	.127
	Predicting raw change[a]		
I. Clinical sample, prognostic ($N = 57, R = .547$)		J. Clinical sample, diagnostic ($N = 59, R = .486$)	
Occupational level	−.454	Job problems	.391
Employment status	.246	Police problems	.186
(high = employed)		Overall volume	.165
Educational level	.233	Spouse problems	−.123
Interpersonal isolation	−.175	Interpersonal problems	.102
(high)			
K. Full sample, prognostic ($N = 504, R = .183$)		L. Full sample, diagnostic ($N = 520, R = .353$)	
Employment status	.127	Job problems	.242
(high = employed)		Police problems	.143
Marital status	−.102	Overall volume	.140
(high = married)			
Interpersonal isolation	−.089		

Note. The signs of the betas have been reversed to indicate the relationship to remission, that is, low Time-2 overall problem scores. The final step was established for each regression when the subsequent step failed to add at least .01 to the multiple correlation coefficient.   Full panel, $N = 521$; "clinical" panel, $N = 59$.

[a]In the direction of improvement.

noteworthy: *low* age predicts *high* Time 2 problem scores but also *high* improvement, and age does not enter in the regression on raw change at all. Clearly, studies of prognosis would come away with quite different impressions of the influence of age, depending on their scoring of the dependent variable. Contrary to the picture of problem drinkers created in clinical studies—where the median age of alcoholics is most often in the mid forties—cross-sectional, general-population surveys repeatedly have shown that drinking problems are largely a young man's game (Cahalan, 1970; Cahalan & Room, 1974). In a sense, this finding merely is replicated in the positive association between youth and Time 2 problem levels. Youth also may emerge as a predictor of improvement because of its influence on initial position in the full sample, an influence that provides younger, rather than older, respondents with more opportunity to remit because of the generally higher mean problem scores of younger men at Time 1. The disappearance of age in the regression equation for raw change suggests, however, that young men are more likely than older men both to acquire and to lose drinking problems. The association between age and raw change is curvilinear, which eliminates age from the regression equation for raw changes. By extension, the positive association between youth and remission becomes a byproduct of the fact that youth predicts greater *instability* in drinking problems over time.

Let us assess the implications of these findings for our larger argument. Ordinarily, the study of remission from alcoholism involves some group of alcoholics, a set of prognostic variables, and some measure of the degree of improvement experienced by each case after some time has passed. We have seen that the particular form of the scoring of improvement is not a big factor in our results in this clinical sample. Nevertheless, most efforts to generalize these findings from a clinical study, either by incorporating them into a theoretical account of the abatement of drinking problems or by applying them to a larger universe of drinkers, seem ill advised. We have seen in the full sample of current drinkers that (1) prognostic variables accounted for much less of the improvement variance than was accounted for by the same variables in the "clinical" sample; (2) substantial differences appeared in the rosters of independent variables called in to account for the improvement variance, as the form of the dependent variable was varied; and (3) the strengths and even the signs of individual predictors within these rosters were susceptible to reversals across the dependent variable forms.

Remission and Diagnostic Variables

Ideally, diagnostic variables should separate nonalcoholics or pseudoalcoholics, whose drinking problems are episodic or transitory, from genuine alcoholics, whose problems persist as long as drinking continues. In a general-population sample, properly functioning diagnostic criteria applied at Time 1 should generate a fan-spread pattern (Armor, 1975) of drinking problem levels at Time 2. Respondents who scored low on diagnostic criteria at Time 1 should score low or lower on drinking problems at Time 2, and respondents who scored high on these criteria should go on to score high or higher on problems.

Like the prognostic factors, particular diagnostic factors revealed a good deal of variation in their predictive strengths, depending on the sample ("clinical" or full) and the form of the dependent variable in the regression. Unlike prognostic variables, however, the interpretation of the diagnostic variables is complicated by their variable associations with initial position in both the "clinical" and the full sample. In the "clinical" sample, Time 1 diagnostic variables show correlations with the

Time 1 overall problem scale that range from a high of .51 (symptomatic behaviors) to a low of −.02 (usual quantity); in the full sample, these correlations
range from .58 (symptomatic behaviors and overall volume) to .39 (spouse problems) (see Appendix C).

When the Time 2 overall problem score was the dependent variable, the regression equation for the full sample (Table 9-4, unit D) generated six variables that
contraindicate *low* outcome scores: symptomatic behaviors, spouse problems, loss
of control, overall volume, interpersonal problems, and usual quantity. Without a
control for initial position, it is difficult to interpret the meaning of this set of
variables. Symptomatic behavior, for example, may anticipate high Time 2 problems by virtue of a strong association with Time 1 problems and a low tendency
toward turnover. Spouse problems, on the other hand, may predict high Time 2
scores because they are often characteristic of respondents with low Time 1 scores,
thereby providing more opportunity for worsening among respondents who report
this drinking problem. In the clinical sample, where initial position is roughly
controlled, job problems predict *low* Time 2 problem scores, whereas symptomatic
behavior, binges, spouse problems, and loss of control contraindicate low Time 2
scores. When *improvement* is predicted in the "clinical" sample, the roster of best
predictors is again revised: job problems, heavy intake, police problems, and interpersonal problems are all associated positively with remission. In general, the
prediction of both improvement and raw change, whether in the full or "clinical"
sample, relied most on job problems, police problems, and either of two indicators
of heavy drinking, heavy intake or (high) overall volume. As we have shown elsewhere (Cahalan & Roizen, 1974), job and police problems are particularly transitory in a general-population sample. To reiterate, the findings of the various
regressions when diagnostic variables are used show considerable variation as the
sample and outcome measures are varied.

DISCUSSION

A corollary to the fact that there is no natural boundary between alcoholic and
nonalcoholic drinkers in our general-population studies is that there will be no
natural boundary between remission and nonremission from alcohol-related problems. Therefore, the notion of remission can be equated with a variety of more or
less arbitrary standards falling between abstinence at one extreme and "any improvement" at the other. In the first part of this chapter, we roughly quantified the
impact of varying both outcome criteria and criteria for defining the problem
drinking group in which remission is to be calculated. In this general-population
sample, these variations in criteria produced improvement rates varying from 11%
to 71%. The abstinence rate was virtually zero.

Although these remission levels are highly responsive to measurement criteria,
the general trend of the figures is clear, and it supports Emrick (1975) and much of
the earlier literature: By most criteria, there was a substantial amount of spontaneous remission of drinking problems in a population in which the overall trend in
drinking problems was stable or even increasing. This suggests that the conventional
clinical picture of drinking problems as relatively stable and lasting phenomena may
need changing. Instead we might picture a great deal of episodic and situational flux
in a relatively large fraction of the population that ever drinks enough to risk
drinking problems.

In taking up the problem of accounting for remission, we have tried to show how the remission problem crosscuts medical conceptualizations of alcohol-related problems. Ordinarily, remission would be handled as a prognostic question. Studies would follow already diagnosed cases over time, exploring the factors associated with improvement and nonimprovement in patients' illnesses. Such studies *presume* rather than *test* the validity of the diagnostic factors that place patients in the study group in the first place. This presumption tends to orient prognostic inquiries around clinical groups, around measures of getting better, and around aspects of patients' circumstances that are not invariant by virtue of the fact that all subjects are diagnosed with the same illness.

In regard to illnesses or putative illnesses that are troublesome for even the best diagnosticians, the remission problem can be transposed into a diagnostic one. In the alcoholism field, the logic of studies of diagnostic criteria has been that of the "criterion-group" test, in which samples of "known" alcoholics are compared to samples made up predominantly of nonalcoholics, in order to uncover criterial attributes of the illness. These tests are cross-sectional rather than longitudinal, in part because they build on the assumption that the diagnosis has been properly assigned to members of the criterion group. At least where the disease being diagnosed is considered a lifelong condition, the more *longitudinal* aspects of diagnosis should become more apparent. Any inventor of a new early-detection test for pregnancy would point out that proof rested, not so much on dissimilarities between a criterion group known to be pregnant and a control group largely unpregnant, but on whether or not women of either group who turned out positive on the test went on to show the more easily seen attributes of that condition. If the diagnosis of a condition involves a temporal dimension, it is a short step to the observation that remission is a diagnostic issue. As a diagnostic issue, the study of remission might involve some modifications in the logic and practice of prognostic studies. A diagnostic approach to remission might be oriented around samples that include both reputedly positive and negative cases, around measures of change that move in both directions, and around independent variables drawn from current diagnostic protocols.

In the latter part of this chapter, we have separated out and systematically varied the dimensions of these alternative research strategies. Although it is certainly true that few actual studies of remission would confine their activities to the requirements and limits of one of the 12 regression studies, this chapter should serve to show some of the varieties of findings when different research designs are used. The differences in these findings show that the substantive results of research on remission are partly by-products of (1) the way the research problem has been defined and (2) the research design that each problem definition commonly implies.

APPENDIX A: OPERATIONAL DEFINITION OF PROBLEM SCALES

I. *Individual Scales.* All scales are based on information about a respondent's behavior within the year preceding the interview. Respondents who qualify at the high-severity level for a given problem have been assigned scores of 5; the score of those who qualify at the minimal level is 1; and a score of 0 is assigned to all other respondents.

A. *Binge.* A respondent's self-report of being drunk for more than 1 day in a row.
   1. *High level.* Reports going on binges within the last year.
   2. *Minimal level.* No minimal score on this variable.
B. *Current intake.* A summary scale of the frequency of drinking relatively high quantities at a sitting.
   1. *High level.* A respondent who drinks 12 or more drinks at one time at least once a week *or* who drinks 8-11 drinks per drinking occasion nearly every day.
   2. *Minimal level.* A respondent who drinks 12 or more drinks at one time 1-3 times per month *or* who drinks 8-11 drinks 1 to 4 times per week *or* who drinks 4-7 drinks nearly every day.
C. *Overall volume.* An estimate of a respondent's monthly overall volume of alcohol consumption, based on his frequencies of drinking beer, wine and liquor and his frequencies of drinking various quantities per sitting.
   1. *High level.* Overall volumes that fall in the top 5 percentiles of the volume distribution. Percentiles are based on the panel subsample of current drinkers who report no treatment for alcohol-related problems.
   2. *Minimal level.* Volumes that fell in the 90th to 94th percentiles.
D. *Usual quantity.* The usual number of drinks a respondent drinks on one occasion.
   1. *High level.* Eight or more drinks per occasion.
   2. *Minimal level.* Six or seven drinks per occasion.
E. *Spouse problems.* Self-reports of alcohol-related problems with current spouse or ex-spouse.
   1. *High level.* Spouse became angry about respondent's drinking *or* threatened to leave *or* actually left respondent because of his drinking.
   2. *Minimal level.* Spouse wished respondent drank less or acted differently when he drank.
F. *Interpersonal problems.* Alcohol-related problems with any relatives (not including spouse) or friends.
   1. *High level.* Relationships with relatives or friends were broken up or threatened *or* relatives or friends got angry about respondent's drinking.
   2. *Minimal level.* Not as severe as above, but relatives or friends would have liked respondent to drink less or act differently when respondent drinks.
G. *Job problems.* Alcohol-related problems regarding respondent's employment.
   1. *High level.* Respondent went to work drunk *or* lost out on a promotion or pay raise *or* was fired or lost chance to be hired because of drinking.
   2. *Minimal level.* No minimal score on this variable.
H. *Police problems.* Alcohol-related problems with the law.
   1. *High level.* Respondent has been stopped or talked to by police because of drinking *or* has been in trouble with the law because of drinking *or* has been arrested for drunk driving.
   2. *Minimal level.* No minimal score on this variable.
 I. *Symptomatic behavior.* An additive score indicating classical Alcoholics Anonymous symptoms. It is constructed by adding 1 point for each of: sometimes take a drink the first thing in the morning when I get up;

sometimes take a few quick drinks before going to a party to make sure I'll have enough; sometimes sneak drinks when no one is looking; when drinking by myself, I tend to drink more than I do when I'm drinking with other people; have taken a drink to get rid of a hangover; and, sometimes wake up the morning after drinking and cannot remember doing some things that I did.

1. *High level.* Respondent indicates three or more of the six symptoms.
2. *Minimal level.* Respondent indicates two of the symptoms.

J. *Coping.* Indications of respondent's reliance or psychological dependence on alcohol. Constructed with 2 points for "very important," 1 point for "somewhat important," for each of the two reasons for drinking: when respondent is tense and nervous and when respondent wants to forget worries; plus 2 points for indicating that there are times when he drinks more than usual to forget everything; and 2 points for indicating that he had gotten high or drunk when upset, unhappy, tense, etc.

1. *High level.* Respondent scores 5 or more on the scale.
2. *Minimal level.* Respondent scores 2-4 on the scale.

K. *Loss of control.* An additive score attempting to measure the core of the classical disease concept of alcoholism. It is constructed by adding 1 point for each of the following: has cut down on drinking or stopped entirely for one week or more; found cutting down or stopping to be fairly or extremely hard; sometimes got drunk even when there was an important reason to stay sober; almost always drinks until he passes out; and has sometimes kept on drinking after he promised himself not to.

1. *High level.* Respondent scores two or more on the scale.
2. *Minimal level.* Respondent scores one on the scale.

II. *Summary Scales.* The three summary scales have been constructed in two stages: summing the individual problems relevant to the summary scale, and collapsing the sums into severity levels of no (scored 0), minimal (scored 1), and high (scored 5). The cutting points are drawn so that a respondent who qualified at the high level on any of the individual scales relevant to a summary scale falls into the high category on the summary scale, and so that a respondent who qualifies at the minimal level on any of the individual scales is assigned to the minimal category.

A. *Problematic intake.* A summary of binge, current intake, overall volume, and usual quantity. Raw summary range = 0-20.

1. *High level.* Raw summary score = 5-20.
2. *Minimal level.* Raw summary score = 1-4.

B. *Interpersonal problems.* A summary of spouse, interpersonal, job, and police problems. Raw summary range = 0-20.

1. *High level.* Raw summary score = 5-20.
2. *Minimal level.* Raw summary score = 1-4.

C. *Subjective problems.* A summary of symptomatic behavior, coping, and loss of control. Raw summary range = 0-15.

1. *High level.* Raw summary score = 5-15.
2. *Minimal level.* Raw summary score = 1-3.

III. *Overall Problem Score (OPS).* The three summary scores are combined into a single score that summarizes scores across all problem areas. The collapsed summary scores (0, 1, 5) have been used to construct the overall problem score so that a respondent's OPS raw score will clearly indicate the number of minimal and high problems on the three summary scores as follows:

OPS score	Number of summary problems
0	None
1	One minimal
2	Two minimal
3	Three minimal
5	One high
6	One high and one minimal
7	One high and two minimal
10	Two high
11	Two high and one minimal
15	Three high

APPENDIX B: TIME 1
"PROGNOSTIC" VARIABLES

- *Age.* Respondent's age collapsed into 5-year categories, ranging from 20 to 24 years (coded low) to 55 to 59 years (coded high).
- *Marital Status.* Respondent's marital status, dichotomized to indicate being unmarried (low) or married (high).
- *Geographical Mobility.* Number of times respondent has moved from one address to another, ranging from at least five times (low) to none (high).
- *Index of Social Position.* Respondent's ranking on a collapsed version of Hollingshead's ISP, a variable constructed from the respondent's educational and occupational levels. ISP ranges from collapsed Category 1 (low ISP) to 4 (high ISP).
- *Educational Level.* Last grade in school completed by respondent, ranging from less than eighth grade (low) to postgraduate study (high).
- *Family Income.* Respondent's gross family income in the year preceding the Time-1 interview, ranging from under $3,000 (low) to more than $20,000 (high).
- *Children at Home.* Respondent's household composition with regard to the absence (low) or presence (high) of children.
- *Occupational Level.* Respondent's occupational level, ranging from blue collar, unskilled (low) to white collar (high).
- *Interpersonal Isolation.* A scale indicating the degree to which the respondent is more (high) or less (low) isolated from people (for example, lives alone, rarely gets together with friends, doesn't enjoy social gatherings).
- *Employment Status.* Respondent's employment status, dichotomized to indicate having unwanted unemployment (low) versus being employed, retired, or a student (high).

APPENDIX C: CORRELATIONS AMONG THE TIME 1 PREDICTORS AND TIME 2 DRINKING PROBLEM LEVEL VARIABLES

Variable	X_1	X_2	X_3	X_4	X_5	X_6	X_7	X_8	X_9	X_{10}	X_{11}	X_{12}	X_{13}	X_{14}	X_{15}	X_{16}	X_{17}	X_{18}	X_{19}	X_{20}	X_{21}	Y_O[a]	Y_I	Y_C
																						Time 2 drinking problem level variable		
				Time 1 predictor variable																				
X_1 Age		-.38	-.03	.18	.09	-.01	.37	-.12	.09	-.02	.23	.16	.10	.04	-.21	-.22	-.11	.05	-.13	.02	.02	-.02	-.14	.00
X_2 Moves	-.48		.05	.08	.10	.10	-.04	.01	.24	-.18	-.16	-.21	-.01	.19	.08	.10	.06	-.03	-.09	-.03	-.04	.01	-.01	-.01
X_3 Education	-.29	.20		.10	-.03	.53	-.16	.27	-.09	.03	-.43	-.40	.11	-.05	.05	.17	.09	-.07	.05	-.17	-.07	.13	.03	.09
X_4 Income	.31	-.17	.14		.13	.33	.02	.22	.16	-.12	-.14	-.10	-.18	.29	-.03	.03	-.05	.01	-.02	-.03	.03	-.01	-.08	.00
X_5 Children	.11	-.17	-.13	.13		.08	.05	-.03	.71	-.03	.19	.07	.09	.30	.16	-.09	-.14	-.07	-.20	-.08	.02	-.06	.08	-.04
X_6 Occupational status																								
X_7 Isolation	-.06	.03	-.10	-.05	-.10			-.33	.10	-.11	-.30	-.23	-.03	.12	.15	-.11	-.09	-.05	-.01	-.01	.00	-.31	-.34	-.32
X_8 Employment status	.16	.03	-.10	-.05	.03		-.08		.03	-.15	.23	.20	.18	-.09	-.25	-.13	-.20	-.05	-.24	-.08	-.16	-.14	-.31	-.23
X_9 Marital status	.01	-.09	.05	.16	.10		-.12	-.16		.03	.05	.30	.01	.11	.01	-.10	.06	.05	.15	.05	.43	.34	.27	.38
X_{10} Binge	.17	-.18	-.03	-.07	-.07		-.02	-.02	.03		.16	.09	.18	-.01	.13	.14	.23	.02	-.04	-.07	.00	-.14	-.02	-.14
X_{11} Intake	-.09	-.01	-.16	-.02	-.07		-.30	.23	-.19	.35		.81	.11	-.17	-.11	-.12	-.14	.01	-.31	-.20	.54	-.20	.13	.06
X_{12} Volume	-.04	.01	-.03	-.16	.02		-.16	.20	.09	.28	.82		.12	-.22	.02	-.14	-.25	.04	-.21	-.18	.58	.02	.19	.09
X_{13} Quantity	-.06	.03	-.03	-.05	.03		-.07	.18	.15	.30	.32	.12		-.19	.01	.15	.17	.03	-.23	-.31	.43	-.04	.11	.09
X_{14} Spouse	-.05	.09	-.05	-.09	.07		.04	-.04	.10	.10	.05	.30	-.19		.11	.09	-.07	.00	-.14	.14	.39	.04	.05	.03
X_{15} Interpersonal	-.14	.08	-.03	-.01	.03		.01	-.06	-.13	.26	.16	.14	-.01	.11		-.10	.06	-.18	.03	-.14	.54	-.28	-.21	-.22
X_{16} Job	-.14	.07	.00	-.02	.00		-.05	-.07	-.10	.31	.08	.20	.26	.29	-.10		.06	.05	.15	.28	.46	-.17	.06	.09
X_{17} Police	-.12	.08	.02	-.05	-.06		-.07	-.07	.06	.25	.05	.04	.21	.03	.06	.06		.07	.17	.51	.40	.31	.41	.37
X_{18} Symptomatic	-.07	.04	-.06	-.05	-.06		.04	-.14	.05	.22	.26	.29	.20	.14	.20	.21	.41		.36	.51	.58	.04	.24	.21
X_{19} Coping	-.13	.10	-.02	-.07	-.17		-.11	-.03	-.20	.15	.06	.11	.04	.03	.15	.29	.03	.41		.18	.43	-.28	-.02	.01
X_{20} Loss of control	-.13	.02	.07	.00	-.06		-.03	.13	.05	.16	.17	.18	.16	.19	.18	.29	.21	.18	.11		.33	.06	.02	.08
X_{21} Overall score	-.18	.12	-.08	-.06	-.13		.04	.12	.43	.16	.54	.58	.43	.39	.54	.46	.40	.58	.43	.52		-.23	-.13	-.09
Y_O Overall score[a]	.11	.12	.14	-.06	-.13		-.11	-.16	-.31	.51	.54	.58	.43	.39	.54	.46	.40	.58	-.25	-.32	-.31		.23	.27
Y_I Improvement	-.17	.11	-.03	-.07	-.06		.34	.25	-.34	.34	.42	.37	.31	.19	.31	.49	.34	.25	.28	.23	.27	.06	.75	.83
Y_C Raw change	-.04	.02	.07	.00	-.03		.17	.19	-.31	.17	.17	.18	.16	.07	.16	.29	.19	.10	.11	.11	.33	.65	.63	.89

Note. Cell entries above the diagonal are for the "clinical sample," $N = 59$; cell entries below the diagonal are for the full sample, $N = 520$.
[a] The signs for the correlations between overall score at Time 2 and other variables have been reversed to indicate relationship to remission (low overall problem score at Time 2).

APPENDIX D: REMISSION FROM DRINKING
PROBLEMS AMONG UNTREATED DRINKERS

Time 1 overall problem scale	N	No problems	Time 2 overall problem scale (%)		
			No or minimal problems only	No or minimal problems or drop of 2+ points in score	No or minimal problems or any drop in score
0	316	72	88	88	88
1	93	48	70	70	70
2–3	26	4	54	54	54
5	27	30	56	56	56
6	30	13	37	37	53
7+	29	14	28	59	66

Note. Scores are noncumulative.

REFERENCES

Armor, D. J. *Measuring the effects of television on aggressive behavior.* Santa Monica: Rand Corporation, 1975.

Armor, D. J., Polich, J. M., & Stambul, H. B. *Alcoholism and treatment.* Santa Monica: Rand Corporation, 1976.

Baekeland, F., Lundwall, L., & Kissin, B. Methods for the treatment of chronic alcoholism: A critical appraisal. In R. J. Gibbins, Y. Israel, H. Kalant, R. E. Popham, W. Schmidt, & R. G. Smart (Eds.), *Research advances in alcohol and drug problems* (Vol. 2). New York: Wiley, 1975.

Blane, H. T., Overton, W. F., & Chafetz, M. E. Social factors in the diagnosis of alcoholism. *Quarterly Journal of Studies on Alcohol,* 1963, *24*, 640–663.

Bruun, K. Outcome of different types of treatment of alcoholics. *Quarterly Journal of Studies on Alcohol,* 1963, *24*, 280–288.

Cahalan, D. *Problem drinkers: A national survey.* San Francisco: Jossey-Bass, 1970.

Cahalan, D., & Roizen, R. *Changes in drinking problems in a national sample of men.* Paper presented at the North American Congress on Alcohol and Drug Problems, San Francisco, December 1974.

Cahalan, D., & Room, R. *Problem drinking among American men* (Monograph No. 7). New Brunswick, N.J.: Rutgers Center of Alcohol Studies, 1974.

Clancy, J. Outpatient treatment of the alcoholic. *Journal of the Iowa State Medical Society,* 1961, *51*, 221–226.

Clancy, J., Vornbrock, R., & Vanderhoof, E. Treatment of alcoholics: A follow-up study. *Diseases of the Nervous System,* 1965, *26*, 555–561.

Davies, D. L., Shepherd, M., & Myers, E. The two years prognosis of 50 alcohol addicts after treatment in hospital. *Quarterly Journal of Studies on Alcohol,* 1956, *17*, 485–502.

Drew, L. R. H. Alcoholism as a self-limiting disease. *Quarterly Journal of Studies on Alcohol,* 1968, *29*, 956–967.

Emrick, C. D. A review of psychologically oriented treatment of alcoholism: II. The relative effectiveness of different treatment approaches and the effectiveness of treatment versus no treatment. *Journal of Studies on Alcohol,* 1975, *36*, 88–108.

Eysenck, H. J., & Beech, R. Counterconditioning and related methods. In A. E. Bergin & S. L. Garfield (Eds.), *Handbook of psychotherapy and behavior change: An empirical analysis.* New York: Wiley, 1971.

Gibbins, R. J. Alcoholism in Ontario: A survey of an Ontario county. *Quarterly Journal of Studies on Alcohol,* 1954, *15*, 47–62.

Gillies, M., Laverty, S. G., Smart, R. G., & Aharan, C. G. Outcomes in treated alcoholics. *The Journal of Alcoholism,* 1974, *9*, 125–134.

Goodwin, D. W., Crane, J. B., & Guze, S. B. Felons who drink: An 8-year follow-up. *Quarterly Journal of Studies on Alcohol*, 1971, *32*, 136–147.

Hirschi, T. Procedural rules and the study of deviant behavior. *Social Problems*, 1973, *21*, 159–172.

Jellinek, E. M. Phases of alcohol addiction. *Quarterly Journal of Studies on Alcohol*, 1952, *13*, 673–684.

Keller, M. Definition of alcoholism. *Quarterly Journal of Studies on Alcohol*, 1960, *21*, 125–134.

Kendell, R. E. Normal drinking by former alcohol addicts. *Quarterly Journal of Studies on Alcohol*, 1965, *26*, 247–257.

Kendell, R. E., & Staton, M. C. The fate of untreated alcoholics. *Quarterly Journal of Studies on Alcohol*, 1966, *27*, 30–41.

Kissin, B., Rosenblatt, S., & Machover, S. Prognostic factors in alcoholism. *Psychiatric Research Report*, 1968, *24*, 22–43.

Knupfer, G. Ex-problem drinkers. In M. A. Roff, L. N. Robins, & M. Pollack (Eds.), *Life history research in psychopathology* (Vol. 2). Minneapolis: University of Minnesota Press, 1972.

Lazarsfeld, P. F. *Problems in the analysis of mutual interaction between two variables.* New York: Columbia University, Bureau of Applied Social Research, 1969.

Lemere, F. What happens to alcoholics. *American Journal of Psychiatry*, 1953, *109*, 674–676.

McCaghy, C. H. Drinking and deviance disavowal: The case of child molesters. *Social Problems*, 1968, *16*, 43–49.

Mindlin, D. F. The characteristics of alcoholics as related to prediction of therapeutic outcome. *Quarterly Journal of Studies on Alcohol*, 1959, *20*, 604–619.

National Council on Alcoholism. Criteria for the diagnosis of alcoholism. *American Journal of Psychiatry*, 1972, *129*, 41–49.

Robson, R. A. H., Paulus, I., & Clarke, G. G. An evaluation of the effect of a clinic treatment program on the rehabilitation of alcoholic patients. *Quarterly Journal of Studies on Alcohol*, 1965, *26*, 264–278.

Ruggels, W. L., Armor, D. J., Polich, J. M., Mothershead, A., Stephen, M., with others. *A follow-up study of clients at selected alcoholism treatment centers funded by NIAAA.* Menlo Park, Calif.: Stanford Research Institute, 1975.

Selzer, M. L. The Michigan alcoholism screening test: The quest for a new diagnostic instrument. *American Journal of Psychiatry*, 1971, *127*, 1653–1658.

Thorpe, J. J., & Perret, J. T. Problem drinking: A follow-up study. *Archives of Industrial Health*, 1959, *19*, 24–32.

Wing, J. K. *A four-year follow-up of 50 alcohol addicts after treatment in hospital.* Dissertation in Psychological Medicine, London University, 1956.

IV

COMMENTARIES

10

Age, Cohorts, and Drug Use

Matilda White Riley
Bowdoin College

Joan Waring
Russell Sage Foundation

In this chapter, we discuss the theoretical issues in the studies in this volume, in particular the college and adult studies, from the viewpoint of our emerging theories of the sociology of age (see Riley, Johnson, & Foner, 1972). We considered the question, how might general theories of aging over the life course help to interpret the findings in the studies? There are several immediately apparent and exciting convergences. Thus, if the studies report use of marihuana as a statistical norm among youths as disparate as students at Berkeley and soldiers in Vietnam, we can bring to bear general understandings of postadolescence as a life stage conducive to drug use. At this stage, roles are transient (college student, worker in entry job, soldier, unemployed) and evoke little commitment; rewards are meager (low pay, low esteem) and provide little leverage for social control; marked age segregation (in barracks, dormitories) encourages peers to influence one another. Or, if the studies hint at maturing out of drug use or alcohol use, then we can counterpose the life-stage challenge to young people of aging into the multiple roles of adulthood, with the multifarious demands imposed by these new roles and also the socially approved potential for prestige, power, and financial reward.

As we continued to speculate about convergences between findings from drug studies and the sociology of aging, however, we recognized that our initial interpretive framework was too narrow. Indeed, we were confining ourselves to the data from these longitudinal studies, even though many of them focused on a single cohort only. Thus, despite our own frequent admonitions to the contrary, we were subjecting our interpretations to all the limitations of *cohort-centrism* (Riley, 1973). It is well established that studies of just a single cohort, while essential for understanding the life-course (aging) patterns of individuals, are insufficient for such understanding. The findings are not generalizable. The life course of any particular individual (or cohort) has unique features produced by "history," that is, by the special historical and environmental events characterizing the era in which the person (or cohort) lives (Baltes, 1968; Riley et al., 1972, pp. 27–90; Ryder, 1965; Schaie, 1970).

Clearly, we needed a broader conceptual framework that would interpret drug use in relation both to aging over the life course and to the exigencies of historical and social change. We needed information about the *past*: How did the new patterns of widespread drug use arise? How were these patterns affected by the Vietnam war? By the affluence of the late 1960s? By more complex social processes? We needed information about the *future*: Will future cohorts of young people continue to adopt drugs? If so, will the practice become institutionalized, no longer illegal nor regarded as deviant (as in the case of alcohol use beyond a certain minimum age)? Will drug use continue "to diffuse through the general population" (chap. 7, p. 160) as older people are influenced by younger users? Will future parents influence their children in new ways if the parents themselves also have drug experience?

Thus we decided to address ourselves in this chapter to the nature and potential of the broader conceptual framework we have been developing. We first outline the nature of this framework (calling it a "cohort model") and then cite a few examples to suggest the possible utility of the model in interpreting the data and in the search for antecedents and consequences. We stress the general principle that cohort-specific longitudinal findings take on new meaning when related to comparable data on adjacent cohorts, both predecessors and successors. In other words, to understand drug use in the cohorts being studied requires longitudinal strategies to see how *individuals* develop the relevant behaviors, attitudes, and norms over the life course; but it also requires juxtaposition of these cohorts with other cohorts to indicate whether and how *societal* factors and changes may be at work. Our examples suggest how observed differences or similarities among cohorts can open new avenues of explanation, and they also suggest how interrelationships among coexisting cohorts can operate as societal antecedents or consequences of drug use.

A COHORT MODEL FOR INTERPRETING LONGITUDINAL DATA

Several rudiments of our conceptual model are indicated by the schematic representation in Figure 10-1. This figure shows the life-spans of three selected cohorts (people all born in the same time interval). Cohort C, representing those born in 1950, approximates the earliest cohort used in these drug studies. The people within each cohort *age*. That is, over time they pass through a sequence of roles from birth to death (such as dependent child, student, worker, spouse, retiree), learning to play new roles and relinquish old ones, accumulating knowledge and attitudes and social experiences, and undergoing biological and psychological development and change. As particular individuals are aging and dying, a second crucial process is taking place concomitantly: New cohorts of people are continually being born. Meanwhile, changes in the social structure—designated as "history" at the bottom of Figure 10-1—are constantly occurring (as society undergoes such events as wars, famines, periods of prosperity and depression, changes in the state of science and the arts, revolutions in tastes and beliefs). As society changes, each new cohort encounters a unique sequence of social and environmental events. Hence it follows that the life-course patterns of people in one cohort will differ in some respects from the life-course patterns of those in other cohorts. Different cohorts age in different ways, and it is these differences that cannot be observed from longitudinal study of a single cohort.

Viewed over time, two different dynamisms are in continuing interplay: human dynamics and social change. Human dynamics, the ways in which people age and

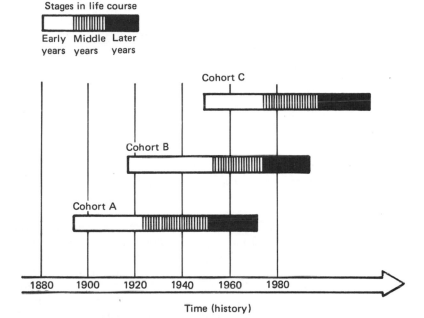

FIGURE 10-1 A cohort model, illustrating processes of aging and cohort flow. *Source.* Matilda White Riley, Marilyn Johnson, and Anne Foner, *Aging and Society, Volume 3: A Sociology of Age Stratification,* New York: Russell Sage Foundation, 1972, p. 10. Copyright © 1972 by Russell Sage Foundation. Reprinted by permission.

cohorts follow one another, are in part caused by changes in society; but they also cause change. The process is two-directional. We often illustrate this point by Waring's (1975) notion of "disordered cohort flow." If one thinks of successive cohorts pushed by aging through the changing structure of age-graded roles, there is often a poor fit between cohorts and the role systems; and the misfit gives impetus to social innovation. For example, an excessively large cohort (like those in the drug studies) may change the whole structure of roles in the schools or in the family, causing strains that encourage drug use. Or social changes may foster a new form of drug behavior in successive cohorts. These cohorts in turn may redefine this behavior as no longer deviant, but, rather, as an established norm. Changes in social norms and social structures thus can operate as both antecedents and consequences of the processes under study.

Uses of the Model

Our suggestion is that, in principle, this model can be valuable for organizing and codifying the steadily accumulating information about drug use and drug attitudes within many successive cohorts. So used, the model would help to redefine and redirect the interpretations of current findings and to generate both new ideas and greater consistency in designs for future research.

Particular studies have special objectives, of course, but reference to Figure 10-1 highlights three strategies for use of this model in any given analysis: (1) tracing the life-course patterns of individuals *within* each cohort; (2) comparing similarities and differences *among* cohorts in these life-course patterns; and (3) showing how the consecutive cohorts, each one lagging behind its predecessor in the process of aging, all *fit together* to form the changing age structure of the society.

Most of the studies under review concern the first of these three strategies, demonstrating the power of the longitudinal approach for analyzing such components of drug use in a single cohort as:

1. Patterns of beginning use (for example, in respect to age, prevalence, and frequency)
2. Duration or discontinuance of use
3. Antecedents and consequences (in terms of individual characteristics or behaviors)

Because of their varied objectives, the studies differ in many respects—in focus on a particular drug or drugs, on definition of use, and on the special components of drug use selected for attention. Not all the researchers relate their analyses directly to age or cohort, and the major treatment of one of the key components—discontinuance of drug use—refers to adult problem drinkers of alcohol (Roizen, Cahalan, & Shanks, chap. 9). The findings of this study are intrinsically important; they show substantial amounts of spontaneous remission among untreated problem drinkers, thus implying that "the conventional clinical picture of drinking problems as relatively stable and lasting phenomena may need changing" (p. 214). Nevertheless it is difficult to integrate these findings on alcohol with those from the other studies on other types of drugs.

Certain of the studies go beyond the single-cohort approach and provide some limited material for use in Strategy 2, comparing cohorts, or Strategy 3, relating coexisting cohorts of differing age. The two major categories of studies in this volume represent different cohorts, after all, with the college students and adults drawn from earlier cohorts (many born around 1951) and the high school students drawn from more recent cohorts (many born around 1956). Smith and Fogg (chap. 4) analyze their data to show that early users of marihuana (in contrast to late users and nonusers) are characterized by such precursors as being rebellious or sociable or having low grade point averages in high school. These data, collected in five waves at yearly intervals, trace cohorts of students entering each school grade from 4 to 12, thus yielding the raw materials for a full-blown cohort analysis (see Nesselroade & Baltes, 1974). Similarly, the Jessors (chap. 2) follow cohorts of junior high school and college students across four annual testings, relating use of marihuana to developmental correlates in terms of environmental, personality, and behavioral antecedents. Kandel, Kessler, and Margulies (chap. 3) include among the antecedents of adolescent entry into drug use the relations of these adolescents with their parents; thus, rather than comparing cohorts, these researchers deal with the interplay between two coexisting cohorts separated in age by a generation.

How, then, can such information on multiple cohorts enhance the understanding of drug use obtained from longitudinal analysis of a single cohort? A few examples from other fields can supplement the limited data from the studies at hand and point the way.

COHORT COMPARISONS

Initiation

Widespread use of illicit drugs is a recent social innovation. Gallup polls show that the proportion of young people 18-25 years of age who had tried marihuana was only 3% in 1964 but has now risen to well over half (see also Johnston, 1973). Such innovation is a striking feature of the topic at hand. It is a phenomenon to be explained, and the search for possible explanations of social innovation requires cohort comparison. Here the question is no longer, Why do some individuals rather than others in the cohort start to use drugs? The question is, rather, Why are members of recent cohorts more likely to begin drug use than their predecessors of like age in earlier cohorts?

A case in point relates to quite a different innovation, the gradual spread of birth control through successive cohorts of Catholic women, contrary to the teaching of the church and the dictates of the pope. A report by Westoff and Bumpass (1973) compares the acceptance of birth control among four cohorts of Catholic women at the age (20-24) of entering adulthood. The percentages accepting birth control rose steadily over time from 30% in the earliest cohort studied (born 1931-1935) to 78% in the most recent cohort (born 1946-1950). How can such cohort differences be explained? Certainly not by longitudinal study of changes in individual women, for the several cohorts comprise entirely different women. In the several cohorts, millions of women make decisions as to the position they will espouse; yet these seemingly personal decisions show marked patterning according to the cohort to which each woman belongs. It is clear that explanations must be sought, not at the individual, but at the *societal*, level—perhaps, as the authors of this study suggest, in terms of technological advances in birth control methods, increasing openness in matters of sex, or shifting norms as to desired numbers and spacing of offspring. The example shows how cohort analysis can supplement the search for explanation by redirecting attention from microscopic personal factors toward macroscopic social changes.

Analysis of such cohort data does not stop with such macro-level comparisons among cohorts entering the system but goes on to examine life-course patterns within each cohort. In an era of innovation, cohort comparisons may show rising levels of initial acceptance of birth control; but do these different beginnings mean different patterns of continuing acceptance as the women in each cohort grow older? In this study the answer is negative. Regardless of the level of initial acceptance, the women in each cohort show a tendency toward increasing acceptance of birth control over the life course; for every cohort, aging seems to coincide, not with greater conformity to the teachings of the church, but with a rising desire not to have more children. Here the cohorts, once their views are established, tend to age in *similar* ways. But note: The fact of similarity could not have been learned from study of a single cohort.

A somewhat parallel finding occurs in the drug study by Jessor and Jessor (chap. 2). In their Figure 2-5, changes in "marihuana involvement" are shown for each of three cohorts at three periods of observation. For each cohort, with boys and girls examined separately, the life-course pattern is upward: Marihuana involvement rises as age advances. When different cohorts are compared, there is also an upward tendency (though here the patterns are not entirely clear, and the figure is not designed to facilitate cohort comparison). For example, if a line is drawn from females in the eighth grade in 1970 to females in the eighth grade in 1971 (the "eighth-grade cohort"), the direction is upward. Similarly, a line from ninth-grade girls in 1970 to ninth-grade girls in 1971 follows an upward course. For boys, the parallel comparisons are similar, save for a dip from ninth graders in 1970 to ninth graders in 1971. Such data, if replicated in more substantial research with a wider time frame, would indicate that more recent cohorts are the more involved with marihuana and that involvement tends to increase over the adolescent years.

Life-course Change

In the examples just cited, cohorts differed at the point of entry or initiation (at beginning use of drugs, for example, or initial attitudes toward birth control), but life-course patterns remained similar across cohorts. In other instances, cohort differences can occur in the shape, rather than the level, of the life-course curve. Here, a striking illustration comes from analysis of long-term changes in labor-force participation of women in the United States (see Riley et al., 1972, pp. 160–197). If one examines a single cohort—say, the cohort born 1896–1905, in which participation peaks at ages 14–24 and again in the middle years 45–54—one tends to phrase interpretations in terms of individual women. One might ask whether, or why, some women drop out of the labor force when they marry and have children, or reenter once the children have left home. But when one examines the entire array of cohorts—from those born in the post–Civil War period to those active in the labor force today—a veritable revolution is uncovered. In the earliest cohort, women on the average tended to join the work force young but to drop out in increasing proportions with advancing age; but in more recent cohorts, the pattern appears to be exactly reversed, with increasing proportions engaging in the work force as they grow older; and the most recent entrants may chart a still different course. Here the interpretation must surely be phrased in societal terms. What *social factors* account for the long-term change in the work cycle of women? To find out, we must examine the secular rise in educational level, for example, or look for a radical restructuring of the feminine role.

Are there such cohort differences in the shape or direction of drug use over the life course? In the length or intensity of use? In any later tendency to mature out or taper off? Potentially different patterns of drug use over the life course may develop depending on the age at which use began. Given the apparent declines in starting age, studies that follow the recent cohorts into their later years might perhaps find new norms and new interconnections between drugs and other life events that distinguish these cohorts from their less accustomed predecessors.

Antecedents and Consequences

Cohort comparisons can also shed light on the antecedents and consequences of drug use. Johnston, O'Malley, and Eveland (chap. 6) provide an example in their search for causal connections between drugs and delinquency. Tracing a nationally representative sample of young men from 1966 (average age of 15 years) to 1974 (average age 23), they find a clear positive relationship between use of nonaddictive illicit drugs and other forms of illegal behavior, particularly crimes against property (contrasted with crimes against people). Beyond this, however, drugs do not seem to play much of a role in leading users to become more delinquent. On the contrary, because most of the delinquency differences between users and nonusers existed *before* drug use began, it may have been the delinquent behavior (and association with deviant peer groups) that led to the use of drugs.

These authors then make the point we are making: In the end, they conclude that their longitudinal analysis of a single cohort cannot suffice to determine the time sequence of drug use and delinquency. For this cohort, as they point out, "the notion of using illicit drugs at all was just rising to consciousness among these young people as they passed through high school. Studies of a more recent class cohort would undoubtedly show less precedence of drug use by other forms of delinquency because the average age of first drug use has declined markedly" (p. 156).

Similar difficulties arise in interpreting the findings by Mellinger and his co-authors (chap. 7) on the possible adverse consequences of illicit drug use among students at the University of California at Berkeley. In their report, also on a single cohort, these researchers examine male freshmen, in 1970 and again $2\frac{1}{2}$ years later, in respect to two outcome criteria: academic performance and clarity of occupational goals. They find that, for most drug users, the generally moderate pattern of use seemed to have few negative consequences, independent of other prior characteristics distinguishing users from nonusers. They do report, however, some evidence of adverse outcomes among small subgroups of "continuing multiple-drug users."

Here too one wonders about the generality of the finding. If, for example, the more recent cohorts are more likely to use drugs, to begin drug use at earlier ages, and to use increasing amounts of some drugs (such as marihuana), is it possible that these more recent cohorts also include more "continuing multiple-drug users"? If so, the adverse consequences might perhaps become increasingly pronounced.

In the search for antecedents, consequences, or other correlates of drug use, these researchers point to possible underlying factors: personal experiences or predispositions, behavior syndromes, or the broader social context. When cohort differences, rather than individual differences, are to be explained, many antecedents and consequences must certainly be sought in the social context. Sources of cohort difference often inhere in the broad sweep of historical, economic, or demographic change, or in the size and composition of the particular cohorts. What, then, is *unique* about these more recent cohorts that may have influenced their increasing use of drugs? Their large size? If so, may we expect a change in drug use as declining fertility begins to produce smaller cohorts of adolescents? The affluence of the late 1960s?—already past. The impact of the Vietnam war? Here Robins's study (chap. 8) seems relevant, for she reports a speeding up of drug initiation (narcotics and marihuana) among youths exposed to the drug-intensive Vietnam setting, in contrast to nonveteran controls. Here again, comparisons with other cohorts might suggest the strength and uniqueness of the Vietnam impact in relation to other social forces.

CROSS-COHORT INFLUENCES

In the attempt to broaden understandings gleaned from longitudinal analysis, we have been discussing possible uses of the cohort model in the search for explanatory clues. Finally, we must consider the coexistence of many cohorts who, despite their differences in age and historical experience, share the same society. Coexisting cohorts, or age strata, can exert profound influence on one another. The extent of this influence markedly affects the rate at which such an innovation as illicit drug use may permeate the society as a whole.

That parents, through socialization, have some effect on the lives of their children is generally assumed. Parental influence, as one of a cluster of antecedents of drug use, is explored in the study by Kandel, Kessler, and Margulies (chap. 3). Isolating three sequential stages of adolescent drug behavior, these researchers point to parents as possible models at the first stage (use of hard liquor) and to poor relations with parents as a factor in the third stage (use of illicit drugs other than marihuana). Parents seem least relevant at the second stage (initiation into marihuana) at which youths adopt associated beliefs and values not prevalent in society at large. It would also be interesting to inquire more directly into the parent cohorts. If many of these parents began life in the great depression and experienced World War II in their youthful years, their own views of youth culture and of the meaning of various drugs might be quite different from those of parents born earlier or later than they (see Kandel & Lesser, 1972). How, then, does the nature of socialization, as well as the vogue for particular drugs, change with history?

Children can, in turn, socialize their parents. There has been much speculation about a possible heightening of reciprocal socialization because of the "permissive" upbringing of the children under scrutiny in these studies. Older children can also influence younger children. Are older children important in the spread of drugs into younger and younger population segments? In short, what is the likelihood that drug use will ramify through the age strata, spreading from the youthful innovators to the middle-aged as well as to the preteens, tending toward rapid institutionalization? Again the answers depend upon supplementing the strategy of cohort-specific longitudinal research.

SOME FEASIBLE COHORT STRATEGIES

Thus, in principle, the cohort model can be broadly useful in drug studies, opening many new avenues of exploration, and guarding against over generalization from single longitudinal designs. But what of the practicalities? Just the few questions we have noted—meager beside those that will occur immediately to the sophisticated students of drug use—could not be approached within the confines of a single study, nor of an entire program of studies over a short span of time.

In advocating the cohort model, our intent is not to call for grandiose new programs of research. Far from it. We are, rather, making two modest pleas for practical research approaches. First, we recommend using a wide range of specific strategies that can illuminate different parts of the model. We heartily endorse longitudinal and panel approaches. How else can one discover what happens to all these drug users as they grow older (see Fillmore, 1974, for a 20-year follow-up study showing decline in alcohol drinking over the life course)? A highly useful modification is the design called "cohort-sequential" (as used by the Jessors, chap. 2, and by Smith & Fogg, chap. 4). Complementing the longitudinal designs is the sequence of age-specific cross-sectional surveys, widely used for analysis of synthetic cohorts. The sequence of cross-sections cannot trace the same individuals over time, but it has compensatory strengths (see Riley et al., 1972, pp. 583–618).

It avoids potential bias from repeated questioning. The samples at each period can meet criteria of representativeness—important in long-term studies, not only because of *panel mortality* (the difficulties reported by Josephson and Rosen, chap. 5, can sometimes be overcome, as in the procedure used by Robins, chap. 8), but also because of relevant changes in the universe under study produced by migration or the birth of new cohorts. The sequence of cross-sections also has the great asset that it makes room for available data from earlier studies—an asset that enables the researcher to delve into the past rather than waiting years or decades for future aging and future social change (see Riley, Foner, Moore, Hess, & Roth, 1968, for a cohort analysis of alcohol drinking). Among the many other useful designs, of course, are those aimed at testing the specific hypotheses or disentangling particular cohort, period, and aging effects that may be suggested, but not confirmed, by the cohort approach (Riley, 1973).

Our second plea is for coordination of research objectives, standardization of key definitions, and complementarity of research designs, making possible the gradual accumulation and codification of knowledge in this important field.

REFERENCES

Baltes, P. B. Longitudinal and cross-sectional sequences in the study of generation effects. *Human Development,* 1968, *11*, 145–171.

Fillmore, K. M. Drinking and problem drinking in early adulthood and middle age: An exploratory 20-year follow-up study. *Quarterly Journal of Studies on Alcohol,* 1974, *35*, 819–840.

Johnston, L. D. *Drugs and American youth.* Ann Arbor: Institute for Social Research, 1973.

Kandel, D. B., & Lesser, G. S. *Youth in two worlds.* San Francisco: Jossey-Bass, 1972.

Nesselroade, J. R., & Baltes, P. B. Adolescent personality development and historical change: 1970–1972. *Monographs of the Society for Research in Child Development,* 1974, *39* (1, Serial No. 154).

Riley, M. W. Aging and cohort succession: Interpretations and misinterpretations. *Public Opinion Quarterly,* 1973, *37*, 35–49.

Riley, M. W., Foner, A., Moore, M. E., Hess, B., & Roth, B. K. *Aging and society,* Vol. 1, *An inventory of research findings.* New York: Russell Sage, 1968.

Riley, M. W., Johnson, M. E., & Foner, A. *Aging and society,* Vol. 3, *A sociology of age stratification.* New York: Russell Sage, 1972.

Ryder, N. B. The cohort as a concept in the study of social change. *American Sociological Review,* 1965, *30*, 843–861.

Schaie, K. W. A reinterpretation of age-related changes in cognitive structure and functioning. In L. R. Goulet & P. B. Baltes (Eds.), *Life-span developmental psychology: Research and theory.* New York: Academic Press, 1970, 485–507.

Waring, J. M. Social replenishment and social change: The problem of disordered cohort flow. *American Behavioral Scientist,* 1975, *19*, 237–256.

Westoff, C. R., & Bumpass, L. The revolution in birth control practices of U.S. Roman Catholics. *Science,* 1973, *179*, 41–44.

11

Longitudinal Studies of Drug Use in the High School: Substantive and Theoretical Issues

John A. Clausen
University of California at Berkeley

Perhaps the most important observation one can make about teenage drug use (especially marihuana use) is that it has gone from being a relatively infrequent and significantly deviant behavior in the period soon after World War II to being a rather widespread behavior, at least on an occasional basis, by the mid-1970s. It is not strongly condemned by adolescents, is regarded ambivalently by many young adults, and is strongly devalued by a large, but decreasing, proportion of older generations. This change in the frequency of marihuana use has entailed changes in the social and personality characteristics of users, especially moderate users in late adolescence, as well as changes in official policy on marihuana. These changes all have implications for research and theory on the causes of drug use.

Few students of drug use would quarrel with the generalization that drug use is in no sense a unitary behavior possessing a single, unequivocal meaning either for users or for nonusers. Drug use in its manifold guises is learned behavior, and it is most often learned by participation in a subculture. The subculture is both incorporated and reshaped by adolescents as they mature in successive cohorts within what is commonly referred to as the "adolescent society" of contemporary America. Most students of drug use would also agree that we are dealing with the developing behaviors of individuals who are embedded in different social matrices (families, peer networks, schools), which are themselves embedded in larger sociocultural milieus, all of which are changing. One deals, then, with the interaction of features of person, network, and culture. One must take into account dimensions of personality of different individuals functioning within particular networks in which they build up shared norms, some of which are unique to the networks, and one must consider the varying meanings of individual behaviors and subgroup norms within the larger normative systems that make up the culture. I examine the implications of these assertions below as I consider the theoretical frameworks of the high school studies reported in this volume.

Until a few years ago, research seeking to delineate the process by which adolescents learn their orientations and behaviors with reference to particular drugs has relied on retrospective reports, sometimes buttressed by participant observation. Retrospective reports enable one both to get at least a rough understanding of the process of learning drug-relevant orientation and to get some notion of changing patterns of association and changing accessibility of the individual to conventional social controls. Valid formulations can only be achieved to the extent that users are both aware of and willing to give reasonably accurate accounts of their changing patterns of association and accessibility to controls. Because retrospective accounts of past attitudes and orientations tend to be recast in the light of the present, if one wants valid assessments of antecedents and correlates of changing patterns of drug use (of changing attitudinal orientations, goals, patterns of association, and role performance), one needs longitudinal data.

Before turning to the specific studies, I want to consider briefly the kinds of general issues that longitudinal studies permit one to address, issues that cannot be unequivocally answered without having observations at more than a single time point:

1. Changes associated with the process of becoming a user—changing orientations toward, and beliefs about, drugs; changing practices with reference to drugs; and changing meanings or functions served by drugs (requiring observations at a minimum of two time points;
2. The antecedents of shifts in drug behavior (onset of use, increased use, stopping use) to be found in personality, in patterns of association, and in social situations encountered; the changes in these antecedent dimensions associated with shifts in drug behaviors (again requiring, at a minimum, two time points;
3. The differential timing (antecedent, concurrent, or subsequent) of shifts in attitudes, values, self-perceptions, situations encountered, and patterns of association relative to changes in drug behavior (requiring a minimum of three data time points). With data on three or more time points, one can focus on predictors of change in subsequent drug behavior, on concurrent correlates, or on consequences either of changes of drug behavior or of social response to the individual's drug behavior. One can also study the circumstances under which some users proceed to heavier drug use, some stabilize at a given type and level of use, and others back away from drug use.

All four longitudinal high school studies are in the tradition of panel studies of public opinion rather than in the tradition of intensive longitudinal studies of human development. Designers of longitudinal and panel studies have to face the basic decision of whether to go after very intensive data on a small sample or less intensive data on a much larger sample. Opting for a relatively large sample, especially if one secures data from more than a single source, seems to me a wise decision in terms of payoff when one is dealing with a topic such as drug use, though obviously one inevitably wishes for more intensive assessments in some areas of behavior and personality. As I consider each study separately, I indicate the particular strengths of each and the points at which one would like to have additional information and analyses.

There is another question of strategy to consider in the presentation of results in this volume. That is the strategy of taking, as a primary index of drug use, whether the individual has *ever* used a given drug. When one is focusing on age at initiation, it is obvious that the first use constitutes a kind of initiation. So long as most individuals have not used a given drug, even a single exposure obviously sets those exposed aside as either precocious or deviant. But in a longitudinal study, the focus of subsequent interest will be on changes in drug behavior, on tendencies to increase usage, on turning to drugs whose use is regarded as more seriously deviant than maintaining some steady level of usage, or on backing away from drug use at all. What I most miss in all of the reports under consideration is the failure at this stage in the analysis to examine changes in levels of drug usage in specified periods antecedent to each contact with the study sample.

Strangely, from most of the reports, one would have only a vague idea of how frequent the use of various drugs is among high school students in the United States. Only one report presents systematic data on the increase in rates of drug use from grade to grade over the high school years, and none of the reports gives even a crude estimate of the level of heavy drug use.[1] Yet the level of drug use prevailing at a given time and place is a statement on certain of the cultural norms of that time and place. The attitudes and behaviors of individuals with reference to drug use take their meaning partly from the *extent* to which they are generally shared and partly from the social reputations and social position of those with *whom* they are shared. This is a basic point to which I return after consideration of the individual studies.

For each of the substantive reports of longitudinal studies, I comment briefly on the theoretical framework employed, the general research design, the ways in which theoretical concepts are operationalized, the research questions posed in the analyses here reported, and the ways in which one might seek further illumination of processes of change in the use of drugs. Discussion of characteristics of the populations and samples studied I defer until my discussion of the Josephson-Rosen report on panel loss.

THE STUDIES

Kandel, Kessler, and Margulies

The study by Denise Kandel and her associates (chap. 3) deals with only two time points 5 or 6 months apart. Its objectives are quite sharply delimited, and they are oriented toward a theory that is quite explicitly spelled out. The adolescent is seen as embedded in a matrix of social relationships, of which parental and peer relationships are most crucial. The generations have different positions with reference to drug use, especially marihuana use, and so the focus of attention is on the differential influence of parents and peers at any given time. The adolescent's responses to social influences are seen as the function of personal characteristics and situational factors. Finally, the process of becoming a user of a given illegal drug is seen as a developmental stage in a progression that may go from cigarettes and wine and beer to hard liquor, marihuana, and multidrug use, or it may stop at any stage along the way.

The aim of their analysis is primarily to determine the relative influence of parents and peers at each of three stages of drug use (hard liquor, marihuana, and multidrug use) and the extent to which the two sources of influence overlap with

[1] *Ed. note*. Purely epidemiological concerns specifically were not to be a focus of the reports.

each other and with other factors (such as characteristics of the focal respondent and the quality of relationships between respondents and sources of influence). This is, then, primarily a search for antecedents and data on relationships within the immediate social matrix. Attributes of the individual and of the social matrix are utilized at a single time point at or shortly after the initial assessment of drug-use status.

Parental and peer behaviors and orientations, like orientations of the focal respondent, are obtained by questionnaire. Fathers and mothers, alternatively selected, report on parent–child relationships. The closest friend's responses are taken as representative of the peer network, but in addition, the focal respondent is also questioned on her or his perception of peer approval of drug use, on peer network conversation about drugs, and about the availability of drugs through persons known to her or him. In my opinion, this study gains greatly in power of explanation by securing data directly from parents and peers rather than relying primarily on the adolescent's own reports of the behavior and orientations of parents and peers. It is apparent from a number of studies, among them the outstanding research of Kandel and Lesser (1972), that adolescents tend to perceive their parents' beliefs and attitudes in terms that best suit the adolescents' own frame of reference and feelings about their parents. My own research with data from families studied intensively in the Berkeley longitudinal studies suggests that adolescents who feel that their parents are understanding and have considerable influence on them are not, in fact, in appreciably closer agreement with their parents on specific values and issues, when the latter are separately assessed for both parties, than are adolescents who feel that their parents are less understanding and have less influence on them. Further, adolescent behavior disapproved of by parents will tend to elicit from the adolescents the perception of a greater gap between the generations than will be the case if there are no issues of this sort between parent and child.

Because the focus of attention in the report is on the transition in drug use from Time 1 to Time 2, the sample is partitioned according to stage of drug use at Time 1. The key question is what information available at Time 1 predicts a given transition to the next highest stage by Time 2? The sample is not partitioned by age or school grade, so one cannot ask whether those who are precocious in progression to a given stage differ in other respects from those who move to that stage when they are several years older. In general, the earlier an individual uses any drug, the more deviant that behavior pattern is, even in terms of peer-group norms. Within some schools, the modal age for making a given transition is substantially earlier than in other schools. Indeed, one finds that classification by school is, in this study, the single most powerful predictor of use of "other illegal drugs" and is one of the most powerful predictors of initiation to marihuana use. Year in school, however, is, in these data, only modestly correlated with any of the transitions: It is most strongly correlated, *negatively*, with marihuana use. Among those who were already using hard liquor, younger students were more likely, in a given period of 6 months, to begin marihuana use than were older users of hard liquor. Part of this difference may be due to gross differences among the populations of the various schools. Part of it may be due to the fact that those younger people who were using liquor at Time 1 were already more sharply distinguishable in terms of deviant orientations and practices.

The strategy of establishing which parental and peer orientations and relationships and what adolescent values, intrapsychic states, and drug-related attitudes best predict each specific transition to the next highest stage is certainly a legitimate one; yet I feel that the confounding of age and cohort experience markedly diminishes the potential for illuminating the process of becoming a drug user in different contexts. I would like to know more about the variations in level of drug use among the 18 schools in the sample and the variations in the proportion of those who have tried a given drug at each age level. What accounts for the extremely high correlation between kind of school and the transition to other illicit drugs? How do individual schools differ in the proportion of youth who make any given transition in a period of 5–6 months? At Time 1, were 8th graders who soon thereafter began to use hard liquor more like 10th graders who thereafter began to use marihuana or 12th graders who thereafter began to use other drugs than they were like 10th or 12th graders who were liquor users at Time 1?

A somewhat related question is How many of those who used a drug only once or twice at Time 1 have gone on at Time 2 to use that drug 10 or more times in the previous 6 months? Although the transition to another form of drug use is significant, I must confess that I would find it more interesting to know how many young people are using hard liquor or marihuana with considerable frequency than to know that on some occasion they were introduced to a given drug. What does a single usage mean, if one knows nothing more? Does one become a marihuana user by virtue of taking three or four drags from a joint of "really high quality grass" at a party? I realize that in a questionnaire it is difficult to delve deeply into the circumstances of initial drug use and the meaning of that use; yet without such delving I would prefer not to put most of my analysis effort on the "have you ever" type of question.

Despite my wish that a somewhat different strategy had been followed, I think that the findings of the analyses here reported do give us a clearer understanding of linkages. The availability of data from parents and peers, in particular, adds greatly to the strength of the study. It is significant to find that despite a tendency to Guttman scaling of stages of drug use, there are somewhat different patterns of antecedents in parental, peer, and subject attitudes and behaviors for the different transitions.

It is especially significant to find that parentally reported attitudes and behaviors are indeed related to the adolescent's attitudes and behaviors and that we are not merely dealing with distorted perceptions on the part of the adolescent. The influence of parental orientations is especially impressive in view of the fact that prior stage of drug use by the adolescent has been held constant. At each stage of initiation there have already been prior moves that reflected a turn toward, or incorporation into, that segment of the peer culture that precociously experiments with sources of pleasure that are regarded as inappropriate for adolescents. Such prior moves undoubtedly have had an impact on parent–child relationships, so the influence of those relationships upon subsequent shifts in drug behavior by individuals in relatively homogeneous groups gives us valuable new knowledge.

The data from peers do, of course, confirm the earliest theoretical formulation of the importance of peer relations in marihuana use (Becker, 1953) and the more recent research of Goode (1969) and Johnson (1973). Earlier reports of the Kandel study indicate that peer agreement on attitudes toward marihuana use tops all other views shared by peers. It would be interesting to know whether those adolescents who differed from their closest friends shifted friendship patterns or drug orientations by Time 2.

Jessor and Jessor

The Jessors (chap. 2) give explicit attention not only to a general theoretical formulation but also to the special relevance of longitudinal or panel studies. They recognize on the one hand that longitudinal studies do not resolve the major issues in causal analysis and on the other hand that such studies "are uniquely important because of the *descriptive information* they can yield about process and change: descriptions of the course of human development, of the trajectories of psychosocial growth, or of the contour of behavioral trends" (p. 41). A major strength of their report is that it traces changes in value orientations and attitudes that have direct implications for, and linkage with, drug use.

The Jessors' conceptual design puts major emphasis on three systems of variables: (1) the personality system, within which they distinguish a motivational-instigation structure, a personal belief structure, and a personal control structure; (2) the perceived environment system, which involves both distal structures (such as perceptions of parental and peer supports, controls, and compatibility) and a proximal structure that involves parental and peer approval and modeling of specific problem behaviors; and, finally (3) the behavior system, which in this instance includes both deviant or problem behaviors and conventional behaviors. Demographic and social structural influences as well as specific patterns of socialization, home climate, and peer and media influence are recognized as potentially important but are considered only as they exert their influences through the personality system and the perceived environment system. The Jessors indicate that implications for change may be derived by elaboration of the notions of age grading, age norms, and age expectations in relation to problem behavior, but they do not in their report attempt to spell out the norms or to conceptualize process beyond suggesting the importance of the developmental concept of transition proneness.

The Jessors developed sets of scale items for the assessment of each of their key variables. These were administered in questionnaires to three cohorts of students, annually over a 3-year period. This gave them a basis for tracing changes in values and other dimensions of personality, in parent–adolescent and adolescent–peer relations and other elements of the perceived environment, and in conforming and deviant behaviors over this 3-year period, all as reported by individuals for themselves.

Much of the analysis presented is a demonstration that the various measures of the personality system and the perceived environment vary significantly and consistently between marihuana users and nonusers for each period of measurement, using the data cross-sectionally. Although the demonstration is impressive, it does not bear upon the questions that longitudinal data alone can answer. Elsewhere (Jessor, Jessor, & Finney, 1973), they report correlations between marihuana behavior involvement and elements of the perceived environment in the fourth measurement year that suggest that some patterns of association vary by age, but one must wait for subsequent reports to assess the meaning of age and cohort shifts in these correlations.

To my mind, the most intriguing findings of this report are those that relate to changing values and perceptions with increasing age in each cohort. The valuing of achievement goes down, the valuing of independence goes up, and "tolerance of deviance" increases, regardless of marihuana use. I put *tolerance of deviance* in italics because I suspect that we are dealing here with a changing definition of deviance as well as an increasing tolerance of a variety of nonconforming behaviors. The Jessors have documented important shifts in features of both the personality system and the perceived environment that add significantly to our understanding of adolescent behavior. If they can assess the circumstances that underlie these shifts, or that tend to inhibit or exacerbate them for some adolescents or in some milieus, they will add a great deal more to our understanding. Pervasive changes in social climates and changing patterns of association and orientation with aging are certainly involved, but it is likely that social structural and situational influences affect the speed of change.

The Jessors' analysis of "transition proneness" strikes me as less fruitful. The meaning of transition proneness at any point in time or age level will depend on both the number of individuals who have already made a given transition and the number who may be expected eventually to make it. To show that there are significant (but modest) differences in attitude or personality between those who will in the next year try marihuana and those who will not, may or may not be useful. What is called transition proneness is a combination of orientations and behaviors that increase the probability of being in the right situation and in the right frame of mind to experiment with drug use or other deviance. Transition proneness in grade 7 is obviously a very different matter from transition proneness in grade 12, especially if one wishes to identify individuals who are candidates for dropping out of school and for serious deviance. Further, a knowledge of the attitudinal antecedents of transition (many of which are fairly obvious, such as having decided that there is nothing wrong with trying marihuana at a party) may be less useful than a knowledge of the circumstances under which people with a low transition probability were in fact inducted into drug use. It would be unfair to ask that the Jessors deal with every facet of the process of becoming a drug user, but I submit that we need solid data on events in the process, not just on attitude change. All of the studies under consideration leave this part of the picture out of their theoretical and empirical domains.

I must also confess a lack of enthusiasm for the perceived environment as a set of explanatory variables. It is certainly important to know how adolescents perceive their parents and peers, but the perceived environment is (as the Jessors themselves have recognized) a product forged in the interaction of personalities and environmental events and relations. The personality system and the perceived environment are conceptually separable but very difficult to separate in assessment. A youngster alienated from his or her parents perceives them very differently than does his or her sibling who is close to the parents. Both sets of perceptions *may* be reflective of parental responses, but then again they may not. This is why one needs assessments of environmental influences and relationships by someone other than the index adolescent whose drug use is under consideration. The elements that have been incorporated in the conceptualization of the perceived environment are likely to be highly predictive, and, indeed, the proximal structure accounts for most of the explained variance in marihuana involvement; but this is largely because of the demands of cognitive consistency in the individual's account of orientations and behaviors. In general, one knows that drug users tend to overstate the amount of drug use among their peers. They tend to be oriented toward peers who approve of their own behaviors rather than toward those who disapprove. Similar value orientations among associates tend to predict close relations, as Newcomb (1961) demonstrated so effectively. Consequently, one may have in the perceived environment less an explanation of deviance than an incorporation of elements of deviance.

The strategy of relating changes in attitude toward deviance to the time of initiation of marihuana use (Figure 2-7) seems to me an excellent one. Because of the relatively small size of the group of initiators each year in the high school study of the Jessors, it was apparently not feasible to carry out this analysis by separate cohorts. Had such an analysis been possible, it might have yielded an even sharper picture of one way in which the developmental course of the precocious user differs from those of modal users and later users.

Despite the reservations I have noted above, the Jessors' approach seems to me to promise the greatest payoff for learning about the meaning of marihuana use and involvement, precisely because it sets marihuana use in the context of the developmental process and attends to other salient features of that process. Like the other researchers represented, the Jessors would like to predict drug use but they have not become so preoccupied with prediction as to eschew other approaches to their data.

Smith and Fogg

Smith and Fogg (chap. 4) report a small segment of data from a 5-year study of cohorts defined by grade placement (from grade 4 to 12) in 1971, the third year of the research. Although the decision of each individual to use or not to use drugs is seen as resting upon social, economic, environmental, and psychological variables, the strategy of the research is to focus on psychological variables, particularly attitudes, personality, and behavior patterns that either (1) differentiate among groups of students having different levels of drug involvement, (2) are precursors of various patterns of drug use, or (3) show changes that become evident after initiation of drug use. No attempt is made to seek data on the process of becoming a user or the consequences of such use.

In this study, then, attention is focused on current attitudes, behaviors, and dimensions of personality rather than on the immediate social matrix and the larger sociocultural environment. The adolescent's attitudes, behaviors, and personality are assessed by both self-report and peer ratings of strategically selected aspects of personality that reflect the individual's past reactions to various circumstances, situations, and people in the environment as assessed by those with whom she or he has most closely interacted in the context of the classroom. School performance is also assessed by data taken directly from school records.

Smith and Fogg, in their report, also deal with preliminary analyses that relate to prediction. Here the predictions are made from data secured in 1969 and relate to drug use within the next 4 years. Two criteria of drug use are used: (1) most important, grade level during first use of marihuana (early use being defined as use by the 9th grade) and (2) whether marihuana has ever been used by grade 12 or the last year of study.

The classification of first use of marihuana presents no real problem, except that this classification cannot be used for Cohort 12; but the definition of "later use" or simply "use" is somewhat problematic in that Cohort 9 is carried only to the 11th grade, whereas Cohorts 10 to 12 are carried through the 12th grade. Because it appears likely that there would be a significant increase in use from grade 11 to 12, and because there is reason to believe that those making this transition to drug use would be less deviant than those who became early users, patterns of association would be expected to change. In general, it appears that nonuse of marihuana at Year 12 does set off early use more sharply from nonuse at Year 11; most of the correlations for Cohort 10 (using early users versus nonusers) are higher than those of Cohort 9, whether one is correlating drug use with self-reports, peer ratings, or grade point average.

The findings, in this relatively homogeneous, middle-income, white population, indicate that both self-reports and peer ratings distinguish users from nonusers and that the most impressive discriminations can be made between early users and those who remain nonusers through the last year of study. Among the attitudinal items, it is the most obvious cluster, relating to obedience and seeing oneself as law abiding, that most sharply distinguishes early marihuana users from their peers. Orientations toward academic achievement and feelings of being self-sufficient and of being valued and accepted also prove to be highly predictive.

Among peer ratings (which prove to be substantially more predictive for males than for females), obedience again tops the list, but close behind are several personality variables of a different sort: impulsive, cannot always be trusted, not tender, and being seen as neither working hard nor thinking hard. The early drug users are also seen as not considerate or courteous. These very negative perceptions of early drug users by their peers seem to me extremely important. They suggest that precocious use of drugs is viewed as strongly deviant within this population of students, whereas those who became users toward the end of high school are much less sharply set off from their nonusing peers.

The dimensions of personality tapped in this study seem to me more salient and more successfully assessed than in any of the other studies, and this is particularly true of those given by the peer ratings. My hunch is that these dimensions will prove especially valuable in differentiating those who go beyond occasional drug use to heavy use, especially heavy use of hard drugs. These dimensions go deeper than either the attitudinal dimensions of personality that the Jessors have tapped or the modest set of items on depression and normlessness that Denise Kandel and her associates included in their battery. It is obviously difficult to assess impulsiveness and tenderness using self-report items alone. The use of peer ratings, so elegantly developed, adds greatly to the power of the study.

Again, one regrets that the analysis of the Smith-Fogg study to date focuses so largely on prediction and that it does not examine changes in self-concept and in social reputation associated with changes in level of drug use. The use of peer ratings as an independent source of assessment of the personality would afford an extremely valuable set of reference points for examining change in social reputation. Ideally, of course, one would like to know something about the actual patterning of peer relationships; in the Smith-Fogg study, the strategy ruled out obtaining such information. Nevertheless, a major strength of these data is that they permit the examination of change in independent data sets relating to the same individuals. The enormous quantity of data collected in this study will obviously require a long period of analysis. One hopes that, during that period, different analysis strategies will be employed to examine change, and particularly to examine change that entails substantial levels of drug use.

Josephson and Rosen

Josephson and Rosen (chap. 5) address themselves, not to theoretical issues, but to a very practical methodological issue that has extremely important implications for generalization. Loss of cases from a potential panel may occur at three separate stages: (1) the point of securing permission from parents for the participation of their adolescents in the study; (2) the initial point of panel measurement, especially if a questionnaire is administered in the school on a single occasion and if the absence rate is high; and (3) the time of follow-up of the panel, where losses may be attributable to such circumstances as transfer from the school, dropping out, absence on the day of the second administration of measurement, inability to follow instructions so as to reproduce a devised code for matching, or unwillingness to reproduce a code that will permit matching.

Josephson and Rosen convincingly document the degree of bias associated with panel attrition as a consequence of absence from school and inability or unwillingness to identify oneself. They do not discuss the problem of panel loss as a consequence of failure to secure permission for the child's participation in the study initially, though in several of the studies, most notably that of the Jessors, the largest segment of loss of the designated sample occurred as a consequence of failure to secure parental permission to participate. It is unfortunate that we do not have more information for each study on exactly the procedures used in order to secure parental permission.[2]

Why did 42% of the parents in Boulder, Colorado withhold consent to their children's participation in the Jessor study while only 4% of New York State parents withheld permission? What was the nature of the loss? We know that social status sometimes markedly influences parental permission for a child to participate in a demonstration or research program. For example, 86% of upper-middle-class parents gave permission for their children to participate in the polio vaccine trials in 1954 against only 43% of working-class parents (Deasy, 1956). Because permission slips contain the family name, it should not be difficult in most instances to establish the rates of permission granted by different segments of the population.

To the extent that the return of permission forms is left to the student whose participation is sought, one might anticipate that personality attributes significantly related to drug use (such as rebelliousness or low sense of responsibility) would lead to a low return rate. One might recommend that permission requests be mailed to parents rather than delivered by students and that they be mailed out well in advance, with return envelopes, and with follow-up when necessary to secure a response.

I should be inclined to argue that maximum payoff would be secured from a thoroughly planned and well-executed study in a single locality rather than from a study of diverse communities in which one must collect data under great time pressure without adequate local arrangements. Further, I would argue for study of a single cohort or relatively few cohorts studied over precisely the same age range, all members being followed up with intense effort, rather than study of a series of cohorts followed over varying age ranges. If it were possible to administer questionnaires to all members of a series of high school classes, without having to seek parental permission, the gains of extending cross-sectional data over many cohorts might well merit the additional data collection. If one must anticipate a major effort to get full participation, however, I would argue for a focused effort in which every potential member would be pursued. Those who cannot be studied should, to the maximum degree possible, be described. If one cannot generalize even to a local

---

[2] *Ed. note.* Not all school systems require such consent.

population, what is the point of trying to carry out a national study? Whatever (in my opinion, limited) argument there may be for a national cross section, it is surely not valid where a panel is concerned.

In a school-based, cross-sectional study, administration of questionnaires on a single day will lead to some underrepresentation of heavy drug users, but overall losses are not likely to be of major consequence. When one wishes to conduct a panel study, however, provision for subsequent administration of questionnaires to absentees would appear essential if major biases are to be avoided. Nonrepresentativeness of a panel seems to me much more serious than possible contamination effects.

Again, after the experience reported by Josephson and Rosen, unequivocal identification by name of all potential and actual panel members seems essential in order that characteristics of nonparticipants and dropouts can be established. Josephson and Rosen suggest that investigators "may wish to consider the desirability of reporting more fully and more uniformly than they have" (p. 132) on attrition and the factors contributing to it; I would put it much more strongly: It is *essential* that investigators in this area of research analyze and report on attrition and the effects of such attrition.

No follow-up study can monitor individuals closely enough to permit the assessment of change as it occurs. Nevertheless, recurrent interviewing may permit one to collect strategic information, not only on contemporary attitudes and practices, but also on recent events and their meaning to the individual. A questionnaire simply does not give the necessary flexibility for such data collection; a partially structured interview might well do so. I am aware of the increase in cost and effort entailed, and yet I believe that the payoff from adding 200 interviews (assuming that one could get a completion rate of 80% or more) would be far greater than adding any number of questionnaires to one's basic cohort.

Ideally, interviews would be used both to supplement questionnaire responses and to reach at least some of those who drop out of the questionnaire panel. One might interview strategically important subsamples selected on the basis of drug-use characteristics derived from the questionnaire. Some subgroups, such as heavy users who are also delinquent, would be more difficult to reach than others, but with well chosen personnel who have earned the trust of the adolescent society, it should be possible to increase greatly our knowledge of the process of change through the use of recurrent interviews. I would be especially interested in those who become users but then back away from use, and they should be relatively easy to interview.

CONCLUDING COMMENTS

Some may see these reports on high school drug use as essentially atheoretical because the theories employed are relatively loose and not formulated in precise terms. I agree that there is far less precision of formulation than would be desired, but I do not believe that the understanding of drug behavior and other forms of deviance will be greatly enhanced primarily by producing more elegant formulations using structural equations.

The primary questions to be addressed, in my opinion, must recognize that the causation and consequences of drug use (as of any other behavior) are to be understood in terms of the (changing) social meanings attached to drug use and in terms of the decisions individuals make with reference to such meanings in the light of drug availability, social ties, and personality orientations and needs. The set of influences that leads a 15-year-old to try, and then to use regularly, hard liquor, marihuana, and other drugs in rapid succession may overlap somewhat with the set that leads an 18-year-old to drink hard liquor and smoke marihuana occasionally; but they are likely to operate under very different circumstances and have very different consequences.

The interesting questions about drug use are not to be encompassed in a single prediction equation or a series of such equations. It may be useful to formulate, for a given time, age group and cultural milieu, the nature of the relationships between, on the one hand, experiences, attitudes, and personality assessed prior to drug use and, on the other hand, the subsequent onset or, better, level of use of legal and illegal drugs. This can be a useful basis for identifying potential users but will not tell one much about the process through which nonusers are transformed into occasional users and occasional users into heavy users.

I must confess that I am not much interested in why an 18-year-old uses marihuana occasionally. Such use remains illegal, it is true, but only the combination of willful ignorance and monumental hypocrisy in our society sustains the illegality while making alcohol and tobacco legal. Inasmuch as most 18-year-olds do not share either the ignorance or the particular hypocrisy, one can hardly fault them for this modest violation of law. I am, however, interested in learning how and when some adolescents turn to very heavy use of marihuana or alcohol, use that seems both symptomatic of serious alienation from the goals of adult society and a self-defeating impairment of functioning.

Once a given drug is tried or used at least occasionally by a majority of members of an age group or any other group not self-selected, one can regard initial use by other members of the group (or by persons who aspire to become members) as instances of cultural or subcultural transmission. It is not drug use per se that constitutes the cultural content, however; it is the set of beliefs and practices in which the drug use is embedded.

All of these studies make abundantly clear that marihuana use is initiated among those who have taken on more favorable attitudes and beliefs about marihuana and its use. Such favorable attitudes are likely to be linked with exposure to high use and to the enthusiasm of prior users. Local availability of marihuana is certainly a prerequisite to use, and local level of use among older youth is surely a major influence on attitudes toward use by younger members. This is why we need data on the frequency, level, and circumstances of drug use at each age level and among socially salient subgroups of the population (including specific school populations) in order to assess the normative structure of drug use.

The several studies I am discussing use somewhat different measures and focus on somewhat different facets of the prediction process; yet all do focus primarily on prediction, and all show gratifying consonance in the most salient variables even though the findings are derived from a substantial range of different populations. The greatest contribution to the prediction, for an individual, of various forms of adolescent behavior regarded as deviant within adult society but widespread in adolescent society, quite clearly derives from the individual's involvement in the adolescent society. The earlier the individual is involved in adolescent society or uses it as a reference group, the earlier he or she is likely to smoke, drink, experience sex, or try illegal drugs. The data of Kandel and her associates suggest that the earlier any one of these transitions takes place, the sooner other transitions will occur.

One surmises that the identification of those who will be precocious in drug behaviors might well be possible in terms of quite early signs of rebelliousness or precocity in other behaviors, but even the high correlations observed in these studies account for no more than half of the variance. They tell us relatively little that we did not know, although they give us much more assurance of what we know.

Figure 11-1 presents an arrangement of the situations and variables that seem to be involved in adolescent drug use. They are arrayed along two dimensions, very crudely conceived. The horizontal dimension represents, at one pole, the

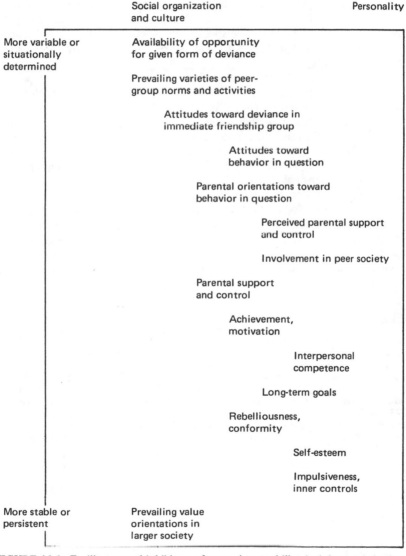

FIGURE 11-1 Facilitators and inhibitors of precocious and illegal adolescent behaviors.

sociocultural order, at the other pole, the characteristics of individual personality most removed from the immediate sociocultural influences. The vertical dimension runs from those aspects of the social, cultural, and personal systems most subject to change (or that exist side by side in alternative, situationally available forms) to those features of social order and personality that exhibit greatest stability.

Drug availability, neighborhood norms, and similar situational features obviously vary tremendously within urban society. Where a given adolescent is located in the urban social structure will influence the particular cultural forms and opportunities available to her or him, will probably influence her or his parents' orientations and behavior, and will influence various portions of her or his personality differentially. Many attitudes will be very largely determined by location; achievement motivation and personal goals will be somewhat less influenced; and interpersonal competence and the organization of inner controls will likely be substantially less influenced by general placement (although they will be responsive to parental behaviors and some situational constraints).

Causal influences on drug-using behaviors may move along different pathways, depending on where in the social structure and where in the distribution of personality tendencies a given individual is located. An impulsive, rebellious, middle-class adolescent who is not getting along with his or her parents may seek out, in the adolescent society, those peer cliques whose behaviors flaunt convention. In so doing, he or she is likely to shift patterns of association in the ways that Becker and Goode have described. Attitudes toward a number of behaviors may shift along with the change in personal network.

I am arguing for an examination of alternative courses of development and for the study of the decision-making processes and considerations that adolescents engage in where drug use and other "problematic" behaviors are entailed. Such an examination will not yield a single model of drug-using behavior. It will, I think, yield some clues as to critical phases of the developmental process that will permit more realistic planning for dealing with the more serious dangers of adolescent drug use.

REFERENCES

Becker, H. S. Becoming a marihuana user. *American Journal of Sociology*, 1953, *59*, 235–242.
Deasy, L. C. Social class and participation in polio vaccine trials. *American Sociological Review*, 1956, *21*, 185–191.
Goode, E. Multiple drug use among marihuana smokers. *Social Problems*, 1969, *17*, 48–64.
Jessor, R., Jessor, S. L., & Finney, J. A social psychology of marihuana use: Longitudinal studies of high school and college youth. *Journal of Personality and Social Psychology*, 1973, *26*, 1–15.
Johnson, B. D. Marihuana users and drug subculture. New York: Wiley, 1973.
Kandel, D. B., & Lesser, G. S. *Youth in two worlds*. San Francisco: Jossey-Bass, 1972.
Newcomb, T. *The acquaintance process*. New York: Holt, 1961.

12

Some Episodes in the History of Panel Analysis

Paul F. Lazarsfeld[1]
University of Pittsburgh

The studies with which I am dealing in this review are based on repeated interviews with, or observations on, the same people. The general problem is what kind of worthwhile knowledge can be gained from such data. Both the kinds of data used and the kinds of questions asked can vary, and such variations can lead to different analytical techniques. My task is to make some observations on the history of some of these techniques and on their relationship to one another at the time they were first developed.

Unavoidably, there is a certain personal element in this review. I have been concerned with the issues discussed here for almost 50 years, and at the beginning of the period under review, the so-called Columbia tradition played a considerable role. The history of the statistical-estimation problem is not included; this is, of course, a crucially important topic, but it is different from a discussion of the ways in which repeated interviews can be analyzed. I am not well enough acquainted with the history of the estimation issue, but it certainly has its place in the history of panel analysis.

At some points in this review, I use examples not derived from the drug studies. Although the drug problem reflects all the issues one faces in today's empirical social research, it is useful to remember from the beginning that the problem is not new. It has been perceived by econometricians in their modern version of business-cycle analysis. Figure 12-1 is characteristic of their approach. Taken from a 1940 review of economic research by the Dutch economist Tinbergen (1940), the schema has been used, in various forms, by other economists and also by me and by Hovland when we discussed the relationship between the repeated-interview approach and the classical controlled experiment (see Hovland, 1959). A long time ago, Richardson raised the question of what happens if a country's expenses for armaments depend on its earlier investment and on the investment in armaments by a competing nation (see Rapaport, 1957). Just for the record, here are the equations that derive from such a problem:

$$X_t = a_{11} X_{t-1} + a_{12} Y_{t-1}$$
$$Y_t = a_{21} X_{t-1} + a_{22} Y_{t-1}$$

[1] Deceased.

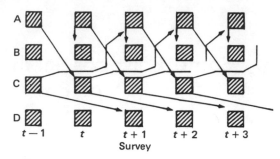

FIGURE 12-1 The basic idea of panel analysis across time and across variables. (From Tinbergen, 1940.)

Now I turn to what I think is the beginning of panel analysis in today's empirical social research. Without further apology, I start with a personal reminiscence.

TIME OF THE 16-FOLD TABLES

The term *panel analysis*, as far as I know, was introduced by me in two short notes in the *Public Opinion Quarterly* in 1938 and 1940 (Lazarsfeld, 1940; Lazarsfeld & Fiske, 1938). In 1937, I was appointed director of a Rockefeller project to study the social effect of radio. I was very soon confronted with commercial studies that showed a correlation between listening to a certain radio program and use of the product advertised. It was obvious to me then that the correlation between listening and buying was not at all conclusive evidence of the effect of radio advertising. It could, for instance, very well be that consumers listened to radio advertisements after having made very expensive purchases in order to be reassured that they had made the right decision. I suggested that this dilemma could be resolved by interviewing the same listeners at two different time periods. In 1939, I obtained a grant from the Rockefeller Foundation to study the 1940 political campaign, using this approach to do repeated interviews with the same sample in

TABLE 12-1 Current Marihuana Use and Depressive Mood over Time

	Wave 2 (spring 1972)				
	Current marihuana user		Not current marihuana user		
Wave 1 (fall 1971)	Depressed N	Not depressed N	Depressed N	Not depressed N	Total N
Current marihuana user					
Depressed	255	110	78	45	488
Not depressed	78	243	15	77	413
Not current marihuana user					
Depressed	159	58	1019	482	1718
Not depressed	44	135	401	1586	2166
Total N	536	546	1513	2190	4785

Note. From Paton, Kessler, and Kandel, 1977.

TABLE 12-2   Current Multiple-drug Use and Depressive Mood over Time

| | Wave 2 (spring 1972) | | | | |
| | Current multiple-drug[a] user | | Not current multiple-drug[a] user | | |
Wave 1 (fall 1971)	Depressed N	Not depressed N	Depressed N	Not depressed N	Total N
Current multiple-drug[a] user					
Depressed	98	38	85	19	240
Not depressed	19	69	20	39	147
Not current multiple-drug[a] user					
Depressed	97	37	238	119	491
Not depressed	19	60	104	292	475
Total N	233	204	447	469	1,353

[a]Indicates use of marihuana and other illicit drugs within last 30 days.

Erie County, Ohio. We made seven such interviews. Now, I want to concentrate on the analysis of two dichotomous response questions at two different time points. We organized these data in the form of the so-called 16-fold table, which was the main innovation of this period (Lazarsfeld, Pasanella, & Rosenberg, 1972). Two such 16-fold tables (Tables 12-1 and 12-2) are used in Kandel's study, in which the two items are current use versus nonuse of drugs and depressed versus not depressed mood (Paton, Kessler, & Kandel, 1977). The simplest level of analysis of these data was to observe the changes over time in each attribute separately. In other words, one should note trends in the relative frequency of depression or in drug use. However, I do not consider these trend data part of a panel analysis and therefore will not discuss them further.

The next level of analysis was to relate all the observations pairwise as in Figure 12-2. If I may leave aside the question of what measure of association is to be used, Figure 12-2 shows the six possible relations that exist on the second stratification level[2]: the stability across time of each item separately; the cross-sectional association at each of the two time periods; and, finally, what Campbell later called "the cross-lagged associations" between one item at Time 1 and the second item at Time 2 (Campbell & Stanley, 1963/1966). Notice that I call one item "odd" and the other time "even." As shown, the odd item is the use of drugs, whereas the even item dichotomizes respondents by depressed or not.

The use of dichotomies stimulated us to raise the obvious question of what would happen if we were to consider not merely pairs of attributes, but *triplets*,

[2] *Ed. note* (Neil W. Henry). Lazarsfeld here uses the terms *stratification level* or simply *level* to refer to the complexity of the data being examined. Thus, the first level is marginal frequencies, the second level involves pairs of items, and so on (Lazarsfeld, 1972). In earlier work (for example, Lazarsfeld & Henry, 1968), he had used the word *order* in much the same way: *Third-order data* referred to the joint distribution of three variables. The latter terminology conflicted with that used in correlation analysis, where a *zero-order correlation* was, of course, based on pairwise distributions, and I believe this was one reason why he chose to use the term *level* in his later writings.

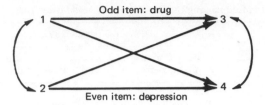

FIGURE 12-2   Pairwise correlations: two waves, two items. (From Lazarsfeld, 1972.)

and finally *quadruplets*. Tables 12-3 and 12-4 show what one gets if one interrelates the drug use and depression questions at Time 1 with drug use at Time 2. My interest here is not in substantively interpreting these tables but in suggesting a comparison of the findings, and most of all, in pointing to the general kind of analysis implied. Using the terminology of dichotomous algebra (Lazarsfeld, 1960), one can put the findings in the following form: The conditional relation between taking drugs at Wave 2 and being depressed at Wave 1 is positive, whereas the same conditional relation is negative for nondrug users. I come back later to a more precise formulation of this difference. There is no difficulty in relating this third-level table to the more detailed figures of the 16-fold table.

If one uses terms in a somewhat figurative way, it is not difficult to interpret the analysis discussed so far in terms of effects. The cross-lagged associations clearly have the character of an earlier position on one item affecting the subsequent position of the other item. In the third-level tables (Tables 12-3 and 12-4), it is easy to think of the findings in terms of *conditional effects*. Nonusers who are depressed at the first interview are more likely to start drug use than those who are not depressed, whereas depressed users slightly decreased their drug use (possibly because of the feeling that the drugs do not relieve their depression). On the other hand, nondepressed people at Time 1 are more likely to maintain their drug use, if users, but are less likely to start, if nonusers. This is a verbalization of the comparison between the first column and the second column in Tables 12-3 and 12-4.

The situation is different when one looks at the full 16-fold table and the information it contains. Then it becomes somewhat difficult to use an effect terminology. Figure 12-3 shows how we looked at it around 1940 when the first such analysis was made. We claimed that examination of the major diagonal and the minor diagonal cannot contribute to the analysis of change, leaving eight critical

TABLE 12-3   Proportion of Marihuana Users at Wave 2 by Depression and Drug Use at Wave 1

		Wave 1			
		Use marihuana		Do not use marihuana	
		%	N	%	N
Wave 1	Depressed	75	488	13	1718
	Not depressed	78	413	8	2166

TABLE 12-4 Proportion of Multiple-drug Users at Wave 2 by Depression and Drug Use at Wave 1

		Wave 1			
		Use multiple drugs		Do not use multiple drugs	
		%	N	%	N
Wave 1 {	Depressed	57	240	27	491
	Not depressed	60	147	17	475

cells. Four of them contain the people who are originally in a consistent state and move to inconsistency. (We assumed that the two attributes O and E are generally positively related so that we could refer to a person in state $++$ as being consistent. This is especially apt if one attribute is an attitude and the other a related behavior.) These cells are marked with a triangle. The other four cells (marked by an asterisk) contain the people who move from inconsistency to consistency. These critical cells can be divided in still another way, according to the contribution they make to maintenance or change in the cross-association. We made the point that the cells marked with O are those that indicate a greater contribution of the odd item to the interrelation between the two. The cells marked E correspondingly indicate a greater contribution of the even item. One does not talk of effects at this point, but of the contributions the two items make to the maintenance of their interrelation. A variety of indexes can be formed to measure the relative contribution of the two items. But any choice of measure in the drug study shows that the contributions of drug use and of depression to their interrelation are about the same.

I might add a remark in retrospect. The interpretation given to the eight cells is,

Time 2

O / E	$+$ $+$	$+$ $-$	$-$ $+$	$-$ $-$	Row total
$+$ $+$		Δ E_1	Δ O_1		p_{12}
$+$ $-$	* O_2			* E_2	$p_{1\bar{2}}$
$-$ $+$	* E_3			* O_3	$p_{\bar{1}2}$
$-$ $-$		Δ O_4	Δ E_4		$p_{\bar{1}\bar{2}}$
Column total	p_{34}	$p_{3\bar{4}}$	$p_{\bar{3}4}$	$p_{\bar{3}\bar{4}}$	1

Time 1 (row label at left)

FIGURE 12-3 Eight critical cells indicating where there is change on one but not on both attributes between two interviews. (From Lazarsfeld, 1972.)

as far as I can see, not in question. I am not so sure whether we were right to disregard the main diagonal. Maybe the staying power of the four original patterns could find an interpretation in terms of process analysis. This deserves further discussion.

I now return to the second-level associations. Their link with the 16-fold table inaugurated a new phase.

TIME OF THE CROSS–LAGGED CORRELATION

Sometime in the late 1950s, Don Campbell discussed 16-fold tables showing concurrent changes in vote intention and political attitudes with special emphasis on the use of the critical cells in the fourth stratification level (Campbell & Clayton, 1961). He pointed out that what I called "mutual effect" could also be obtained by comparing what he called the two "cross-lagged correlations." In the symbolism introduced in Figure 12-3, these would be r_{14} and r_{23}. It so happens that, with the data at hand, the two measures lead to the same substantive results as the analysis of the full table. It is easy to give numerical examples where this would not be the case, but this is quite irrelevant. The main point is that variations on the theme of cross-lagged correlation analysis inaugurated a new direction in the analysis of panel data.

Clearly the six pairwise correlations available on the second stratification level should be divided into the three groups I mentioned above, following Figure 12-2. Authors began to discuss the large number of configurations that can be derived from this information. Campbell was impressed by data in which five correlations were positive, but one cross-lag was negative (Campbell, 1969). Pelz and Andrews (1964) were especially interested in situations in which the cross-lags (r_{14} and r_{23}) were higher than the stability of each variable (r_{13} and r_{24}). They also introduced partial cross-lagged correlations, for example, $r_{14.2}$, in which Variable 2 was partialed out of the 1–4 relation. Yee and Gage (1968) introduced correlations between one variable and the change in the other. In an unpublished paper by David Armor (1975) of the Rand Corporation, this idea was extended toward correlating the change in one variable with the average of the other. As can be seen from some of the reports in this volume, the Campbell tradition remains alive when more than two panel waves are available.

All these efforts brought about new ideas, too numerous to be discussed here. They have, however, one attribute in common. They all can be reduced to the manipulation of correlations between pairs of variables only. Presently, I have some doubts to raise on this point.

Another aspect of this tradition is more difficult to articulate. Increasingly, the literature in this field talks about panel analysis as a substitute for controlled experiments designed to answer the question, What causes what? As mentioned above, my own work began with this same problem in mind. But as I was forced to consider higher levels of stratification, I began to wonder whether the issue should not be looked at differently. We are really studying ongoing processes in which a number of variables continuously interact and thus propel the process. An effect at one time is a cause at the next. Is this only a difference in imagery and verbalization, or has it a bearing on our actual procedures?

The emphasis on pairwise correlations raises still another question of which all modern authors are well aware. Suppose the correlations between the same variable observed at two different times are fairly low. Is this a substantive observation or the result of measurement error? Kendall (1955) has analyzed data where students were asked to rate their mood of the moment on a graphic rating scale. Her subjects used their concrete experiences to determine where they put themselves on the rating scale. Yet, we know that moods are actually quite unstable. How does one separate "true" changes from measurement error? As far as I can tell, three approaches have been taken. One is to use, as a standard for error, empirical findings on topics that in principle should be stable over time, for instance, answers to the question, In which month were you born? This would give an idea of the error due primarily to the data-processing technique. Another possibility is to introduce various assumptions about the magnitude of measurement error and then to see how robust the findings of the panel study remain. Probably the most promising approach is the introduction of "unobserved" variables as explicit indicators of the presence of error in an analytic model. As we shall see, this requires a large increase in the data needed for panel study, and the results may well depend upon the specific theoretical assumptions (see sec. IV of Blalock, 1971; Kendall, 1955).

I will not pursue the measurement problem but instead elaborate on the question of what the consequences are if one only uses pairwise correlation when dealing with panel studies. I propose to do this in a somewhat oblique and historical way. As I mentioned before, this restriction may be overcome by looking at higher order frequencies, whereas the tradition of quantitative variables requires a more strenuous effort to realize their implications. My next section therefore is a digression from my historical task.

A DIGRESSION ON THE ALTERNATIVE USE
OF DICHOTOMIES AND QUANTITATIVE VARIABLES

The prevailing form of correlation analysis goes back to Karl Pearson and his then assistant, Yule. Around the turn of the century, Yule got interested in the work of the economist and logician Jevons and spent several years on what he came to call "attribute statistics." As a matter of fact, in the first edition of Yule's (1911) famous textbook on statistics, a quarter of the book was devoted to this topic. Yule repeatedly pointed out that attribute statistics should be developed in their own right because they were so close to the way logicians talked about causal relations. He repeatedly referred to pertinent procedures as "mental arithmetic." For quite a while, this part of Yule's work was not further developed, but it was revived when quantitative social-research attention turned to such dichotomies as sex, right or wrong answers to a test item, and graduation from high school. As can be seen from the story of the 16-fold tables, my own work was in the Yule tradition from the beginning. So is Leo Goodman's work, to which I turn presently.

The early authors, writing in the tradition of classical correlation analysis, also had to face the problem of how to deal with dichotomies. Their solution was to consider them "dummy variables" that would have only two values, 0 and 1. This approach dates from the discovery by Yule that the phi-coefficient of association between two dichotomies is identical to the Pearson-r correlation computed on the scaled dummy variables (Yule, 1912). There is a large literature on this topic into which I do not want to enter except to stress one point (see, for example, Henry, 1973). The Pearsonian tradition forced attention to the kinds of problems and topics that were appropriate for its algebraic machinery. This distracted concern from topics and procedures that are implicit in many of the reports in this volume.

In Table 12-5, I present the raw figures on which Table 12-4 was based. The respondents are here divided according to whether they were drug users at Time 1. For each of these two groups separately, there is a *conditional* cross-lagged association. One can easily see that the conditional lagged association is negative for Time 1 users and positive for Time 1 nonusers ($\varnothing = -.03$ and .13 respectively). If the two tables are added cell by cell, one gets the unconditional cross-lag table, and it turns out to be positive ($\varnothing = .11$). The reason for that can easily be seen from an algebraic formulation of the whole situation. One represents the association in a fourfold table by the difference of the cross products ($[ij] = (n_{++}n_{--} - n_{+-}n_{-+})/N^2$), which incidentally, contrary to textbook tradition, was Yule's preferred "measure." Then, in an obvious symbolism, the following relation exists:

$$[23] = \frac{[23;1]}{p_1} + \frac{[23;\bar{1}]}{p_{\bar{1}}} + \frac{[12]\,[13]}{p_1 p_{\bar{1}}} \tag{12-1}$$

The negative conditional association $[23;1]$ is obliterated because $[12]$ and $[13]$ are highly positive.

Equation 12-1 can also immediately represent the idea of *partial association*. As the weighted average of the two conditionals, one denotes this partial association by

$$[23;\hat{1}] = \frac{[23;1]}{p_1} + \frac{[23;\bar{1}]}{p_{\bar{1}}}$$

which is by Equation 12-1 simply a function of the second-order association:

$$[23;\hat{1}] = \frac{[23]p_1 p_{\bar{1}} - [13]\,[12]}{p_1 p_{\bar{1}}} \tag{12-2}$$

The expression $[23;\hat{1}]$, when appropriately normalized, becomes the partial cross-lagged correlation that was stressed by Pelz and Andrews (1964) (for example, $[23;\hat{1}] = 0$ whenever $r_{23.1} = 0$).

But what about the fact that the two conditional associations, $[23;1]$ and $[23;\bar{1}]$, are not equal? There is little literature available as to how they would be treated

TABLE 12-5 Relation between Depression at Wave 1 and Multiple-drug Use at Wave 2 Controlling for Initial Drug Use at Wave 1

		Use multiple drugs at Wave 1			Do not use multiple drugs at Wave 1		
		Use at Wave 2	No use at Wave 2	Total	Use at Wave 2	No use at Wave 2	Total
	Depressed	136	104	240	134	357	491
Wave 1	Not depressed	88	59	147	79	396	475
	Total	224	163	387	213	753	966

in classical Pearsonian terms. Let me make a suggestion on how the most primitive model could take care of the matter. I quote from a paper by Birren (1974), who deals with two tests given to people of various ages. He reports: "The correlation between the Wechsler Memory Scale and speed in young subjects was not significantly different from zero. In fact it was minus .01. In elderly subjects, i.e., those over 60 years, the correlation between the Wechsler Memory Scale and speed of copying digits was .52" (p. 811).

Now make the following assumption. One deals with children of various ages: Test x_2 is a memory test; test x_3 is a measure of speed of writing digits; and x_1 is age. The two test scores and the age of a group of children are standardized. The test performances (x_2 & x_3) of the children increase linearly with age; the slopes of the two regression lines are, respectively, a_2 and a_3. Suppose, in addition, that the covariance of the two tests also increases linearly with age, and let c be the rate of change. If the data on memory and speed were plotted, one would see that the scatter around the regression line is less for older people than for younger, corresponding to Birren's finding of higher correlations in the older group.

With a few more simplifications added, the coefficient c turns out to be as follows:

$$c = \frac{\Sigma x_1 x_2 x_3}{N} - \frac{a_2 a_3 \Sigma(x_3)^3}{N} \tag{12-3}$$

The summation goes over all N children. The computation of c requires the third mixed moment of all three variables; one also needs the third moment of the age distribution, which, of course, can be controlled by the selection of children.

The slope c in this simple case was defined to be the rate of increase in the test covariance. It corresponds to the *difference* between the two conditional cross-lags in the dichotomous case of Equation 12-1. This difference can be expressed in terms of the so-called symmetric parameters that appear in Goodman's and my work, and which are closely related to the third mixed moment in Equation 12-3. The fact that such third moments do not appear in Pearsonian tradition is of course due to an implicit assumption of multivariate normal distribution. (The pattern of relations discussed above could not occur, of course, if the three variables had a jointly normal distribution.) It also explains why the difference between conditional cross-lags has had so little attention.

In the early formalization of survey analysis, this difference played a considerable role. The pertinent textbooks usually make a distinction between three modes of analysis that could be called, in Weberian terms, "ideal types." If both conditional relations vanish, one is dealing with either an intervening variable ("interpretation") or a spurious factor; if they are nonzero and unequal, however, attention is focused on the difference between the two conditional relations, which is called the mode of "specification." (See Hyman, 1955, pp. 275–329; Rosenberg, 1968.)

RESURRECTION OF PATH ANALYSIS

In 1954, Herbert Simon published a paper on spurious correlations. He observed that publications in the tradition of the dichotomous variable and survey analysis "have made important contributions to our understanding of the phenomenon of causal analysis" (p. 467). He did not discuss the mode of specification that I stress in the preceding section. Rather, he concentrated on the difference between "interpretation" and spurious relations where the controlled variable in Equation 12-1 was antecedent to the two others. Simon showed that these two modes of analysis could be represented by two systems of recursive linear equations linking three quantitative variables. The method had been developed by him and other members of the Cowles Commission, although Simon did not explicitly refer to them. Because this paper appeared originally in the *Journal of the American Statistical Association,* it did not become known to sociologists until it was included in Simon's (1957) collection, *Models of Man.* Even then, general circulation of this approach in the social-research community had to wait for Hubert Blalock's (1961/1964) *Causal Inferences in Nonexperimental Research.*

Blalock gave credit to Simon and Wold and was aware that he made two critical choices. He definitely voted against the idea that dichotomous algebra was an appropriate starting point:

> But if we confine our conception of causality to these attributes, we shall encounter considerable difficulties with continuous variates. On the other hand, we can always take a continuous variable and dichotomize it if we wish. In effect, this means that *we can do whatever formal and theoretical thinking we please in terms of continuous variables and then dichotomize these later if we choose to do so* [emphasis added]. (p. 32)

A few pages later, he described the price he had to pay:

> For simplicity, we shall assume that causal relationships can be represented by *linear regression models*, though theoretically we can handle nonlinear relationships in a similar manner. Realistically, however, the more variables with which we must deal, and the more complex the causal model, the simpler our assumptions must be concerning the manner in which the variables are combined. We shall also *assume that the effects of the several variables are additive* [emphases added]. (p. 44)

Blalock is not explicitly aware of the connection between these two decisions. Actually, as mentioned above, basic conceptual ideas get lost, especially the notion of specification and other aspects of conditional relations. On the other hand, as is now well known, the testing of simple causal structures becomes manageable. (The historical connection between Simon's article and path analysis, developed 25 years earlier by Sewall Wright, was demonstrated in a paper by Raymond Boudon, 1965, followed by an impressive collection of additional examples by O. D. Duncan, 1966.) Path analysis rapidly became the leading orientation of quantitatively inclined, empirical, social researchers (Goldberger & Duncan, 1973). The new trend was reinforced by the arrow notation of path analysis and by the availability of computer programs. It was also supported by a new generation of able mathematical sociologists who affected the policy of journal editors. All this greatly accelerated the swing toward path analysis.

No one would want to pit path analysis against panel analysis. Each has its advantages and its difficulties; their relative merits might depend upon the problem at hand. I want, however, to bring up two problems for discussion. One is exemplified by reference to Figure 12-2. Panel analysis arose because of the idea that cross-sectional correlations by themselves cannot contribute anything to a dynamic analysis. An initial correlation between the odd and the even variable has to be taken as a given. Changes in this correlation can be accounted for by turnover in each item, by conditional and unconditional cross-lags, and by exogenous factors. No simultaneous correlations should be introduced into an explanation. This position can, of course, be challenged and O. D. Duncan has done exactly this. In a paper (1969) discussing the relation between 16-fold tables and path analysis, he added arrows between 3 and 4 in my Figure 12-2; then he showed that in such a model not all path coefficients could be identified. This, of course, is not surprising; one can always add enough arrows to show unidentified path coefficients. Whether Duncan's approach is a fruitful new development is an interesting question.[3] Whether the issue of simultaneous effects can be settled by thinking of additional panel waves is again something I am not quite clear about.

Another analytic problem has been raised, especially by some recent work of Pelz (Pelz & Faith, 1970; Pelz & Lew, 1970). There is no reason to assume that the causal interval (the period over which variable x has a maximum influence on variable y) coincides with the period between our interview waves. One may not assume that the causal interval is the same as the interval of maximum cross-correlation between variable x and variable y. Pelz and his associates have demonstrated that the delay in maximum cross-correlation between variable x and variable y does not necessarily correspond to the true causal interval. Goldberger (personal correspondence) has also derived this effect algebraically.

ROLE OF NONOBSERVABLES

The use of latent elements is, of course, an old standby. Factor analysis, the "true score" in test theory, and latent-structure analysis are some typical examples. The explicit application of this idea to panel analysis is, however, much rarer. If I am not mistaken, the following is the first example. It is taken from Volume 4 of *The American Soldier* (Stouffer, Guttman, Suchman, Lazarsfeld, Star, & Clausen, 1950). The problem was to see how the attitudes of enlisted men toward their officers changed over time. Originally, three questions were asked at each interview wave. For my purpose, however, two questions suffice, which I call O and E. The wording of the questions and the marginal frequencies at the two interview waves are as follows:

Percentage of Positive Answers

Question	Interview	
	Time 1	Time 2
Item O: How many officers you now serve under are the kind you would want to serve under in combat? Positive answer: all or most	65	36
Item E: How many of your company officers do you think would be willing to go through anything they ask their men to go through? Positive answer: all or most	65	49

[3] Heise, who wrote a major paper on panel and path analysis (1970), explicitly excludes cross-sectional arrows. He cites Duncan's paper from the *Psychological Bulletin* (1969) in his bibliography but does not comment on the contradiction in his text.

TABLE 12-6   Association Matrix for Two Waves of Items O and E

Parameter	(1)	(2)	(3)	(4)
Time 1				
Item O (1)		.111	.059	.046
Item E (2)			.061	.067
Time 2				
Item O (3)				.144
Item E (4)				

Note. From *The American Soldier,* Vol. 4, *Measurement and Prediction* by S. Stouffer, L. Guttman, E. A. Suchman, P. F. Lazarsfeld, S. A. Star, and J. A. Clausen, p. 450. Copyright 1950, © 1978 by Princeton University Press. Reprinted by permission of Princeton University Press.   Entries are crossproducts [*ij*], which are equivalent to covariances of the dummy variables corresponding to the items.

There are six associations possible between the four questions, and I use the cross-product difference divided by the square of the sample size (in other words, [*ij*]) to represent them. The numerical result is as in Table 12-6.

Latent-structure analysis makes the following assumption: A latent disposition (good or bad) of the responding soldiers to their officers can change over time. To get at this "true" disposition, questions O and E are asked at Time 1 and Time 2. The joint frequencies of the replies permit the derivation of *latent frequencies*: the number of soldiers who have a good or bad attitude at the two waves respectively, and the number who shift in the interim.

I do not propose to include here the details of a latent-structure analysis. Like any model used to specify the effects of an unobserved construct, it puts certain restrictions on the manifest data. In this case, the requirement is that [13] [24] = [14] [23]. In different terms, the determinant of the figures in the right upper corner of the table should vanish. This condition is only approximated in my example, but the approximation is not too bad in view of another condition that the values of [12] and of [34] should be considerably greater than the other four cross-product differences. The configuration required by the model is easily stated in terms of my discussion in previous sections: The product of the stabilities for the two items should equal the product of the two cross-lags, and the association of indicators that belong to the same latent attribute should be relatively high. If these conditions are satisfied, it can be shown that the phi-coefficient characterizing the latent-turnover table is given by the following formulas:

$$\varphi^2 = \frac{[12]\ [34]}{[13]\ [24]} = \frac{[14]\ [23]}{[13]\ [24]}$$

For sample data, the geometric mean of these two ratios might be used to estimate φ^2. This association is all one can get from second-level data. If one takes into account the triple frequencies, however, one can derive the full turnover table for the latent attribute. In this special case, the figures happen to be as follows:

Latent Turnover for Soldier Example

		Disposition at Wave 1		
		+	−	Total
Disposition at Wave 2	+	135	4	139
	−	95	90	185
	Total	230	94	324

(Incidentally, these figures show that the attitude of the soldier is deteriorating, which one would have guessed from the marginal frequencies of the two items at the two waves.)

Let me compare this whole example with data taken from Coleman's *The Adolescent Society* (1961) and discussed in Coleman (1964). He asked high school students two questions at two time points. The marginal answers for boys are as follows:

Percentage of Positive Answers

		Interview	
Question		Time 1	Time 2
Item *O*:	Would you say you are part of the leading crowd?	37	41
Item *E*:	Being in the leading crowd makes one go against one's principles.	46	43

In the discussion that follows and in Tables 12-7, 12-8, and 12-9, the responses to Item *O* at different times are denoted by odd numbers: 1 (Time 1) and 3 (Time 2); and responses to Item *E* by even numbers: 2 (Time 1) and 4 (Time 2). The association matrix for the four questions is given in Table 12-7. Notice that now the items are arranged in different order from the previous example. The condition for the four cross-product differences [12] [34] = [23] [14] is almost perfectly satisfied, but the rearrangement of items suggests a different interpretation from Table 12-6. Items 1 and 3 now are clearly the indicators of one latent attribute, and 2 and

TABLE 12-7 Association Matrix for Two Waves of Items *O* and *E*

Parameter	(1)	(3)	(2)	(4)
Item *O*				
Time 1 (1)		.128	.024	.024
Time 2 (3)			.032	.031
Item *E*				
Time 1 (2)				.071
Time 2 (4)				

Note. Based on data from Coleman, 1964, p. 396.

TABLE 12-8   Association Matrix for Marihuana Use (Item O) and Depression (Item E)

Parameter	(1)	(3)	(2)	(4)
Item O				
Time 1 (1)	·	.100	.015	.008
Time 2 (3)		·	.017	.015
Item E				
Time 1 (2)			·	.118
Time 2 (4)				·

4 of the other. This means that in this example the appropriate model does not involve latent turnover between the two waves. One deals instead with the association between two latent attributes, each measured by the same question asked twice.[4]

Where does Kandel's material fit into this picture? Is there a latent disposition— say, mental imbalance—that can oscillate but that can be made visible by two indicators, *use* and *depression*? Or do the data show that the latent association between these two factors is only more securely measured by asking the same questions twice? Let me present, in Tables 12-8 and 12-9, the association matrices corresponding to the two initial tables, using, of course, only the second- and first-level frequencies that can be taken from the marginals, and by adding pertinent rows and columns. Neither of the two structures fits perfectly, but the data certainly come nearer to the idea of latent association (like Coleman) than of latent turnover (like the case in *The American Soldier*).

I do not know of any concrete example in which path analysts have analyzed unobservable turnover, although Heise (1970) is clearly aware of the problem and discusses an interesting case of simulated data. In Kenny's paper (1973) on common factors in panel analysis, a "Model I" is discussed mathematically. It is based on a system of linear equations, but its results are isomorphic with the parameters obtained from a latent-attribute model. Heise and Kenny and many

[4] Goodman (1973) has analyzed the same data in a paper on panels and latent-structure analysis. As far as I can tell, he is not aware of the basic difference between the models appropriate for these two sets of panel data. There are also differences in the way Goodman and I continue the analysis as we move to higher level data, but this is irrelevant to my discussion.

TABLE 12-9   Association Matrix for Multiple-drug Use (Item O) and Depression (Item E)

Parameter	(1)	(3)	(2)	(4)
Item O				
Time 1 (1)	·	.073	.023	.020
Time 2 (3)		·	.025	.010
Item E				
Time 1 (2)			·	.111
Time 2 (4)				·

others in their tradition discuss in detail problems of measurement errors and estimation not covered by my review.[5]

The study of unobservables is certainly an interesting topic in itself, but I am not sure whether it contributes much to understanding the dynamics of a process.

TIME OF THE MARKOV CHAIN

It is a pleasure to end this review with a recent development that does not require me to mention my own work. As far as I can tell, the application of transition probabilities to panel data begins with T. W. Anderson's "Probability Models for Analyzing Time Changes in Attitudes" (1954). In social-mobility studies, the idea of stayer–mover models was introduced about the same time by Blumen, Kogan, and McCarthy (1955). The most extensive recent elaboration of transition analysis is the work of Singer and Spilerman (1974, 1976).

Ed. note. This section is concluded by Neil W. Henry.

This section is obviously incomplete, and we can imagine that Lazarsfeld would have wanted to add a final integrative section based on his reaction to the papers delivered at the Conference on Strategies of Longitudinal Research on Drug Use. The following remarks are not meant as a substitute for the unwritten conclusions but may be useful to the reader nonetheless.

Anderson's (1954) work (which originally appeared as a Rand Corporation memorandum in 1951) includes a "model for several attitudes," which is illustrated through the analysis of a 16-fold table of the kind discussed here. He showed how the hypothesis that change on one attribute is independent of change on the other could be tested using a chi-square test. This, of course, serves as a starting point for the analyses discussed above, which presume that a link between the variables does exist. Anderson also reanalyzed the seven-wave Erie County data, mentioned earlier, using Markov chains.

Coleman (1964, pp. 132–188) introduced the continuous-time Markov process as a model for the 16-fold table, analyzing data from his study *The Adolescent Society*. Singer and Spilerman (see, for example, Singer & Spilerman, 1974) in a series of papers beginning in 1974 have refined Coleman's methodology and considered more complex process models.

It is interesting to note that all of the work cited by Lazarsfeld that deals with dichotomies (and, more generally, discrete variables) can be cast within the framework of Markov chain models. Included among these are the Kendall–Lazarsfeld model for response errors in the appendix to *Conflict and Mood* (Kendall, 1955) as well as Wiggins's (1973) work involving latent variables changing through time. The full implications of a time-series model only become evident, however, when more than two interviews are available. In this sense, the final section on Markov chains is an anomaly, inasmuch as the work in that area served as a stimulus and model for

[5] A latent-structure analysis gives more than just a latent fourfold table. It permits one to compute the probabilities that any of the four indicators would be answered positively by occupants of both sides of the latent class at both panel waves. This is due to the use of third-level frequencies. For a detailed and highly competent discussion of latent-process analysis, see Wiggins (1973).

the analyses discussed earlier in the chapter, where the "process" only extended for two waves.—Neil W. Henry

REFERENCES

Anderson, T. W. Probability models for analyzing time changes in attitudes. In P. F. Lazarsfeld (Ed.), *Mathematical thinking in the social sciences*. New York: Free Press, 1954.

Armor, D. J. *Measuring the effects of television on aggressive behavior*. Santa Monica: Rand Corporation, 1975.

Birren, J. E. Translations in gerontology—from lab to life: Psychophysiology and speed of response. *American Psychologist*, 1974, *29*, 808–815.

Blalock, H. M., Jr. *Causal inferences in nonexperimental research*. Chapel Hill: University of North Carolina Press, 1964. (Originally published, 1961.)

Blalock, H. M., Jr. (Ed.). *Causal models in the social sciences*. Chicago: Aldine, 1971.

Blumen, I., Kogan, M., & McCarthy, P. J. *The industrial mobility of labor as a probability process*. Ithaca, N.Y.: Cornell University Press, 1955.

Boudon, R. B. A method of linear causal analysis: Dependence analysis. *American Sociological Review*, 1965, *30*, 365–374.

Campbell, D. T. More plausible rival hypotheses in the cross-lagged panel correlation technique. *Psychological Bulletin*, 1969, *71*, 74–80.

Campbell, D. T., & Clayton, K. N. Avoiding regression effects in panel studies of communication impact. *Studies in Public Communication*, 1961, *3*, 99–118.

Campbell, D. T., & Stanley, J. C. *Experimental and quasi-experimental designs for research*. Chicago: Rand McNally, 1966. (Originally published, 1963.)

Coleman, J. S. *The adolescent society*. New York: Free Press, 1961.

Coleman, J. S. *Introduction to mathematical sociology*. New York: Free Press, 1964.

Duncan, O. D. Path analysis: Sociological examples. *American Journal of Sociology*, 1966, *72*, 1–16.

Duncan, O. D. Some linear models for two-wave, two variable panel analysis. *Psychological Bulletin*, 1969, *77*, 177–182.

Goldberger, A. S., & Duncan, O. D. (Eds.). *Structural equation models in the social sciences*. New York: Academic, Seminar, 1973.

Goodman, L. A. Causal analysis of data from panel studies and other kinds of surveys. *American Journal of Sociology*, 1973, *78*, 1135–1191.

Heise, D. R., *Causal inference from panel data*. In E. F. Borgatta & G. W. Bohrnstedt (Eds.), *Sociological methodology 1970*. San Francisco: Jossey-Bass, 1970.

Henry, N. W. Measurement models for continuous and discrete variables. In A. S. Goldberger & O. D. Duncan (Eds.), *Structural equation models in the social sciences*. New York: Academic, Seminar, 1973.

Hovland, C. I. Reconciling conflicting results derived from experimental and survey studies of attitude change. *American Psychologist*, 1959, *14*, 8–17. (Reprinted in Lazarsfeld, Pasanella, & Rosenberg, 1972.)

Hyman, H. *Survey design and analysis*. New York: Free Press, 1955.

Kendall, P. *Conflict and mood*. New York: Free Press, 1955.

Kenny, D. A. Cross-lagged and synchronous common factors in panel data. In A. S. Goldberger & O. D. Duncan (Eds.), *Structured equation models in the social sciences*. New York: Academic, Seminar, 1973.

Lazarsfeld, P. F. Panel studies. *Public Opinion Quarterly*, 1940, *4*, 122–128.

Lazarsfeld, P. F. The algebra of dichotomous systems. In H. Solomon (Ed.), *Studies in item analysis and prediction*. Stanford, Calif.: Stanford University Press, 1960. (Reprinted in Lazarsfeld, Pasanella, & Rosenberg, 1972.)

Lazarsfeld, P. F. Mutual relations over time of two attributes: A review and integration of various approaches. In M. Hammer, K. Salzinger, & S. Sutton (Eds.), *Psychopathology*. New York: Wiley, 1972.

Lazarsfeld, P. F., & Fiske, M. The "panel" as a new tool for measuring opinion. *Public Opinion Quarterly*, 1938, *2*, 596–612.

Lazarsfeld, P. F., & Henry, N. W. *Latent structure analysis*. Boston: Houghton Mifflin, 1968.

Lazarsfeld, P. F., Pasanella, A., & Rosenberg, M. *Continuities in the language of social research*. New York: Free Press, 1972.

Paton, S., Kessler, R. C., & Kandel, D. B. Depressive mood and illegal drug use: A longitudinal analysis. *Journal of Genetic Psychology,* 1977, *131,* 267–289.

Pelz, D. C., & Andrews, F. M. Detecting causal priorities in panel study data. *American Sociological Review,* 1964, *29,* 836–848.

Pelz, D. C., & Faith, R. E. *Some effects of causal connection in simulated time-series data* (Causal Analysis Project, Interim Report No. 2). Ann Arbor: Institute for Social Research, 1970. (Published without the technical appendix in *Proceedings of the social statistics section of the Annual Meeting of the American Statistical Association,* December 1970.)

Pelz, D. C., & Lew, R. A. Heise's causal model applied. In E. F. Borgatta & G. W. Bohrnstedt (Eds.), *Sociological methodology 1970.* San Francisco: Jossey-Bass, 1970.

Rapaport, A. Lewis F. Richardson's mathematical theory of war. *Journal of Conflict Resolution,* 1957, *1,* 249–299.

Rosenberg, M. *The logic of survey analysis.* New York: Basic, 1968.

Simon, H. A. Spurious correlation: A causal interpretation. *Journal of the American Statistical Association,* 1954, *49,* 467–479.

Simon, H. A. *Models of man.* New York: Wiley, 1957.

Singer, B., & Spilerman, S. Social mobility models for heterogeneous populations. In H. L. Costner (Ed.), *Sociological Methodology 1973–1974.* San Francisco: Jossey-Bass, 1974.

Singer, B., & Spilerman, S. The representation of social processes by Markov models. *American Journal of Sociology,* 1976, *82,* 1–54.

Stouffer, S., Guttman, L., Suchman, E. A., Lazarsfeld, P. F., Star, S. A., & Clausen, J. A. *The American soldier,* Vol. 4, *Measurement and prediction.* Princeton: Princeton University Press, 1950.

Tinbergen, J. Econometric business cycle research. *Review of Economic Studies,* 1940, *1,* 73–90.

Wiggins, L. M. *Panel analysis.* San Francisco: Jossey-Bass and New York: American Elsevier, 1973.

Yee, A. H., & Gage, N. L. Techniques for estimating the source and direction of causal influence in panel data. *Psychological Bulletin,* 1968, *70,* 113–126.

Yule, G. U. *An introduction to the theory of statistics.* London: Griffin, 1911.

Yule, G. U. On the methods of measuring association between two attributes. *Journal of the Royal Statistical Society,* 1912, *75,* 579–642.

13

The Interdependence of Theory, Methodology, and Empirical Data: Causal Modeling as an Approach to Construct Validation

Peter M. Bentler
University of California at Los Angeles

There exists a fundamental interdependence between substantive social science theory, the theory of methodology and statistics, and empirical data: Each realizes its fullest potential by incorporating the best of the other. Substantive theory remains little more than speculation without sound data gathered in the context of an appropriate methodology to exploit both theory and data. Theoretical development in methodology, mathematical modeling, or statistics cannot rise above purely formal development, however elegant such development may be, without an important problem to tackle and without substantive theory to guide analyses of viable empirical data. Even the best empirical data cannot reveal their secrets without a scientist's careful attention to their inherent methodological and theoretical deficiencies as well as to their strengths.

The interrelations among theory, methodology, and data have been pointed out many times previously, particularly in the philosophy of science literature as it relates to the social sciences. In this chapter, I am pursuing the theme in the context of *construct validation,* an idea developed by Cronbach and Meehl (1955). Construct validation refers to the scientific confirmation of tests and measures as indexes of postulated attributes or qualities. I propose that construct validation can be operationalized and assessed by some recent developments in causal modeling. This newly developed set of methodological tools can help to foster and to evaluate substantive theory as it is applied to appropriately gathered empirical data.

Although construct validation by causal modeling represents a potentially fruitful approach to a variety of empirical data, it is particularly relevant to the understanding of repeated-measurements data such as the longitudinal research on drug abuse described in this volume. In such research, one typically deals with multiple indicators of various important constructs, measured sequentially, to be

Work on this chapter was supported in part by Research Scientist Development Award KO2-DA00017 and research grant DA01070 from the U.S. Public Health Service.

understood in the context of various background or control variables. Meaningful analysis of the research data requires evaluating the causal influences of the background variables on the constructs at various time points, the effects of various constructs on each other, the effects of a construct on itself across time, and such potential effects as indicator errors correlated across time. Repeated measurements automatically generate correlational data, so that methods for drawing causal inferences from correlational data immediately become relevant to longitudinal research. Although a variety of analytic strategies can be employed to deal with various aspects of such longitudinal data, the causal-modeling approach allows the entire system to be analyzed simultaneously in the context of theory. In principle, this approach is also appropriate to more complex longitudinal designs such as the cohort-sequential data obtained by Jessor and Jessor (chap. 2) and by Smith and Fogg (chap. 4), but although theory has clearly pointed to the need for understanding cohort effects in longitudinal research (Riley & Waring, chap. 10), no appropriate general methodology has yet been developed for this purpose.

Before proceeding to explicate construct validation and how it can be operationalized, I review the roles of description and explanation in social science; then I turn to understanding methodological approaches—descriptive, exploratory and model building, and hypothesis testing—in substantive research, assessing the interaction of data and theory in each case. Thereupon, I review the concept of construct validity and propose to use a causal-modeling approach to implement it. I then describe some recent developments in the analysis of mean and covariance structures, developments that have intertwined the best of psychometric, econometric, and statistical theory. Finally, I deal with the generality and scope of mathematical models as they interrelate to social science theory and data.

Is a review of traditional thinking necessary in the context of a description of newer methodological developments and their implications? I think it is essential in order to provide a perspective on what may reasonably be expected from the newer methods, as well as to reinforce the virtues of some older ways when considered in relation to research goals. The belief must be resisted that a new concept or procedure will have momentous impact, finally making social and behavioral research truly scientific in molds approved by philosophers of science or by practitioners in the successful physical sciences. Seldom are such expectations realized. The concept of construct validity, for example, was heralded as a useful advance over previous concepts of validity (APA Committee on Psychological Tests, 1954), but its novelty, usefulness, and clarity were soon considered controversial (for example, Bechtold, 1959; Cronbach, 1971, pp. 480–484), and its potential contributions were reformulated (for example, Campbell, 1960; Loevinger, 1957). Thus, in this chapter, I do not propose a revolutionary methodological panacea for the social sciences; rather, I suggest the importance of combining tried and novel methods according to the goals of an investigation.

DESCRIPTION AND EXPLANATION
IN SOCIAL SCIENCE

Describing a phenomenon or an effect is a task that generally precedes the theoretical understanding or explanation of the phenomenon or effect. In the earliest stages of investigation, the description itself may be quite crude and unsophisticated, using neither elegant research methods nor constructs in approaching the problem. Clinical observation might provide an important example of the initial stages of description. Adequate description, carried out with due regard for methodological issues such as sampling, measurement, artifacts, and the like, will generally replace unsystematic description. But even at this stage, substantive knowledge must be consulted for hypotheses or partial theories of the phenomenon. This consultation is necessary at the very least to define the domain of relevance of the phenomenon and to identify variables that might be measured or environmental conditions that might be necessary to observation of the phenomenon. Statistical methods that might be consulted are descriptive in nature, and statistical inference may be limited to the problem of drawing specialized parametric inferences about a subject population from the given sample.

Explanation of a phenomenon is a step further removed from description. Certainly adequate description is a necessary precursor to the development of effective or useful explanations of the phenomenon. Explanation typically involves going beyond the data: drawing deductions from a model, making predictions based on prior experience and theory, and testing hypotheses. Although it can be argued that complete and thorough description may suffice in some domains of inquiry (for example, history, anatomy), the development of principles that can be applied to changing circumstances typically involves going beyond the data. Similar considerations make it obvious that there are levels of explanation, from simple, highly specific hypotheses that may have received thorough empirical support, to complex and elaborate theoretical systems that interrelate and explain numerous specific phenomena in various contexts. Certainly explanation at any level represents an important goal of science.

Research on the psychosocial aspects of alcohol and drug abuse is now primarily in the descriptive phase of scientific inquiry. As with the renowned blind men approaching their elephant, researchers in this area are oriented toward getting a descriptive hold on the phenomenon. What kind of people are affected, under what circumstances, with what kind of consequence? Questions like these represent the dominant status of the field—not surprising in view of the relative newness of the research area, the shifting nature of the phenomenon, and the difficulty of the material. Although there exists in the field some data exploration and model building, few if any theories of substance abuse are formalized enough to represent testable models that can be evaluated and compared for adequacy. Model testing is still a task for the future.

Experimentation and Explanation

An ideal method of going from description to explanation involves experimentally manipulating independent variables, randomly assigning subjects to treatment conditions, and observing the outcome on univariate or multivariate dependent variables. True experiments provide the surest means to development of theory through confirmation and rejection of hypotheses because potentially confounding extraneous variables will, through randomization, be uncorrelated with treatment outcome in large samples (for example, Fisher, 1935). Obviously, there must be a continuous interchange between substantive theory and experimentation, for the choice of independent variables to be manipulated must be dictated by substantive knowledge; similarly, the choice of appropriate dependent variables depends upon substantive theory and prior empirical results. As model building proceeds through a variety of manipulations and observation of effects, substantive theory can gain in effectiveness and range.

It is possible for substantive theory to play a relatively minor role in experimentation when rather arbitrary values are chosen for independent variables and when only single dependent variables are measured. In such simple univariate analysis-of-variance situations, the role of theory may be limited to defining both the manipulations and the relevance of a given observed dependent variable to each manipulation. Because of the inherent virtues of the experimental method, any relation between independent and dependent variables will become empirically verified or disconfirmed, thus providing an impetus to the revision of substantive theory if wrong or confirmation of theory if right. When several independent variables have been manipulated simultaneously, their interaction can be investigated by exploratory means even in the absence of theory, but theory can focus upon the relevant analyses to the exclusion of the irrelevant ones.

There is, of necessity, a stronger interrelationship between theory and empirical data via quantitative techniques when experimentation is concerned either with the manipulation of variables that are themselves based on parameters and embedded within a theory or with the measurement of multiple dependent variables. In such situations there must be a greater reliance on theory to develop the data-analytic strategy. The data provide feedback for the modification and further development of theory. Thus with dozens of dependent variables in an experiment, it will be desirable to develop a model of the relationship of these variables to the constructs being experimentally modified in the experiment because it is unlikely that the variables will reflect the treatment equally. A discriminant-function analysis, for example, will provide useful information beyond the basic multivariate analysis-of-variance results, which is itself in need of theoretical guidance when independent-variable interactions are too complex or numerous to investigate routinely (for example, Bock, 1975; Tatsuoka, 1976).

When randomization is not perfect, it may be possible to apply adjustment techniques such as analysis of covariance to control for the unwanted effects of nuisance variables (for example, Cronbach, Rogosa, Floden, & Price, 1976; Overall & Woodward, 1977a, 1977b). In recent developments, theory has a particularly important role (Sörbom, 1976). With such methods, causal hypotheses can be sharpened.

In the social sciences, unfortunately, true experimentation is difficult, if not impossible, to execute. Thus, whereas experimentation may be possible as a means of determining the acute effects of certain drugs, the psychosocial basis of drug abuse and dependency cannot similarly be investigated. It is not an accident that research into etiologies and consequences of substance abuse, as reported in this volume, for example, must rely upon nonexperimental means. Consequently, moving from description to explanation remains difficult at best in this field. The data obtained are correlational in nature, and are obtained perhaps under a variety of nonexperimental conditions.

Correlation and Causation

Every researcher who has studied philosophy of science or statistical methods has learned that correlation does not imply causation. Do there exist any means of making causal statements from correlational data? The specific idea of analyzing causation by analysis of correlations was introduced years ago via path analysis (Wright, 1921), but the best single general source on inference in nonexperimental research remains the work of Campbell and Stanley (1963), who discuss a variety of alternative quasi-experimental designs for data gathering as well as the associated strengths and weaknesses of each. Clearly, different data-gathering methods will yield results with different attributes, and no method approaches the virtues of the true experiment. The possibilities for alternative explanations of given results are immense in naturalistic settings because confounding cannot be unraveled through control variables when there is an absence both of theory and of knowledge of sampling conditions. There is no point in repeating the Campbell–Stanley discussion here, although it should be noted that the literature on nonexperimental designs is growing rapidly (for example, Cook & Campbell, 1976; Kenny, 1975; Linn & Werts, 1977).

It is often stated that the associational nature of correlational data—the measurement of response–response interrelations rather than stimulus–response relationships (Bergmann & Spence, 1944)—represents its fatal flaw. It can, however, be proposed that there is a different, but equally severe, problem with correlational techniques as traditionally developed: They are simply descriptive and exploratory in nature rather than hypothesis testing or confirmatory. Although it is possible to test hypotheses about population values of observed correlations, or sets of such correlations (for example, Larzelere & Mulaik, 1977), such tests are only rarely incorporated into a reasonably developed theoretical framework; and the information gleaned from such simple tests represents a rather minor improvement over the data themselves. Correlational results, like psychological tests, are hardly ever used as instruments of social science theory (for example, Loevinger, 1957; Underwood, 1975). This is not a necessary state of affairs and it is changing.

Methodologists have recently introduced mathematical models and methods of statistical analysis, such as causal modeling, that have made it possible to test relatively complex theories that could be actualized in nonexperimental data (for example, Duncan, 1975; Heise, 1975). Correlational data can be inspected with these techniques to determine whether the data are consistent with a given theory or whether, given the data, the theory must be inadequate. Although there is no methodology for proving a theory to be correct and although multiple theories may equally well describe the data, an incorrect theory can be rejected if the data logically (theoretically) provide a reasonable test of the theory. I have more to say about causal modeling later because I propose it as a method of construct validation and evaluation.

Integration of Experimentation and Correlational Methods

In the ideal situation, correlational data as well as experimental data would be relevant to the building and testing of substantive theory. In spite of Cronbach's (1957) 2-decades-old classic plea for the integration of these two "disciplines," however, their integration remains a task for the future (Cronbach, 1975). The methodology for integration may finally be developing in the form of extensions of nonexperimental hypothesis-testing procedures about correlational structures to situations that require drawing inferences about group means as well (Bentler, 1976b; Jackson & Alwin, 1976; Jöreskog, 1971a, 1973a; Keesling & Wiley, 1975; Sörbom, 1974, 1976). There is nothing in such methods that demands the use of strict experimentation, so their usefulness will extend to the analysis of quasi-experimental data. The procedures are causal-modeling methods that require fairly detailed specifications of interrelationships among observed data and hypothetical constructs and that can be put to test if the statistical assumptions of the methods are met. In the absence of reasonable theory or hypotheses, the methods cannot be used effectively.

Traditional methods of analysis of variance make strong assumptions about homogeneity of correlations and covariances in order to draw inferences about means without undue difficulty (these assumptions may be put to the test, of course). Most analysis of approaches to covariance structure grow out of the factor-analytic tradition and therefore make the strong assumption that means are unstructured in terms of the covariance parameters in order to be able to draw inferences about the covariance parameters without undue difficulty. The newer methods, aimed at explaining mean and covariance data simultaneously, make fewer assumptions, but use of these techniques requires stronger substantive knowledge and more complicated methods of parameter estimation.

Longitudinal Methods and Explanation

In the absence of true experimentation, researchers have turned to longitudinal methods in an attempt to eliminate certain explanations for given data. In contrast to cross-sectional research, longitudinal research involves the passage of time, and as Western philosophy has almost universally agreed that causal processes must work forward in time, not backward, time-dependent events can help to eliminate otherwise plausible explanations of data.

Whereas repeated measurement of a set of subjects provides potentially important information that simply cannot be obtained any other way, namely, intra-individual change and individual differences therein, or information about the stability of attributes, and whereas it eliminates potential bias problems associated with retrospective recall, simple longitudinal designs without appropriate control groups leave much to be desired in internal and external validity (for example, Labouvie, 1976; Labouvie, Bartsch, Nesselroade, & Baltes, 1974). Even with such controls, implicit assumptions regarding relevant, a priori, substantive knowledge are required, assumptions whose utilization may make causal interpretation rest upon a shaky base. For example, in order to obtain a reasonable causal model to test longitudinality, one must be measuring all relevant causal variables and be assessing their effects at appropriate, rather than arbitrary, times (for example, Heise, 1975). One must know quite accurately the causal lag, that is, the time required for an influence to occur. As Davis (1976) states, "If weather influences one's mood, the influence probably occurs the same day; but if a college degree influences income, the effect cannot be detected the evening of Commencement" (p. 30). Measuring the right variables at the wrong time is as useless as measuring the wrong variables at the right time. Substantive theory is clearly called for, but even reasonably well-developed theory may be unable to exclude alternative explanations as reasonable. Of course, longitudinal research itself may be necessary to help determine the information on lag time that may be required for effective use of longitudinal methods, in other words, use that increases the scope and power of a substantive theory.

There is no denying the possible virtues of the longitudinal method for drug-abuse research, but in this application its limitations must also be appreciated. After reviewing three converging lines of longitudinal evidence for their models of drug and alcohol use, including descriptive, predictive, and associative data, Jessor and Jessor (chap. 2) conclude that

> It is only fair to say . . . that the causal texture of the relationships we have been dealing with remains very much a matter of presumption. None of our strategies, not even the prediction of onset [of drug use] where a time lag was involved, can do more than document an association and the temporal order of the events or processes involved. That the subsequent events were "produced" by those that were antecedent still eludes direct demonstration. (p. 67)

Baltes (1976) has elegantly noted the dilemma of explanation through longitudinal methods: "Longitudinal research has the disturbing feature of appearing both as a panacea to the designer and a Pandora's box to the interpreter. . . . The Pandora's box quality of longitudinal work is often more apparent than the panacea-like quality (p. 2).

There are, of course, a wide variety of fairly traditional research approaches to longitudinal data and their analyses (including newer ways to carry out traditional analyses, for example, Pedhazur, 1977), but statistical models for the analysis of such data are growing at a rate that makes it difficult for substantive researchers to keep up with their development. Among these techniques are general ones that can be applied to longitudinal binary or categorial data (Bishop, Fienberg, & Holland, 1975; Davis, 1975, 1976; Goodman, 1975a, 1975b; Hildebrand, Laing, & Rosenthal, 1976; Muthén, 1976, 1977; Nerlove & Press, 1973; Roberts, 1976; Shaffer, 1973, 1977) and to continuous data (Bentler, 1976a; Jöreskog, 1973a; Simonton, 1977; Tucker, 1966) or to discrete-time or continuous-time models in the time-series context (Glass, Willson, & Gottman, 1975; Hannan & Young, 1977; Hibbs, 1976; Land & Felson, 1976; Land & Spilerman, 1975; Singer & Spilerman, 1975; Swaminathan & Algina, 1977). The class of models for continuous data known as structural-equation models seems to be particularly appropriate to the causal modeling of social phenomena (Bentler, 1973, 1976a; Corballis & Traub, 1970; Geraci, 1976; Hsiao, 1976; Jöreskog, 1973b, 1977; Wiley, 1973). These models are similar to models developed in the econometric literature but go beyond it by incorporating factor-analytic models as measurement models. There now exist discussions of these models as applied specifically to longitudinal data (for example, Jöreskog & Sörbom, 1976, 1977; Wheaton, Muthén, Alwin, & Summers, 1977). Being general models, however, they can deal with cross-sectional as well as longitudinal data. Their utilization is likely to increase in the future because of recent evidence that linear models for interval-scale data represent reasonable approximations even in circumstances in which the linearity and scale properties of the data may be open to question (for example, Havlicek & Peterson, 1977; Kruskal & Shepard, 1974). Although nonlinearities cannot always be ignored, and should not be if theoretical considerations dictate their understanding (for example, Anderson, 1977), linearity is often an acceptable assumption in the absence of well-developed theory. In the next section, I discuss the basic idea behind this kind of causal modeling.

Causal Modeling

Methodological and statistical theorists in the social sciences have not failed to note the dilemma faced by substantive researchers in moving from description to explanation without the availability of experimental methods. As pointed out above, they have recently formulated quantitative techniques that would accept correlational data as well as causally ambiguous longitudinal data as input to a process of analysis that has come to be known as "causal modeling," "structural-equation modeling," "confirmatory factor analysis," or "analysis of covariance structures." What is the basis of techniques like these?

Causal modeling attempts to translate theoretical statements regarding the influences of certain sets of variables on others into a complete systems framework that yields testable statistical consequences. It amounts to a procedure for transforming assumptions into predictions. If the predictions are consistent with data, the assumptions become more plausible, but if the data reject the prediction, the assumptions must be reformulated or abandoned. The procedure for translating assumptions into predictions can be illustrated in a simple way, using the formula for partial correlation given in most statistics texts. It states that

$$r_{12.3} = \frac{r_{12} - r_{13}r_{23}}{\sqrt{(1 - r_{13}{}^2)(1 - r_{23}{}^2)}}$$

where the concern is with the correlation between Variables 1 and 2, holding 3 constant. A simple rearrangement of this formula yields

$$r_{12.3}\sqrt{(1 - r_{13}{}^2)(1 - r_{23}{}^2)} = r_{12} - r_{13}r_{23}$$

One now makes a causal-modeling assumption and attempts to make a data prediction based on this assumption. Assume the causal model is true, namely, that Variable 3 is the only "cause" of Variables 1 and 2. If this were exactly true, then when one partials out the causal effect of Variable 3, Variables 1 and 2 should no longer be correlated (the correlational similarity between these variables is presumed to be caused by Variable 3). Thus, the substantive theory translates into the assumption that the partial correlation $r_{12.3}$ would equal 0. In that case, the right-hand side of the above equation would equal 0, and the terms could be rearranged to yield $r_{12} = r_{13}r_{23}$. Thus, the correlation between Variables 1 and 2 would be given by the product of the two other correlations; this is the data prediction. If my simple causal model were exactly true, then this is the effect one should observe in the data. If the data were of some other form, the causal model would have to be rejected or reformulated in some other way. For example, there may be other causal influences at work or the equations may not appropriately represent the effect of random or systematic errors. New assumptions would need to be specified.

If the data are consistent with the deduction drawn from a causal model, as in the final equation above, the causal model is plausible. It can by no means be proven, however, and there may in general be many models that might be consistent with a given set of data. Ideally, one would have substantive reasons for developing competing causal models, based on differing assumptions, so that the data might be evaluated relative to a set of models under consideration. For the simplified example, one might have reasons for considering the effects of Variable 1 on 2 and 3, proceeding through the partial correlation $r_{23.1}$ to yield the deduction $r_{23} = r_{12}r_{13}$. Rearranging terms, one finds that $r_{12} = r_{23}/r_{13}$. From the vantage point of this model, the correlation between Variables 1 and 2 is now given as the ratio of the remaining correlations rather than as their product as in the previous example. It may well be that the data confirm one model but not the other.

To make the hypothetical example more concrete, one might let Variable 1 represent drug use, Variable 2 represent criminal behavior, and Variable 3 represent unconventional attitudes. The first mathematical model above would express the idea that unconventional attitudes cause both drug use and criminal behavior. The second model, in constrast, would suggest that drug use causes both criminal behavior and unconventional attitudes. The data might confirm one or the other model, or neither.

Although this example provides an idea about how causal modeling can be applied to social science research and specifically to drug-use research, it should not be taken as a realistic substantive example. There are numerous reasons for this reservation. They include the concepts that such models should be evaluated with respect to latent, rather than observed, variables and that such models should always be specified with respect to all known relevant variables simultaneously (certainly other variables besides unconventionality will affect the relationship of drugs to crime). In addition, one must always recognize the importance of appropriately defining and measuring the various variables involved: Are we, in this instance, talking about property crime, violent crime, or both? Are we talking about marihuana use or true addiction? Are we talking about right and left political ideology, or problem behavior? There is no substitute for specific substantive research experience as a prerequisite to the appropriate use of causal modeling. An introductory discussion of early path-analytic approaches to causal modeling can be found in Werts and Linn (1970) and Naditch (1976). Naditch also provides some drug-abuse examples.

Causal modeling can be applied with equal force to longitudinal data and to cross-sectional data and also to models concerned with means of variables as well as with the interrelations of variables. Actually, longitudinal data may be particularly amenable to causal modeling because the time-ordered sequence of events not only ean make results of causal-modeling studies more interpretable but can also provide a basis for questioning a result that may work statistically but may be implausible logically. For example, suppose that the correlational structure $r_{12} = r_{13}r_{23}$, described above, were found to be consistent with certain data. Most investigators would nonetheless be suspicious of any imputed causal interpretation of the result if Variable 3, the causal variable, was measured some months after Variables 1 and 2. Unless it could be demonstrated that the standing of subjects on Variable 3 was extremely stable for a lengthy period of time that included prior measurement of the other variables, the data would be causally suspect. Clearly, the longitudinal method has something to offer to causal modeling. Before exploring causal modeling more fully, I must first evaluate whether causal modeling is the only effective way for substantive theory, methodology, and empirical data to interact.

MATCHING METHODOLOGY TO SUBSTANTIVE RESEARCH GOALS

Causal modeling cannot easily be applied to domains of inquiry that are still purely descriptive in nature and in which research has not progressed beyond data exploration. Some preliminary model building, of a sort potentially translatable into testable propositions, must exist. To illustrate, substance abuse as a research area appears to be ready for causal modeling. Although not all conceptual and measurement issues in the area are agreed upon (see Clausen, chap. 11), the definition of substance abuse and its manifestations have become clarified and reasonably agreed upon, and some antecedents and consequences of abuse have been empirically documented and theoretically dissected. It would now be possible to translate the variety of findings and hypotheses of the field into preliminary causal models, but it is my impression that an active interchange between substantive and methodological experts will be required before such an effort will come to fruition. There must exist an appropriate match between the methodology utilized and the substantive question being addressed. It would seem useful to review the variety of methodological contributions that are necessary precursors to construct evaluation through causal modeling.

Domain Definition

Before methodology can contribute to meaningful research, minimal substantive knowledge must exist. Any field of inquiry must have its limits defined, including at the very least the specification of relevant variables, subject populations, and environmental contexts of operation of subjects and variables. Whatever the level of sophistication in a given field of inquiry, without a minimal amount of consensual agreement by relevant experts as to these fundamental aspects of description of the field, it would be impossible to design rational data-gathering strategies or proposals for experimental manipulation of independent variables. Obviously the domain of a field as perceived by experts will be continuously changing as new data are obtained and new theories are developed either to explain the data or to suggest further ideas for research. Although it may not be appropriate to describe domain definition as an important part of theory building, it does represent the minimal contribution of a substantive sort to guide methodology and data gathering. The value of a methodology cannot be determined in the absence of some consensus about the substantive domain.

As witnessed by the numerous substantive contributions described in this volume, the fields of drug and alcohol abuse have been able to arrive at some consensus on their research domains. Although not every researcher has subscribed to the same definitions of relevance to the area, there are substantial areas of agreement (Elinson & Nurco, 1975). For example, there is agreement about the existence of a continuum of alcohol and drug use, with abuse representing an end point of the continuum; there is agreement about the relevance of the abuse concept to such diverse populations as teenagers and homemakers; it is recognized that environmental circumstances such as drug availability, peer values, and peer behavior are relevant to the expression of use; and there is a hint that certain social, environmental, and individual precursors to use exist. Of course, as the varying operational definitions of use and abuse in this volume have demonstrated, there is by no means complete agreement. Psychological, sociological, economic, biomedical, and legal considerations at times dictate different focuses on the phenomenon.

Data Description

In the absence of theoretical understanding of a given research field beyond some agreement on the domain of relevance and in the absence of specific propositions, hypotheses, or theories to test, methodology can contribute most effectively to substantive research through its developed methods of descriptive statistics. Such an approach is well illustrated in this volume by Josephson and Rosen (chap. 5). Univariate statistical descriptions such as means and standard deviations, or frequency distributions, can describe the phenomenon under study in given populations. When there are numerous variables, univariate techniques can be repetitively applied, and although this is an important aspect of data analysis, univariate data-analytic methods will need supplementation by bivariate and multivariate description. Cross-tabulations, correlations, chi-squares, and other methods, as outlined in statistics texts, are appropriate and useful. Univariate and bivariate descriptions can be used in conjunction with inferential statistics if there is an attempt to draw inferences from the samples to some population. (It may not be necessary to use statistical tests at all, however, when the sample size is exceedingly large, inasmuch as almost any null hypothesis is likely to be rejected.)

Multivariate data description is somewhat more complex by the very nature of the vastness of the possibilities. When the data do not have any particularly elegant and simple form, at least approximately, it may be necessary to use descriptive levels beyond first- and second-order moment statistics, such as means and covariances. Decisions will have to be made that allow for simpler summary methods to be adopted, for example, for the level of measurement scale utilized in the variables, for linearity versus more complex joint distributions of the variables, or for the potential classification of variables as independent or dependent. When decisions such as these have been made (and, perhaps, tested for adequacy), standard methods of multivariate analysis (Bentler, Lettieri, & Austin, 1976; Bishop, Fienberg, & Holland, 1975; Bock, 1975; Kendall, 1975; Morrison, 1976; Timm, 1975) can be utilized to describe the data. These might include such techniques as multiple regression, principal-components analysis, factor analysis, discriminant functions, or Guttman-scale analysis—techniques that have been extensively and effectively utilized in the studies in this volume.

By and large, these univariate and multivariate methods can be utilized for their ability to summarize and describe data even in the absence of any hypothesis testing based on substantive ideas. Of course, because accuracy of description is traded off against the ability of a technique to describe even chance features of the data, some decisions may be necessary to simplify the data in a reasonable way without distorting their essential features. For example, having very many variables in a regression equation will allow greater precision in predicting a dependent variable, but the use of too many variables may lead the equation to describe chance interrelations among data; it may be more sensible to eliminate some predictors, as Smith and Fogg (chap. 4) did. Similarly, accuracy of description is enhanced when many principal components are utilized to describe the intercorrelations among variables, but extraction of too many components may lead to poor replicability in new samples. Although data description may be the main concern, statistical methods of inference may be called upon to help make decisions. Data description may also be modified by the use of methods that eliminate the effects of unusual observations (for example, Bentler & Woodward, 1977b; Wainer, 1976b; Wainer & Thissen, 1976), although both substantive and methodological considerations must help in evaluating whether an observation is a peripheral one of no significance or a significant clue about the phenomenon under study.

The use of statistical descriptions based on simpler, rather than more complicated, parameters provides the first logical movement toward model building. For example, stepwise regression may be used as a clue to find important antecedents of a phenomenon even though it represents a somewhat arbitrary procedure that is not guaranteed to find an optimal predictor set (for example, Beale, Kendall, & Mann, 1967). Substantive theory building may proceed from multiple data sets that converge and confirm such descriptive findings. The drug and alcohol research reports described in this volume have made generally appropriate and informative use of descriptive methods. For example, the technique of stepwise regression was used effectively by Roizen, Cahalan, and Shanks (chap. 9) to select a parsimonious set of prognostic and diagnostic indicators of problem drinking. Jessor and Jessor (chap. 2) made a more systematic, theory-based use of the same technique in their sequential selection of variables into their regression equations on the basis of their model of drug use. Perhaps the distributional statistical assumptions necessary to use the methods as inferential tools have not been met in all cases (for example, Mellinger, Somers, Bazell, and Manheimer, chap. 7, and Kandel, Kessler, and Margulies, chap. 3, use a binary dependent variable in multiple regression); but when description, rather than hypothesis testing, is desired, only the dedicated statistician will object. Bentler, Lettieri, and Austin (1976) have provided a handbook for substance-abuse research that covers a variety of designs and multivariate data-analytic strategies, including descriptive, exploratory, and hypothesis-testing procedures.

There are potential dangers inherent in the use of purely descriptive methods, for although they lead one to stay close to the data, they also may make it difficult to abstract adequately the important features of the data. Discussion of four major difficulties follows.

Excessive Redundancy in Communication

There exists a delicate balance between a simple description repeated many times and a complex technique used sparingly. Frequency distributions, cross-tabulations, and intercorrelations are simple to understand and to present, but when used repetitively for multitudes of variables, the redundancy in communication may make it difficult to focus on the truly important aspects of the data. A complex multivariate method, such as multiple-group discriminant analysis, may provide a useful single summary of the essential features of the data, but the results may not communicate easily to researchers untrained in the method; there may be too little redundancy in such analyses. In general, however, raw multivariate data will be so massive and excessively redundant that some method of simplification would be desirable even at the expense of bending some assumptions associated with statistical inference (such as a normal distribution of the dependent variable). Most well-known multivariate methods are reasonably robust with regard to violation of assumptions. For example, principal-components analysis is most appropriately utilized when data are linearly related, but violation of this assumption is generally not very important (for example, Kruskal & Shepard, 1974). One simply needs to know that the typical consequence is one of generating small "artifactual" components (*artifacts* when considered in relation to a simpler, nonlinear data description; *real* as linear components).

Inappropriate Level of Analysis

The operant behavioristic tradition in psychology would consider description at the level of the individual subject essential and would consider the use of summary data for groups of subjects as distortions of essential features of the data. Shontz (1976) reviews some methods for studying data at the individual level. Whether a given level of analysis—individual, subgroup, well-defined sample—is appropriate depends upon the features of the data the researcher considers important. In the classical experimental situation, the researcher may consider individual data relatively meaningless ("error variance") because emphasis may be placed on mean results only. Another researcher, however, may consider the individual differences to be of crucial importance to theory development and to the research domain as defined. The role of individual differences, considered in relation to situational and other determinants of behavior, represents, for example, a current area of substantive theoretical debate (for example, Hogan, DeSoto, & Solano, 1977; Mischel, 1977). This debate extends directly into the areas of substance abuse, where Roizen, Cahalan, and Shanks (chap. 9) question the traitlike aspects of problem drinking. Clearly, decisions as to appropriateness of level of analysis in data aggregation depend upon substantive considerations, as in Robins's (chap. 8) effective use of rates and ratios. Of course, when one goes beyond the data to inferential statistical questions, statistical theory may demand analysis at a particular level.

The same considerations that require thought to be given to the aggregation of data across subjects suggest that attention be given to problems of data aggregation across variables. Although data must be gathered on particular variables as decided on in advance of an investigation, the presentation of results may appropriately focus upon levels of analysis other than that of the individual variables. For example, several variables may represent essentially interchangeable indicators of a possibly multidimensional construct, so that more coherent results could be presented on the composite composed of a sum of the component variables (Bentler, 1972; Bentler & Woodward, 1977a). In the drug-abuse area, one would have to decide whether presentation of data on specific drugs was essential or irrelevant; depending upon the purpose, different choices would be made. It is possible, for example, that Mellinger and his co-workers (chap. 7), and Kandel and her co-workers (chap. 3) could have developed alternative analyses based on variable aggregation, a technique used effectively by Johnston, O'Malley, and Eveland (chap. 6), Jessor and Jessor (chap. 2), and Smith and Fogg (chap. 4). Of course, a concern for correlates of a given kind of substance use, as in the work of Kandel and co-workers (chap. 3), requires a different measurement orientation.

Overgeneralization of Results

A major danger of descriptive methods lies in the precision that they imply about the observations. Without a statistical method and substantive theory to guide choice of data-analytic questions to be asked, there may exist a strong tendency to consider the observed data as truth that could equally well be uncovered by other investigators in other circumstances. Data replicability may be a will-of-the-wisp, however, if the conditions of data gathering are not well understood. Without either knowledge of sampling parameters involving subjects or some idea about selection of variables from the potential "universe" of variables, the generalizability of conclusions based on given data may be unknowable. For example, sampling loss or volunteer bias may make the results unrepresentative of a well-defined population (see, for example, Josephson & Rosen, chap. 5); cohort, age, or other effects may contribute to the results in unknown ways (see, for example, Riley & Waring, chap. 10); methods of measurement, such as self-report, may make generalization to other methods difficult (self-reports were used in almost all studies in this volume, but see the contrast provided by Kandel and co-workers, chap. 3, and by Smith and Fogg, chap. 4, for example); environmental contexts may not be measured or understood (but see the creative analysis of Robins's post-Vietnam data, chap. 8, for an approach to environmental impact). Although any quasi-experimental study will always be limited in internal and external validity, and experimental research will always be similarly limited to the conditions of experimental situations, researchers primarily concerned with data description may not pay the same attention to experimental and data-gathering design considerations as they otherwise would in a hypothesis-testing framework. Cross-validation and the use of large samples may mitigate problems of overgeneralization, but they do not eliminate them.

Focus on the Irrelevant

When data gathering and analysis are not intergrated with a theory, it is easy to overemphasize the value of wrong variables, and it may be difficult to incorporate data on such variables into theory. It is highly likely that variables will differ in their importance to a research domain, but gathering data requires only a simple binary decision to include a variable or exclude it from the data-gathering procedures. Once measured, the descriptive analysis of even unimportant variables, by easily implemented computer programs, may become irresistible. It may be easy to forget that the data have differential quality regarding their ability to answer certain substantive questions, and it may be difficult to separate the forest from the trees. Careful substantive consideration before data gathering will make data more meaningful.

A more difficult interpretive problem is faced when the research methods used impose unknown but definite distortions on the data or when they produce results that are better interpreted as methodological artifacts than as meaningful empirical results. It may be difficult to ignore such artifactual sources of results. For example, certain designs, involving either matching or the selection of subjects who have extreme standings on given variables, may well demonstrate regression to the mean, but in the absence of knowledge about this phenomenon, such results could be interpreted as substantively meaningful. While it is entirely possible that artifacts and theory would predict similar results, as in the physiological law of initial values, only careful attention to design pitfalls can minimize interpretive dangers. It is also quite easy for the apparent precision of a complex methodology to lull an investigator into ignoring the real possibility of artifacts. The example of unnecessarily many principal components extracted from nonlinear data has been given. Similarly, a result produced by the analysis of covariance, controlling for irrelevant variance, may be substantively meaningless (for example, Lord, 1967).

The reverse phenomenon, of using a simple technique inappropriately when a more complex technique is called for, also has potential dangers. For example, linear regression may make data description simple, but if the variables are truly nonlinear, important effects may be hidden from discovery. In this case, however, there is typically less chance for overemphasizing irrelevant effects.

Data Exploration and Model Building

Quantitative techniques play an important role, not only in describing existing data by way of summary statistics and significance tests, but in making it possible for an investigator to play with the data using alternative formulations to obtain a better understanding of the phenomenon under investigation. Indeed, such data exploration makes it possible for the investigator to build on hunches and guesses to develop more complicated models of the phenomenon being studied, models that could be evaluated statistically through hypothesis testing in new samples. Several substance-abuse research reports incorporated in this volume, such as Roizen, Cahalan, and Shanks (chap. 9); Johnston, O'Malley, and Eveland (chap. 6); Kandel, Kessler, and Margulies (chap. 3); and Smith and Fogg (chap. 4), used analytical methods in the service of model building.

There is a wide variety of methods available for data exploration. The type of greatest interest to the substantive researcher will typically be multivariate in nature, to be applied when a large number of variables and subjects have generated data. As in the case of multivariate data description, the researcher will have to decide such things as the choice of measurement scale of the variables (that is, nominal, ordinal, interval), the use of linear versus nonlinear models, the possibility of data aggregation across variables or subjects, and the use of decision rules (for example, statistical methods) for deciding on the acceptance of a result or for performing additional analyses. In contrast to data description, however, the goal in data exploration and model building is to make some tentative decisions on what information must be retained in future work because of its essential nature and what information appears to be redundant or irrelevant to the phenomenon under study. For example, one may be interested in locating predictor variables that account for a significant amount of variance in a dependent variable and in separating such predictors from other variables that either are redundant with the previous set or account for only a small proportion of variance (see Kandel, Kessler, & Margulies, chap. 3). Similarly, one may be interested in discovering the major sources of variance underlying the intercorrelation of a set of variables; large sources of variance may be retained as reliable dimensions of interest, and smaller sources of variance may be rejected. The hope, of course, is that decisions made according to the amount of variance a discovered variable (or dimension) might "explain" would be synonymous with the importance of that variable (or dimension) in the budding substantive theory. As always, rules of statistical decision might be invoked to help isolate the important from the trivial, but well-rationalized nonstatistical methods can be used as well. For this purpose, the methods previously mentioned are as applicable to data exploration as they are to data description, particularly when one has hunches and hypotheses that can be put to test. Some additional methods and ideas are, however, relevant to this situation.

There do not seem to exist many techniques for the exploratory analysis of categorical multivariate data, particularly in situations in which a mix of independent and dependent variables is to be analyzed. Even in the most simple situations, it seems to be helpful to have a model (for example, Kenny, 1976a; Kessler, 1977; Lazarsfeld, chap. 12). One of the most popular search methods is automatic interaction detection (Sonquist & Morgan, 1964), which represents a model for forming statistical tree diagrams allowing for interaction among variables. The relevance of this technique to drug-abuse research is described by Somers, Mellinger, and Davidson (1976). Methods of actuarial prediction, regression using categorical predictors, and multivariate analysis of variance based on categories are also described by Bentler, Lettieri, and Austin (1976). Ordinary linear regression can work quite well, including stepwise procedures to select a subset of predictors from the complete set. Goodman (1975b); Hildebrand, Laing, and Rosenthal (1976); Nerlove and Press (1973); Robinson (1974); and Rock, Werts, Linn, and Jöreskog (1977) describe some alternative methods. In view of the popular use of multiple regression even in circumstances when the dependent variable is not on an approximate interval scale, it must be pointed out that the results will reflect the scale distortion as well as the distribution on the variable. When all variables are binary, the distribution effect is more pronounced. At the very least, the investigator must be reluctant to place too much emphasis on the resulting predictor weights, which are in any case often not optimal on cross-validation and need not be relied upon too heavily (for example, Bentler & Woodward, 1977b; Wainer, 1976a).

Analysis of the internal structure of variables, for the sake of discovering redundancies or poorly measured concepts, or for obtaining the latent dimensionality of the objects, is a difficult matter in an exploratory situation with discrete variables (for example, Bishop, Fienberg, & Holland, 1975). In the absence of a reasonable model to test, one could utilize the ordinal analogue to principal components developed by Bentler (1970). A new factor-analytic method has recently been developed by Muthén (1977). When only a few components are of interest and one is willing to reject small dimensions as irrelevant, standard principal components may be utilized. A similar statement can be made when ordinal variables are analyzed. Certainly there is no need to utilize the expensive variety of nonmetric factor analysis described by Kruskal and Shepard (1974) in view of the results of Woodward and Overall (1976) that ordinary principal components based on ranks seem to work effectively, and in view of Kruskal and Shepard's results that demonstrate that the assumptions of interval data and linearity do not do much violence to ordinal, but error-contaminated, data. Indeed, in the presence of error, principal components analysis seems to outperform the more appropriate ordinal model.

The most widely used method of exploratory multivariate data analysis is almost certainly the technique of factor analysis. Principal components analysis, mentioned previously, is a close competitor. A choice among methods must be determined according to the investigator's goals. In general, there are few circumstances in which principal components analysis has the better rationale. This is because the results of factor analysis need not depend on the variance of the variables, whereas results of principal components are specific thereto (which explains why it is typically essential to standardize variables in this situation, in the absence of some true or natural meaning associated with the nonstandardized variables). In addition, the investigator typically searches for latent dimensions that account for the interrelations among variables, a situation whose mathematical statement demands the use of the factor model with its ability to separate error variance from the recovered dimensions (this is not possible with components). It might be said that the main general reason for using component analysis rather than factor analysis lies in pragmatism rather than theory: It is cheaper to implement and yields virtually the same results when large sets of variables are analyzed. In the context of discovery, such a pragmatic rationale is acceptable. An introductory chapter on this topic may be found in Bentler, Lettieri, and Austin (1976). Various drug research projects in this volume utilized factor analysis to purify measures (for example, Smith & Fogg, chap. 4; Kandel et al., chap. 3).

There are situations when interest lies, not in the variables, but in the subjects, and one desires to investigate whether subjects can be organized into more homogeneous groups. Cluster analysis is then an appropriate technique; it is discussed, for example, by Lorr (1976) and Hartigan (1975). Similarly, data may consist, not of the traditional subjects-by-variables data matrix, but rather of dissimilarities among objects obtained either individually or from other techniques such as sorting or categorization tasks. In situations such as these, new data-analytic techniques of an exploratory nature are being generated quite regularly, as described, for example, by Carroll (1976) or Takane, Young, and DeLeeuw (1977).

In general, it must be stated that the possibilities for exploratory, model-building data analysis are so immense that an overview chapter like this cannot do justice to their description. The main purposes of my discussion must be to provide the reader with an introduction to the range of existing methods and to survey the possible limitations of exploratory data analysis, a topic to which I now turn.

Reification of Decision Rules

Model-building techniques by their very nature cannot test clean statistical hypotheses because the data are artificially "massaged." Numerous models tend to be tried, in succession, on the same data, with the intent of achieving an ever better fit between model and data. Similarly, rules of statistical decision are used repetitively in an interlaced manner without regard to the required independence of data. Nonetheless, because the point of the analysis is to separate the data into its essential and nonessential aspects, some decision rule must be utilized. For example, in principal components or factor analysis, there is the widely known Guttman–Kaiser rule of eigenvalues of the correlation matrix greater than 1 that is used to determine the number of factors; in regression, an F test may be used for deciding when to stop adding variables to a stepwise prediction equation. Although rules such as these are both necessary and reasonably rationalized, in general they cannot be defended against the criticism that they are arbitrary. Similarly, in stepwise regression, variables are selected according to their ability to assist in predicting a criterion incrementally. Yet the order of inclusion of variables may be quite arbitrary, determined for example by the reliability of the predictor rather than by any fundamental relationship to the dependent variable. Related to the reification problem is the issue of cross-validation.

Absence of Cross-validation

One way to demonstrate that the decision rules being utilized are reasonable would be to cross-validate the procedure and the resulting parameter estimates in a new sample. When data sets are large, it is wise to randomly split the sample prior to analysis so as to verify that the results obtained in the exploratory sample can be confirmed in the independent sample. A statistical test would be highly desirable in this context. For example, although factor analysis may have been utilized in a model-building way in one sample, it is possible to use confirmatory factor analysis in another sample (Jöreskog, 1969). This provides a chi-square test to determine the adequacy of the model. Such cross-validation is not only highly desirable but essential when highly efficient computerized procedures have been utilized to grind every last ounce of interrelation or predictability out of a given set of data. The very effectiveness of such search methods makes it highly likely that chance associations are processed as if they were real. New data, however, could clarify whether *overfitting*, that is, fitting a model to random features of the data, had occurred. About the only time that cross-validation would not seem to be essential is when the sample size is so large as to represent effectively the entire population without much distortion, as in the work of Josephson and Rosen (chap. 5). Other research reports in this volume, such as Roizen and co-workers' (chap. 9) "clinical" sample results, could certainly have benefited from cross-validation.

It must be recognized that cross-validation is itself a complicated procedure that is not carefully enough analyzed in the literature. The specific method to be utilized would depend on the particular question to be answered. For example, if the number of factors is the only issue to be raised in the exploratory factor model, then ordinary exploratory maximum-likelihood factor analysis would be appropriate. If, however, the actual factor structure, with its particular factors, is to be interpreted, the given set of loadings must be used in the new sample. Similarly, with stepwise regression, one may question whether the chosen variables do in fact significantly predict the criterion; in that case, the optimal weights can be reestimated. But if the question revolves around the particular combination of weights chosen, the weights themselves must be used in the new sample. The procedure of using given weights in various subsamples could have been used to advantage by Jessor and Jessor (chap. 2). In the light of the findings of Wainer (1976a), one could also inquire about the efficacy of equal weights; typically, there is minimal, if any, loss on cross-validation. Bentler and Woodward (1977b) obtain the optimal binary weights for regression and provide an analysis-of-variance test for their significance. They also provide a test for the increment in predictability possible by using differential weights. Gunst, Webster, and Mason (1976) provide a set of weights that are superior to least-squares weights when the predictors are multicollinear.

Virtue would seem to lie with methods of cross-validation that are entirely different from those chosen for initial data exploration. For example, if automatic interaction detection were used to identify interacting variables, ordinary regression with an appropriate design might be able to verify its reality. Similarly, if factor analysis were used to identify variables that defined sets of factors, it would be possible on cross-validation to assess the internal consistency of the composites formed on the basis of the factor results and to verify the relative independence of composites so formed. Such a change of methods in confirmatory samples is particularly important if certain assumptions of a method are not met, for example, factor analysis of binary data; the internal consistency of items marking a factor could then be assessed by a nondimensional index (Bentler, 1972; Bentler & Woodward, 1977a). Such a method change might convince skeptics who did not happen to believe strongly in a given methodology but who could appreciate the reason for its use. In any case, substantive theory would seem more likely to be fostered if the phenomenon being described could be adequately captured with a variety of methodological approaches.

Inattention to Analytic Distortions

Although analytic methods can be utilized for data exploration even when their statistical assumptions are not met, and although techniques can be utilized even though the data are not optimal for their use, there are consequences to these decisions. These consequences should be spelled out to the consumer of reports based on exploratory methods so that their importance can be appreciated. For example, interval-level linear models may be used in data exploration in spite of the inevitable distortions due to nonlinearities in the data or failure of the variables to meet the measurement requirements of the techniques. The consequence, even in clean cross-validation samples, may well be that a given model may not fit the data within statistical error; this may not reflect the inaccuracy of the substantive theory as much as the distorting effect of the chosen analytic method. This consequence may not suffice as a reason to give up use of the technique, however, particularly when alternative models can be evaluated on the same data. In that case, the distorting effects might be similar in all models, and choice among the models would not be biased. A comparison of models is the procedure advocated in confirmatory factor analysis. For example, even though, strictly speaking, no known model of certain data may fit adequately, as indexed by a chi-square test, chi-square comparisons among competing models may show one model to be statistically superior to others. Unfortunately there is no generally accepted way of deciding whether a substantive theory is wrong or the measurement model is inadequate when only a single model is evaluated and found not to fit the data.

The emphasis placed, in this discussion, on cross-validation of exploratory results in model building leads quite directly to the issue of model evaluation, which is concerned with procedures for testing strict, a priori hypotheses on data.

Model Evaluation

When substantive theory can be translated into an appropriate mathematical model and when reasonable assumptions can be made regarding both measurement level and distributions of variables, then strict model evaluation through hypothesis-testing statistical procedures is possible. Substantive theory or prior model building must have developed to the point that explicit expectations regarding the data can be formulated and null hypotheses can be tested. Hypothesis testing is the basic goal of statistical methods as taught in social science and is exemplified particularly by true experimentation. A perusal of the drug-abuse research reports in this volume suggests that the state of this art is only slowly approaching the hypothesis-testing phase. Data description and exploration dominate the methodologies. Not a single report explicitly tests alternative models, though Johnston, O'Malley, and Eveland (chap. 6) use the cross-lagged correlation technique to draw causal inferences about drugs and delinquency.

In the ideal case, as is often emphasized in the philosophy of science literature, competing models and explanations would be pitted against each other for their ability to explain the very same data. The *crucial experiment idea* represents this concept: One theory will receive support; the others will be rejected. Social science seems, however, to have great difficulty formulating theories that are sufficiently explicit to yield contradictory predictions that can be tested in given situations. An example of competing explanations for the same data base was provided in drug research by Kandel (1973), who pitted parental influence against peer influence in accounting for adolescent drug use; peer influence won out. In model building, such as in exploratory factor analysis, one may, in some sense, be pitting one model against another; for example, the number of dimensions might be determined by such a comparison. In this instance, however, there is no strict process of model acceptance or rejection because the analyses really represent ways of building on one another to yield a final representation that seems to be substantively meaningful, and, it may be hoped, statistically acceptable as well.

In the absence of competing models, the adequacy of a given model might be evaluated by its ability to account for a significant amount of variance in some dependent variable. This might be exemplified by a significantly nonzero multiple correlation coefficient or discriminant function. A more stringent test of a model might lie in the use of specific coefficients, such as beta weights, in a statistical method, with verification of reliable prediction. A still more stringent test of a model would lie in its ability to account for essentially all relevant data. This is the goal of causal modeling (discussed below) and of confirmatory factor analysis in which the latent factors underlying a covariance matrix, if adequately understood, would account for all the observed variances and covariances to a reasonable degree of statistical approximation. It might be noted that the goal here is not one of rejecting a null hypothesis, but rather of accepting it; then the model is plausible because it cannot be rejected. Of course, as in traditional methods of statistical hypothesis testing, a given model that does not fit the data would be rejected as inadequate.

A good example of model evaluation with covariance data lies in the analysis of a set of variables that hypothetically measure the same construct. Typically, as in the report of Jessor and Jessor (chap. 2), an internal-consistency coefficient is presented for such data; its value is supposed to reflect the extent to which the variables reliably measure the same attribute. Such a descriptive statistic, however, tests no measurement model. One can test such hypotheses as unidimensionality or equal error variances for variables, however, using confirmatory factor analysis (for example, Jöreskog, 1971a).

As with all good things, there may be problems. These arise, not particularly because of statistical inadequacies, but because of the possible mismatch between substantive concerns and statistical evaluation.

Selection of Inappropriate Statistical Method

Despite the many classes of statistical methods suitable to different combinations of data level, distributions, and data-gathering designs, it may be difficult to find a method that suitably represents the substantive theory involved. The correctness of the statistical model to the task must always be verified, and the assumptions of the model must be adequately rationalized (in the absence of data that show the technique to be quite robust with respect to violations of assumptions).

Undue Reliance on Statistical Tests

Although statistical tests of hypotheses represent an important advance over data exploration, it must be recognized that statistics alone cannot answer questions about the meaningfulness of substantive results. There are situations in which a theory may be essentially correct, but it may be insufficient in scope to handle all sources of variance in data; the statistical test may reject the theory. For example, it is well known that, in factor analysis involving very large samples, the rules of statistical decision may require the extraction of factors that cannot be rationalized or understood. Focus on rejection of one's theory in such a circumstance may be substantively inappropriate, though technically correct. The important issue is one of being able to understand and predict the major sources of variance in the data, not necessarily all such sources.

There is a closely related issue: too heavy reliance on a global test of significance when specific comparisons might provide better suggestions as to how to improve a model. The situation is analogous conceptually to analysis of variance. Granting that there may exist significant overall mean differences, just where are the important ones? Smith and Fogg (chap. 4), for example, performed a discriminant-function analysis to predict onset of adolescent marihuana use. Because specific comparisons among groups verified the relevance of the function to all individual group comparisons, no model modifications were necessary. In contrast, in causal modeling, where models often fail to account successfully for the data, it may not be very important to know that a model does not fit given data unless one can also diagnose the nature of the inadequacies (for example, Costner & Schoenberg, 1973). The problem of detecting correlated errors in longitudinal data is relevant to this volume (see, for example, Sörbom, 1975). It must be emphasized that, even in the true hypothesis-testing context, there is positive value to understanding the data beyond the simple knowledge that one's model of the data is adequate or insufficient.

In the previous several sections, I have discussed the relationship, as mediated by methodological considerations, of substantive model to empirical data. I have noted that there are a wide variety of purposes associated with the interaction of methodology and substantive theory, from pure description to hypothesis testing. Most substantive researchers are quite well aware of these interrelationships and are able to match their levels of investigation reasonably well to the methodology being utilized. My own approach to construct validity emphasizes the data-exploration and hypothesis-testing aspects of construct validity, a topic to which I finally turn. I also attempt to explore somewhat more fully the terms *model* and *theory* that I have until now been using in undefined ways.

CONSTRUCT VALIDATION

Concept

The idea of construct validation, as introduced by Cronbach and Meehl (1955), represented an attempt to broaden the conceptualization of the validation process for psychological tests and measures. It had become customary to focus on content validity, concerned with the adequacy of a hypothetical universe of content of interest to the substantive researcher, and on criterion-oriented validation procedures, concerned with describing the relation of the given test to externally chosen criteria. No comprehensive conceptualization of validation had been proposed, however. It was obvious that there might never be a single, universally agreed-on criterion for a test and that multiple sources of evidence would have to be considered in arriving at a decision on the validity of a test. Cronbach and Meehl proposed that measurement instruments would have to be evaluated with regard to such data as group differences, correlational results, evidence on the internal structure of measures, studies of change over occasion, and studies of process. In addition, inasmuch as instruments are typically designed to reflect a given construct—or postulated attribute—whose meaning must be determined according to its relationship to other theoretical constructs and observable variables, construct validation was construed to represent a process of a continuing sort that would ultimately tie down the given construct in a more complete *nomological network*. The concept of construct validation provided a useful antidote to the simplistic view of validation as represented by a correlation coefficient. It reinforced the importance of separating statements about theoretical relationships from statements about measurement operations. This very same distinction was to be picked up years later in the causal-modeling literature without any reference to the important prior history of this idea.

The Cronbach–Meehl emphasis on constructs represented an important attempt to make substantive theory relevant to the typical process of test construction and evaluation. Loevinger (1957) appreciated the concept proposed by Cronbach and Meehl, but she felt that the Cronbach–Meehl statement was too vague to help in the task of test construction; she suggested that more specific attention be given to certain substantive, structural, and external components of construct validity. (She also objected to the term itself, suggesting that "traits," not "constructs," exist in people; constructs, she felt, are constructions of psychologists.) Bechtold (1959), on the other hand, objected to the whole concept and its implementation, arguing that the phrase and its meaning contributed little of any value to the process of theory building. He suggested that an empirically oriented methodology using explicit operational definitions would serve the goals of research better than the vague concern with "constructs." The value of the concept has remained a source of some contention (for example, Campbell, 1960; Cronbach, 1971). A philosophical orientation to theory and measurement quite similar to that of Cronbach and Meehl was proposed by Margenau (1950); it was based on the more operational and specifiable concepts and on the measurement operations of physics. As adopted and described by Torgerson (1958), the approach generated little controversy, perhaps because of its origin in physics, and perhaps because of the different readership served by Torgerson.

It seems to me that one major source of confusion regarding the concept of construct validation and its possible contribution to social science lies in the difficulties associated with operationalizing the procedure. If a more concrete methodology to implement the concept could be devised, many of the controversies surrounding the idea might be eliminated. In the next section, I propose a causal-modeling approach to construct validation. Although this approach would not incorporate all lines of reasoning and evidence relevant to the evaluation of substantive theory, it would represent a fruitful way to implement construct validation as a methodology.

A Causal-Modeling Approach

In the previous sections of this chapter, I surveyed the interrelations between methodology and substantive theory. I proposed that description, data exploration and model building, and hypothesis testing represent equally important aspects of the scientific enterprise each of whose particular value would have to be determined by the substantive questions being asked as well as by the field's level of theoretical sophistication. I do not abandon this view when proposing a causal-modeling approach to construct validation. This approach will require both explication of a nomological net and establishment of the relation of observed measures to such a net. Along with previous writers, I consider such explication to be necessary to evaluation of theory, but I also think that this approach has some value, albeit limited, for the process of model or theory building. The field of substance-abuse research may be ready to attempt such an approach; it can only succeed if concerted effort is made to translate theory into testable propositions.

In view of the fact that Cronbach and Meehl did not provide a formal definition of *construct validity,* I have some freedom to propose my own, tailor-made to the concerns of this chapter. I try to be explicit about all terms, but I propose that the phrase *substantive theory* be left undefined, to be supplied by the knowledgeable researcher.

- The *construct validity* of a substantive theory refers to the empirical adequacy of a causal model, evaluated on relevant data by appropriate statistical methods.
- A *causal model* is the representation of a substantive theory by a structural model and by a measurement model.
- A *structural model* is a representation of the interrelations among constructs through mathematical equations.
- A *measurement model* is a representation of the interrelations between constructs and variables through mathematical equations.
- A *construct* is a postulated attribute of a measured object.

I propose these definitions as ones that are reasonably consistent with previous writings on construct validity (as cited above) and also with the burgeoning literature on structural-equation models in the social sciences. Thus, they represent a bridge between traditional and more modern methodological concerns. A construct can typically be represented mathematically as a latent (unobserved) random variable, whereas the manifest data on the measured object can be represented as observed random variables. The construct validity of a substantive theory refers, then, to the adequacy of the model that interrelates various latent random variables to each other as well as to observed random variables, the entire representation for the population being evaluated by statistical means. In a given application, the researcher must be able to specify the causal model and to decide which mathematical aspects of the model need to be determined from the data (parameter estimation) and which aspects are to be given in mathematical form by the substantive theory (fixed, known parameters).

In one sense, the current approach to construct validation is different from the Cronbach–Meehl approach. I am concerned with the construct validity of a substantive theory, focusing immediate attention on the entire nomological network of associations of a given construct to other constructs and manifest variables; my goal is to evaluate a theory. The Cronbach–Meehl approach, on the other hand, focuses greater attention on the problem of understanding a given test or measure; their primary goal is to evaluate the construct validity of a test.

The causal-modeling literature has been strongly oriented to the statistical testing of the adequacy of a proposed model. In view of the prior discussion of model building versus hypothesis testing, can the causal-modeling approach to construct validation help improve inadequate theories? I propose that it can be an effective aid to theory building in ways not derivable from previous discussions of construct validity: through an analysis of the identification problem, through alternative relaxation and imposition of parametric constraints, and through analysis of lack of fit of the model.

The identification problem is not easy to explain in nontechnical terms, and it is difficult to find technical generalizations that hold for a wide variety of circumstances and models. The idea is as follows: A given causal model includes as part of its specification a set of parameters that govern the structural and measurement models. These parameters may be known or they may be unknown, to be estimated from the data. Under a given specification, the parameters, along with the random variables, will generate one and only one observed data structure, for example, means and a covariance matrix. If there are two or more different structures generating the same data structure, the structures are equivalent. If a parameter has the same value in all equivalent structures, the parameter is identified, and if all parameters are identified, the whole model is said to be identified. The model must be identified in order for statistical estimation to be successful.

If a causal model has deficiencies in identification, it cannot be evaluated empirically. The possibility and problems of empirically evaluating a theory were discussed by Cronbach and Meehl (1955), and by Torgerson (1958), who emphasized that a sufficient number of constructs must be appropriately defined operationally for a theory to have empirical meaning. Evaluating the identification of a specific causal model provides a test of the possibilities for its empirical evaluation. If the model is "overidentified," meaning, loosely speaking, that there are fewer parameters than data points (for example, means and covariances), the model is scientifically useful because it can be rejected by the data. If the model is "just identified," meaning, loosely speaking, that there is a one-to-one transformation possible between the data and the parameters, the model is not scientifically interesting because it can never be rejected (no matter what the data). If some parameters of the model are "underidentified," meaning, loosely speaking, that they can take on many values rather than be uniquely defined, the model is not statistically testable. This makes the model useless as well. A technical analysis of under-identification may provide clues to various methods for improving the model to make it testable. Sometimes, such an analysis may not be practically feasible, but the methods of causal modeling discussed below provide an index, consequent to a computer analysis, that informs the user whether the model was in fact statistically testable. Thus, the concept of identification and its application in a given situation provides insights to construct validity that were not previously available.

The causal-modeling procedures described below allow one to choose quite freely which parameters of the model are to be treated as known or as estimated from the data. Such a decision can be modified in accordance with the results of data analysis. To illustrate, parameters that were thought to be quite different may turn out to be almost identical; the model could be reestimated subject to the constraint that the parameters be exactly the same. Another illustration might involve modifying the nomological network itself, that is, setting some parameters to a known zero and testing the adequacy of such a restriction. Obviously, causal modeling makes improvement of theories possible through the ability to compare alternatives. In some situations, such model comparisons are completely legitimate and open to a statistical test that compares the two models and has its own chi-square fit value. In other circumstances, as previously pointed out, the statistical assumptions may no longer be met, and cross-validation becomes essential.

If a proposed causal model does not fit the data, one has the possibility of evaluating alternative ways of modifying the model (for example, Costner & Schoenberg, 1973). The measurement model, for example, may need refinement, or the fault may lie with the structural model. It may be possible to obtain clues about lack of fit by examining the residuals, that is, specific areas of lack of fit between model and data. Alternatively, the suggestion has been made to look at certain derivatives whose size would provide a clue to model modification (for example, Sörbom, 1975). Although I am not entirely satisfied with the latter technique, which is dependent on the variance of the variables involved, and which can provide a clue only to minor (local) modifications of the proposed model, clearly, any ability to modify favorably one's initial causal model represents an improvement over previous approaches to construct validity.

I am now ready to provide a short, nontechnical overview of some recent developments in econometrics, psychometrics, sociometrics, and statistics. These developments, based primarily on the pioneering work of Karl Jöreskog and his students, can be directly applied to the problem of evaluating the construct validity of a substantive theory, such as one developed in drug-abuse research. For example, causal modeling can make more elegant the search for connections between drugs and crime, which were studied by Johnston, O'Malley, and Eveland (chap. 6) using cross-lagged panel correlations.

THEORY TESTING VIA ANALYSIS OF MEAN AND COVARIANCE STRUCTURE

I now describe some basic assumptions of these newer methods, review confirmatory factor analysis, discuss higher order factor methods and models with structured means, describe the structural-equation approach, and conclude with mention of an analysis of covariance having a measurement model. All of the techniques described separate a measurement model from a structural model, as defined, but the role of the structural model is more explicit and extensive in the latter approaches. The factor-analytic models tend to be primarily measurement models, though certainly not exclusively so.

Basic Assumptions

Although causal modeling, as defined above, is appropriate with nonlinear data as well as with the simpler linear forms, the assumption of linearity in variables has made the development of a variety of models and the relevant statistical theory much simpler. I am concentrating entirely on these simpler linear models, but the researcher will have to evaluate whether the linearity assumption is reasonable in a given situation. Linearity can often be justified on pragmatic grounds, robustness with respect to violation, and availability of statistical results, as already pointed out.

Although no particular distributional assumptions are necessary to utilize causal models as representations of substantive theory, testing the adequacy of fit of a given model to empirical data generally requires the assumption of multivariate normality, which can be evaluated (Andrews, Gnanadesikan, & Warner, 1973). If the data are not approximately normal, the significance test may well be indicative, not only of lack of fit of model to data, but of departures of the data from normality. Although recent statistical developments have made it possible to dispense with the assumption of normality (Lee, 1977), the newer results are unclear about exactly what forms variable distributions may take. For now, it seems safer to accept the normality requirement and to realize its potential impact. Although the use of "robustifying" techniques can be recommended to smooth out irregularities in the observed data (for example, Wainer, 1976b), the impact of such manipulations on statistical hypothesis testing is yet to be determined. The assumptions of normality and linearity make it possible to focus attention entirely on the means and covariances inasmuch as they convey all the essential information of the causal model. The adequacy of a given model is thus assessed in terms of its ability to represent or provide a model for the sample means and covariance matrix, within statistical sampling error. In many applications, the means are irrelevant and not structured in terms of the causal model, so that the phrase "analysis of covariance structures" (Jöreskog, 1970) can be used.

Confirmatory Factor Analysis

Factor analysis seeks to resolve covariances or intercorrelations among variables into latent dimensions, or factors, that account for the intercorrelations. In my introduction to causal modeling, I analyzed the formula $r_{12.3}$. Factor analysis generalizes this equation to $r_{ij.12...m}$, sets it equal to 0, and solves for the correlation between any pair of variables i and j in terms of the latent common factors, $1 - m$. The variance not accounted for by these common factors is accounted for by the unique variance, which includes error variance and reliable variance unshared by other variables.

The factor-analytic model utilizes a specific type of causal model. There is a measurement model, which relates the observed variables to the latent factors. Its information is typically summarized in the factor-loading matrix, whose rank provides information on the number of factors. The structural model represents the interrelations among the latent constructs, or factors. These are symmetrical, with all factors having an equal causal status in the system. If these factors do not affect each other, the model is said to be "orthogonal"; if they do affect each other, reciprocally, with the direction of influence unspecified, it is said to be "oblique."

The problem posed by exploratory factor analysis, as traditionally developed and well known in social research, is to find a measurement structure consistent with the observed data. The only hypothesis that is typically tested revolves around the number of factors that might be necessary to this task. After this number is found, the solution may be modified into an alternative, mathematically equivalent, orthogonal or oblique solution through rotation or transformation.

It had been recognized for some time that there might be important hypotheses to test other than the number of factors (for example, Anderson & Rubin, 1956). Bechtold (1958) suggested the name "confirmatory" factor analysis for this purpose. No statistical methodology for evaluating factor models that restrict parameters was available, however, until Jöreskog (1969) published his classic paper on the topic and made a computer program available. One may, for example, have knowledge or hypotheses regarding a particular set of values for the factor-loading parameters. Values of 0, for example, would specify that certain factors could not influence certain variables. The process of confirmatory factor analysis involves translating substantive theory into restrictions on parameters in the factor model and then evaluating whether the given causal model could successfully account for the observed intercorrelations. If so, the model could be accepted; if not, it would be rejected and would require modification as an appropriate mathematical description of the data. Confirmatory factor analysis represents far more, however, than an alternative way of fitting the factor model to data, inasmuch as analyses that could never be achieved with the exploratory model can be carried out. To illustrate, a far larger number of factors with fewer numbers of parameters can be obtained than would be possible under the traditional model. Because of the wide range of possibilities, however, substantive theory must play a much greater role in guiding the analyses. If one is attempting to find the factors that account for given data, the confirmatory approach is not the appropriate one; there are simply too many possibilities.

One of the most informative uses of confirmatory factor analysis lies in its ability to quantify and evaluate models for multitrait-multimethod matrices (Campbell & Fiske, 1959; Jöreskog, 1974; see Kenny, 1976b, for an example). It may be remembered that Campbell and Fiske proposed various rules for evaluating the role of method or trait variance in data obtained on similar variables measured under quite different circumstances, in order to determine the convergent and discriminant validity of the measures. With confirmatory factor analysis, the measurement model can be set up to reflect the presence of pure trait factors, pure method factors, or mixture factors, by the judicious selection of fixed 0s in the factor-loading matrix; various models can be tested for adequacy. A similarly interesting application involves testing the adequacy of various unidimensional measurement models, for example, a model involving equal error variances for the variables, leading to an appropriate model-based internal consistency coefficient (Jöreskog, 1971b). (Internal consistency based on no assumptions about dimensionality cannot be obtained by confirmatory factor analysis; see Bentler, 1972.)

Higher Order Factor Models

It was recognized by Thurstone (1947) that factors could themselves be inter-correlated (oblique), and their intercorrelations could be analyzed by a factor-analytic model. Indeed, numerous researchers had taken the results of exploratory factor analyses and subjected the factor-correlation matrix resulting from an oblique solution to a further factor-analytic decomposition. These procedures were entirely exploratory, however, until Jöreskog (1970) proposed to treat the first-order and second-order factor models simultaneously in estimation. As a result, it becomes possible to test more complicated measurement and structural models. In such models, the constructs themselves can be categorized into first-order and second-order constructs. The first-order constructs are related to the observed variables by a measurement model. The structural model, however, consists, not only of the interrelations among constructs as before, but of the relations between first-order and second-order constructs and the relations among second-order constructs. As in the basic factor model, these interrelations are symmetrical so that no causal ordering is assumed among the second-order constructs. The second-order constructs, however, help to generate the first-order constructs. Such models take space to describe in detail, and the reader is referred to Jöreskog (1974) for illustrative applications. The most general higher order factor model is provided by Bentler

(1976b); the previously discussed factor models and several later ones represent special cases thereof.

Factor Analysis with Structured Means

In the basic factor-analytic model, the means of the variables are not of particular interest, and they are not structured or explained by the constructs. As a consequence, estimation of population means is simply executed by use of sample means, and the causal model deals primarily with the covariance structure. In some situations, this approach is not entirely satisfactory. In particular, when there are several groups of subjects who may be drawn from populations with different means but possibly similar measurement or structural parameters, the mean and covariance structure for all groups must be estimated simultaneously. Consequently, estimation is somewhat more complicated. The basic work in this area is given by Jöreskog (1971a) and Sörbom (1974), with Bentler (1973) providing an alternative conceptualization of the problem as applied to longitudinal data. In longitudinal data in particular, it might be desirable to determine whether the measurement and structural models are stationary across time, with only the means shifting.

Structural-Equation Models

Although approaches to the simultaneous analysis of sets of interrelationships have been proposed in various disciplines, econometrics has provided the most explicit development of causal models in which one set of variables, after transformation, can be expressed as linear functions of another set of variables. These "structural-equation" models are appropriate to the analysis of data concerned with unidirectional causal influences as well as with reciprocal causation in which each set of variables influences the others. As developed in econometrics, however, structural-equation causal models were generally formulated at the level of overt variables. Consequently, random errors in variables could provide biasing effects that might lead to erroneous conclusions about the causal influences of latent constructs on each other in a given situation. Thus, the early work on structural-equation models did not take seriously the Cronbach–Meehl (1955) arguments regarding the importance of separating the nomological net of theoretical relationships of constructs from the operational definition of manifest variables as related to latent constructs through measurement operations. In the context of longitudinal research, Corballis and Traub (1970) did realize that the measurement of change should be described at the level of the purified constructs, or factors, rather than at the level of overt variables, but their model was a very specialized one not capable of dealing with a wide variety of causal influences. It took Jöreskog (1973b) and Wiley (1973) to recognize that general structural-equation models could be improved by distinguishing between the measurement and structural models, thus strengthening the idea that theoretical relations should be cleanly distinguished from empirical relations (for example, Block, 1963; Rock et al., 1977). In these more general developments, the measurement model typically involves a confirmatory factor-analytic model that relates manifest variables to latent constructs. The latent constructs are related to each other, in turn, by linear structural equations of the econometric sort; basically, these are regression models among unobserved variables. The entire structure consisting of both measurement and structural models, Jöreskog and Wiley further realized, represented a class of covariance structure models. Consequently, the principles and methods of estimation developed with such models (for example, Jöreskog, 1970) could be applied to structural equations.

The most well-known structural-equation model is currently the LISREL approach of Jöreskog (1977). It can be described as follows: There are two sets of variables. Each set of variables is assumed to have a confirmatory factor-analytic measurement structure; yet the common factors of one set of variables (perhaps after a transformation) represent dependent variables in their linear regression on the common factors of the other set. The consequence of such a model at the level of the covariances is that both sets of variables have a simple confirmatory factor structure composed of factor loadings, factor intercorrelations, and uniquenesses. The dependent set of variables, however, has its factor intercorrelations represented by another, relatively complicated, structural model. The idea of such a model, of course, is that the common-factor constructs of one set of variables cause or lead to the common-factor constructs in the other set. This model also has the useful feature of allowing the indicators of constructs to be correlated across sets of variables, a useful feature in the longitudinal context in which a test–retest correlation may consist in part of correlated errors. An example of Jöreskog's approach to the longitudinal data situation can be found in the work of Olsson and Bergman (1977), who studied ability structure in children between the ages of 10 and 13. A more comprehensive discussion of the value of the model in longitudinal contexts can be found in Jöreskog and Sörbom (1976, 1977) and in Wheaton et al. (1977).

A still more general structural-equation model is that of Bentler (1976a). It includes Jöreskog's (1977) model as a special case. In Jöreskog's model, only the common-factor constructs are related to each other by a structural equation. Bentler's measurement model is more complicated, and the structural model allows the unique and common-factor constructs of one set to be represented as functions of the unique and common-factor constructs of the other set. This type of model would seem to be particularly appropriate to longitudinal data, in which a single common factor may split across time into two factors. For example, general intelligence separates into verbal and quantitative factors. In such situations, one could imagine that the unique (specific) factors on the first occasion could causally influence the split common factors on the second occasion.

Analysis of Covariance with Measurement Model

In the situation in which data exist on several groups, ideally, randomly assigned to treatment conditions, and in which one is interested in drawing inferences about group means when preexisting differences exist between the groups, one rather naturally turns to the analysis of covariance. Analysis of covariance is, however, an inappropriate technique when the covariates are measured with error—the typical situation in the social sciences. On the one hand, random error can have the effect of implying a treatment effect when in fact there is no such effect; on the other hand, the analysis may fail to detect an actual treatment effect. More generally, there is a biasing effect of random error, as has been noted many times (for example, Lord, 1960). The only simple correction would be to use a type of correction of attenuation (for example, Cochran, 1968), but this would require knowledge of the reliabilities of the variables in several groups.

Sörbom (1976) has recently proposed an interesting combination of the LISREL structural-equation model with his method (described above) of factor analysis with several groups, taking means into account. That is, a measurement model is constructed that relates the observed dependent and covariate measures to some latent factors. The latent factors in the dependent variables are regressed on the latent factors of the covariates, and the observed means are structured in terms of the latent factors. The result is a LISREL type of model whose parameters influence both the covariance matrices and the means in dependent variables and covariates. The parameters of the model are first estimated by maximum likelihood, and the ability of the model to fit the data is evaluated by chi-square test. If the model does not fit the data, no further inferences about means can be drawn. If the model does fit the data, a variety of covariance models can be tested, such as a model that might assume equal dependent-covariate slopes. Obviously, it will be important to modify the measurement and structural models if they are not adequate to reproducing the observed data within sampling errors, inasmuch as the goal of the whole enterprise is to evaluate the mean effects generated by the latent factors. The methods of model modification discussed previously are obviously relevant here.

GENERALITY AND SCOPE OF THEORY, METHODS, AND DATA

This concludes my survey of descriptive, exploratory, and hypothesis-testing uses of data, as integrated into substantive theory, and potentially evaluated by a causal-modeling approach to construct validity. The methods of analysis of mean and covariance structure viewed above are obviously growing very rapidly. Potentially, they have a lot to offer social science research. I would like, however, to remind the reader that causal modeling as a hypothesis-testing approach to research is not necessarily superior to alternative approaches to research. It may be that data description or exploratory model building are more appropriate to the level of theoretical sophistication of a given research area and to its data base.

Nonetheless, when an area is capable of formulating a fairly complete nomological network relating constructs to each other and to observed variables, the causal-modeling approach to hypothesis testing with its ability to analyze even nonexperimental, response–response relationships, has great potential. Not the least of its benefits might be that researchers will be stimulated into developing substantive theory, with a goal of making it amenable to evaluation by causal modeling.

Although causal modeling appears to have a useful future in social science research, the causal-modeling methodology itself will need further research and improvement. It is clear that both substantive theory and empirical data make demands on this methodology that it cannot currently meet. For example, substantive theories whose mathematical realization might be expressed nonlinearly in variables and parameters cannot be dealt with effectively. It would be desirable to be able to utilize construct means and interactions among latent constructs in a greater range of models. Data whose measurement level is nominal or ordinal, rather than interval, are as yet severely limited in their ability to contribute to the growth and evaluation of theory. Finally, the assumption of multivariate normality, as typically required in the statistical analysis of causal modeling, is too severe for many data sets.

If causal modeling becomes integrated into social science research, the issue of comparing competing causal models will certainly arise. Which theory has the highest construct validity? When competing models are being evaluated on a given set of data, the comparison may be relatively easy; but when the data bases are different, the problem is much more complicated. In the context of two competing theories attempting to explain the same data, the causal model that fits more adequately would be superior; if two models happen to account for the data equally well, in the absence of other considerations, one could consider the more parsimonious model—the one with the least number of parameters—as the superior model. It might be tempting to utilize the chi-square test, or a similar index derivable from causal models when comparing models across differing data bases, even when the data are only minimally different (as when certain manifest variables are substituted for others). Although such an approach may sometimes work, particularly when the manifest variables are extremely well understood as manifestations of latent constructs, a fit index, in general, cannot provide a sufficient rationale for comparing the maturity and scope of alternative theories. Everything else being equal, including ability to account for data, the theory whose nomological network is richer would seem to be more mature. The richness of the network would be difficult to quantify, however, because at issue would be such considerations as the total number of variables, the number of parameters, the ratio of variables to parameters, the ratio of known to estimated parameters, the richness of the structural model (evaluated perhaps by the number of parameters or the number of dimensions), and the richness of the measurement model (similarly evaluated). In view of the likelihood of disagreement about the necessary trade-offs involved, however, it might be impossible to find a general formula for combining such information. How might one weight, for example, the value of adding a variety of methods of measurement (in the sense of Campbell and Fiske, 1959) to a given structural model, compared to the value of increasing the number of parameters in a measurement model by increasing the number of monomethod (single data-source) variables measuring a given construct? Clearly, one might more easily be able to increase the number of parameters in a model by adding, say, additional self-report variables, but many researchers would feel that greater understanding might be obtained by adding the more remote heteromethod (multiple data-source) variables. In the drug-use area, for example, the approach of Kandel, Kessler, and Margulies (chap. 3) and of Smith and Fogg (chap. 4) reflects the virtue of avoiding method artifacts by using independent data sources. Unfortunately, I have no general solution to the quandary of comparing causal models so as to determine in some abstract way whether one is superior to another. I do propose, however, that a certain degree of skepticism regarding causal-modeling reports is in order. It is entirely possible for statistically acceptable causal models to represent theoretical trivia. The substantively meaningful use of such models must incorporate theoretical sophistication as well as high-quality empirical data. Judging by the scope of the reports in this volume, the drug-abuse research area may have the requisite empirical and theoretical base to be able to engage in meaningful causal-modeling research.

REFERENCES

Anderson, N. H. Note on functional measurement and data analysis. *Perception and Psychophysics*, 1977, *21*, 201–215.

Anderson, T. W., & Rubin, H. Statistical inference in factor analysis. *Proceedings, 3rd Berkeley Symposium of Mathematical Statistics and Probability*, 1956, *5*, 111–150.

Andrews, D. F., Gnanadesikan, R., & Warner, J. L. Methods for assessing multivariate normality. In P. R. Krishnaiah (Ed.), *Multivariate analysis: Proceedings of Third International Symposium*. New York: Academic, 1973.

APA Committee on Psychological Tests. *Technical recommendations for psychological tests and diagnostic techniques*. Washington, 1954.

Baltes, P. B. *Methodological notes on three longitudinal studies on drug behavior*. Mimeograph, the Pennsylvania State University, 1976.

Beale, E. M. L., Kendall, M. G., & Mann, D. W. The discarding of variables in multivariate analysis. *Biometrika*, 1967, *54*, 357–366.

Bechtold, H. P. Statistical tests of hypotheses in confirmatory factor analysis. *American Psychologist*, 1958, *13*, 380. (Abstract)

Bechtold, H. P. Construct validity: A critique. *American Psychologist*, 1959, *14*, 619–629.

Bentler, P. M. A comparison of monotonicity analysis with factor analysis. *Educational and Psychological Measurement*, 1970, *30*, 241–250.

Bentler, P. M. A lower-bound method for the dimension-free measurement of internal consistency. *Social Science Research*, 1972, *1*, 343–357.

Bentler, P. M. Assessment of developmental factor change at the individual and group level. In J. R. Nesselroade & H. W. Reese (Eds.), *Life-span developmental psychology: Methodological issues*. New York: Academic, 1973.

Bentler, P. M. Development and assessment of models for substance abuse etiologies (U.S. Public Health Service grant DA01070). University of California at Los Angeles, 1976. (Available in mimeo.) (a)

Bentler, P. M. Multistructure statistical model applied to factor analysis. *Multivariate Behavioral Research*, 1976, *11*, 3–25. (b)

Bentler, P. M., Lettieri, D. J., & Austin, G. A. (Eds.). *Data analysis strategies and designs for substance abuse research* (National Institute on Drug Abuse). Washington: U.S. Government Printing Office, 1976.

Bentler, P. M., & Woodward, J. A. *Inequalities among lower bounds to reliability: With applications to test construction and factor analysis*. University of California at Los Angeles, 1977. (Available in mimeo.) (a)

Bentler, P. M., & Woodward, J. A. The partition of regression variance for optimal prediction. University of California at Los Angeles, 1977. (Available in mimeo.) (b)

Bergmann, G., & Spence, K. W. The logic of psychophysical measurement. *Psychological Review*, 1944, *51*, 1–24.

Bishop, Y. M. M., Fienberg, S. E., & Holland, P. W. *Discrete multivariate analysis: Theory and practice*. Cambridge: M.I.T. Press, 1975.

Block, J. The equivalence of measures and the correction for attenuation. *Psychological Bulletin*, 1963, *60*, 152–156.

Bock, R. D. *Multivariate statistical methods in behavioral research*. New York: McGraw-Hill, 1975.

Campbell, D. T. Recommendations for APA test standards regarding construct, trait, or discriminant validity. *American Psychologist*, 1960, *15*, 546–553.

Campbell, D. T., & Fiske, D. W. Convergent and discriminant validation by the multitrait-multimethod matrix. *Psychological Bulletin*, 1959, *56*, 81–105.

Campbell, D. T., & Stanley, J. C. Experimental and quasi-experimental designs for research on teaching. In N. L. Gage (Ed.), *Handbook of research on teaching*. Chicago: Rand McNally, 1963.

Carroll, J. D. Spatial, non-spatial and hybrid models for scaling. *Psychometrika*, 1976, *41*, 439–463.

Cochran, W. G. Errors of measurement in statistics. *Technometrics*, 1968, *10*, 637–666.

Cook, T. D., & Campbell, D. T. The design and conduct of quasi-experiments and true experiments in field settings. In M. D. Dunnette (Ed.), *Handbook of industrial and organizational research*. Chicago: Rand McNally, 1976.

Corballis, M. C., & Traub, R. E. Longitudinal factor analysis. *Psychometrika*, 1970, *35*, 79–93.
Costner, H. L., & Schoenberg, R. Diagnosing indicator ills in multiple indicator models. In A. S. Goldberger & O. D. Duncan (Eds.), *Structural equation models in the social sciences*. New York: Academic, Seminar, 1973.
Cronbach, L. J. The two disciplines of scientific psychology. *American Psychologist*, 1957, *12*, 671–684.
Cronbach, L. J. Test validation. In R. L. Thorndike (Ed.), *Educational measurement*. Washington: American Council on Education, 1971.
Cronbach, L. J. Beyond the two disciplines of scientific psychology. *American Psychologist*, 1975, *30*, 116–127.
Cronbach, L. J., & Meehl, P. E. Construct validity in psychological tests. *Psychological Bulletin*, 1955, *52*, 281–302.
Cronbach, L. J., Rogosa, D. R., Floden, R. E., & Price, G. G. *Analysis of covariance: Angel of salvation, or temptress and deluder*. Stanford University, 1976. (Available in mimeo.)
Davis, J. A. Analyzing contingency tables with linear flow graphs: D Systems. In D. R. Heise (Ed.), *Sociological methodology 1976*. San Francisco: Jossey-Bass, 1975.
Davis, J. A. *Studying categorical data over time*. Dartmouth College, 1976. (Available in mimeo.)
Duncan, O. D. *Introduction to structural equation models*. New York: Academic, 1975.
Elinson, J., & Nurco, D. N. (Eds.). *Operational definitions in socio-behavioral drug use research 1975* (National Institute on Drug Abuse Research Monograph Series 2). Washington: U.S. Government Printing Office, 1975.
Fisher, R. A. *The design of experiments*. Edinburgh: Oliver and Boyd, 1935.
Geraci, V. J. Identification of simultaneous equation models with measurement error. *Journal of Econometrics*, 1976, *4*, 263–283.
Glass, G. V., Willson, V. K., & Gottman, J. M. *Design and analysis of time series experiments*. Boulder, Colorado Associated University Press, 1975.
Goodman, L. A. A new model for scaling response patterns: An application of the quasi-independence concept. *Journal of the American Statistical Association*, 1975, *70*, 755–768. (a)
Goodman, L. A. The relationship between modified and usual multiple-regression approaches to the analysis of dichotomous variables. In D. R. Heise (Ed.), *Sociological methodology 1976*. San Francisco: Jossey-Bass, 1975. (b)
Gunst, R. F., Webster, J. T., & Mason, R. L. A comparison of least squares and latent root regression estimators. *Technometrics*, 1976, *18*, 75–83.
Hannan, M. T., & Young, A. A. Estimation in panel models: Results on pooling cross-sections and time series. In D. R. Heise (Ed.), *Sociological methodology 1977*. San Francisco: Jossey-Bass, 1976.
Hartigan, J. A. *Clustering algorithms*. New York: Wiley, 1975.
Havlicek, L. L., & Peterson, N. L. Effect of violation of assumptions upon significance levels of the Pearson *r*. *Psychological Bulletin*, 1977, *84*, 373–377.
Heise, D. R. *Causal analysis*. New York: Wiley, 1975.
Hibbs, D. A. On analyzing the effects of policy interventions: Box-Jenkins and Box-Tiao versus structural equation models. In D. R. Heise (Ed.), *Sociological methodology 1977*. San Francisco: Jossey-Bass, 1976.
Hildebrand, D. K., Laing, J. D., & Rosenthal, H. *Prediction analysis of cross-classifications*. New York: Wiley, 1976.
Hogan, R., DeSoto, C. B., & Solano, C. Traits, tests, and personality research. *American Psychologist*, 1977, *32*, 255–264.
Hsiao, C. Identification and estimation of simultaneous equation models with measurement error. *International Economic Review*, 1976, *17*, 319–339.
Jackson, D. J., & Alwin, D. F. *Estimating experimental effects on factors*. Rockville, Md.: National Institute of Mental Health, 1976. (Available in mimeo.)
Jöreskog, K. G. A general approach to confirmatory maximum likelihood factor analsyis. *Psychometrika*, 1969, *34*, 183–202.
Jöreskog, K. G. A general method for analysis of covariance structures. *Biometrika*, 1970, *57*, 239–251.
Jöreskog, K. G. Simultaneous factor analysis in several populations. *Psychometrika*, 1971, *36*, 409–426. (a)
Jöreskog, K. G. Statistical analysis of sets of congeneric tests. *Psychometrika*, 1971, *36*, 109–133. (b)

Jöreskog, K. G. Analysis of covariance structures. In P. R. Krishnaiah (Ed.), *Multivariate analysis: Proceedings of Third International Symposium.* New York: Academic, 1973. (a)

Jöreskog, K. G. A general method for estimating a linear structural equation system. In A. S. Goldberger & O. D. Duncan (Eds.), *Structural equation models in the social sciences.* New York: Academic, Seminar, 1973. (b)

Jöreskog, K. G. Analyzing psychological data by structural analysis of covariance matrix. In D. H. Krantz, R. C. Atkinson, R. D. Luce, & P. Suppes (Eds.), *Contemporary developments in mathematical psychology* (Vol. 2). San Francisco: W. H. Freeman, 1974.

Jöreskog, K. G. Structural equation models in the social sciences: Specification, estimation and testing. In P. R. Krishnaiah (Ed.), *Proceedings of the Symposium on Applications of Statistics.* Amsterdam: North-Holland, 1977.

Jöreskog, K. G., & Sörbom, D. Statistical models and methods for test-retest situations. In D. N. M. Gruijter, L. J. Th. VanderKamp, & H. F. Crombag (Eds.), *Advances in psychological and educational measurement.* New York: Wiley, 1976.

Jöreskog, K. G., & Sörbom, D. Some models and estimation methods for analysis of longitudinal data. In D. J. Aigner & A. S. Goldberger (Eds.), *Latent variables in socioeconomic models.* Amsterdam: North-Holland, 1977.

Kandel, D. Adolescent marihuana use: Role of parents and peers. *Science,* 1973, *181,* 1067–1070.

Keesling, J. W., & Wiley, D. E. *Measurement error and the analysis of quasi-experimental data.* University of Chicago, 1975. (Available in mimeo.)

Kendall, M. *Multivariate analysis.* New York: Macmillan, Hafner, 1975.

Kenny, D. A. A quasi-experimental approach to assessing treatment effects in the nonequivalent control group design. *Psychological Bulletin,* 1975, *82,* 345–362.

Kenny, D. A. *A cross-lagged panel correlation approach to the sixteen-fold table.* Harvard University, 1976. (Available in mimeo.) (a)

Kenny, D. A. An empirical application of confirmatory factor analysis to the multitrait-multimethod matrix. *Journal of Experimental Social Psychology,* 1976, *12,* 247–252. (b)

Kessler, R. C. Rethinking the 16-fold table problem. *Social Science Research,* 1977, *6,* 84–107.

Kruskal, J. B., & Shepard, R. N. A nonmetric variety of linear factor analysis. *Psychometrika,* 1974, *39,* 123–157.

Labouvie, E. W. Longitudinal designs. In P. M. Bentler, D. J. Lettieri, & G. A. Austin (Eds.), *Data analysis strategies and designs for substance abuse research* (National Institute on Drug Abuse). Washington: U.S. Government Printing Office, 1976.

Labouvie, E. W., Bartsch, T. W., Nesselroade, J. R., & Baltes, P. B. On the internal and external validity of simple longitudinal designs. *Child Development,* 1974, *45,* 282–290.

Land, K. C., & Felson, M. A general framework for building dynamic macro social indicator models: Including an analysis of changes in crime rates and police expenditures. *American Journal of Sociology,* 1976, *82,* 565–604.

Land, K. C., & Spilerman, S. (Eds.), *Social indicator models.* New York: Russell Sage, 1975.

Larzelere, R. F., & Mulaik, S. A. Single sample tests for many correlations. *Psychological Bulletin,* 1977, *84,* 557–569.

Lee, S. Y. *Some algorithms for covariance structure analysis.* (Doctoral dissertation, University of California at Los Angeles, 1977. University Microfilms No. 77-17, 230.)

Linn, R. L., & Werts, C. E. Analysis implications of the choice of a structural model in the nonequivalent control group design. *Psychological Bulletin,* 1977, *84,* 229–234.

Loevinger, J. Objective tests as instruments of psychological theory. *Psychological Reports,* 1957, *3,* 635–694.

Lord, F. M. Large sample covariance analysis when the control variable is fallible. *Journal of the American Statistical Association,* 1960, *55,* 307–321.

Lord, F. M. A paradox in the interpretation of group comparisons. *Psychological Bulletin,* 1967, *68,* 304–305.

Lorr, M. M. Cluster and typological analysis. In P. M. Bentler, D. J. Lettieri, G. A. Austin (Eds.), *Data analysis strategies and designs for substance abuse research* (National Institute on Drug Abuse). Washington: U.S. Government Printing Office, 1976.

Margenau, H. *The nature of physical reality.* New York: McGraw-Hill, 1950.

Mischel, W. On the future of personality measurement. *American Psychologist,* 1977, *32,* 246–254.

Morrison, D. F. *Multivariate statistical methods.* New York: McGraw-Hill, 1976.

Muthén, B. *Structural equation models with dichotomous dependent variables.* University of Uppsala, 1976. (Available in mimeo.)

Muthén, B. *Contributions to factor analysis of dichotomous variables.* University of Uppsala, 1977. (Available in mimeo.)

Naditch, M. P. Path analysis. In P. M. Bentler, D. J. Lettieri, & G. A. Austin (Eds.), *Data analysis strategies and designs for substance abuse research* (National Institute on Drug Abuse). Washington: U.S. Government Printing Office, 1976.

Nerlove, M., & Press, S. J. *Univariate and multivariate log linear and logistic models.* Santa Monica: Rand Corporation, 1973.

Olsson, U., & Bergman, L. R. A longitudinal factor model for studying change in ability structure. *Multivariate Behavioral Research,* 1977, *12,* 221–241.

Overall, J. E., & Woodward, J. A. Common misconceptions concerning the analysis of covariance. *Multivariate Behavioral Research,* 1977, *12,* 171–185. (a)

Overall, J. E., & Woodward, J. A. Nonrandom assignment and the analysis of covariance. *Psychological Bulletin,* 1977, *84,* 588–594. (b)

Pedhazur, E. J. Coding subjects in repeated measures designs. *Psychological Bulletin,* 1977, *84,* 298–305.

Roberts, F. S. *Discrete mathematical models.* Englewood Cliffs, N.J.: Prentice-Hall, 1976.

Robinson, P. M. Identification, estimation and large-sample theory for regressions containing unobservable variables. *International Economic Review,* 1974, *15,* 680–692.

Rock, D. A., Werts, C. E., Linn, R. E., & Jöreskog, K. G. A maximum likelihood solution to the errors in variables and errors in equations model. *Multivariate Behavioral Research,* 1977, *12,* 187–197.

Shaffer, J. P. Defining and testing hypotheses in multidimensional contingency tables. *Psychological Bulletin,* 1973, *79,* 127–141.

Shaffer, J. P. Reorganization of variables in analysis of variance and multidimensional contingency tables. *Psychological Bulletin,* 1977, *84,* 220–228.

Shontz, F. C. Single-organism designs. In P. M. Bentler, D. J. Lettieri, & G. A. Austin (Eds.), *Data analysis strategies and designs for substance abuse research* (National Institute on Drug Abuse). Washington: U.S. Government Printing Office, 1976.

Simonton, D. K. Cross-sectional time-series experiments: Some suggested statistical analyses. *Psychological Bulletin,* 1977, *84,* 489–502.

Singer, B., & Spilerman, S. *The representation of social processes by Markov models.* University of Wisconsin at Madison, 1975. (Available in mimeo.)

Somers, R. H., Mellinger, G. D., & Davidson, S. T. Automatic interaction detection. In P. M. Bentler, D. J. Lettieri, & G. A. Austin (Eds.), *Data analysis strategies and designs for substance abuse research* (National Institute on Drug Abuse). Washington: U.S. Government Printing Office, 1976.

Sonquist, J. A., & Morgan, J. N. *The detection of interaction effects.* Ann Arbor: Institute for Social Research, 1964.

Sörbom, D. A general method for studying differences in factor means and factor structure between groups. *British Journal of Mathematical and Statistical Psychology,* 1974, *27,* 229–239.

Sörbom, D. Detection of correlated errors in longitudinal data. *British Journal of Mathematical and Statistical Psychology,* 1975, *28,* 138–151.

Sörbom, D. *A statistical model for the analysis of covariance with fallible covariates.* University of Uppsala, 1976. (Available in mimeo.)

Swaminathan, H., & Algina, J. Analysis of quasi-experimental time-series designs. *Multivariate Behavioral Research,* 1977, *12,* 111–131.

Takane, Y., Young, F. W., & DeLeeuw, J. Nonmetric individual difference multidimensional scaling: An alternating least-squares method with optimal scaling features. *Psychometrika,* 1977, *42,* 7–67.

Tatsuoka, M. M. Discriminant analysis. In P. M. Bentler, D. J. Lettieri, & G. A. Austin (Eds.), *Data analysis strategies and designs for substance abuse research* (National Institute on Drug Abuse). Washington: U.S. Government Printing Office, 1976.

Timm, H. *Multivariate analysis with applications in education and psychology.* Monterey, Calif.: Brooks/Cole, 1975.

Thurstone, L. L. *Multiple-factor analysis.* Chicago: University of Chicago Press, 1947.

Torgerson, W. S. *Theory and methods of scaling.* New York: Wiley, 1958.

Tucker, L. R. Some mathematical notes on three-mode factor analysis. *Psychometrika,* 1966, *31*, 279–311.

Underwood, B. J. Individual differences as a crucible in theory construction. *American Psychologist,* 1975, *30*, 128–134.

Wainer, H. Estimating coefficients in linear models: It don't make no nevermind. *Psychological Bulletin,* 1976, *83*, 213–217. (a)

Wainer, H. Robust statistics: A survey and some prescriptions. *Journal of Educational Statistics,* 1976, *1*, 285–312. (b)

Wainer, H., & Thissen, D. Three steps towards robust regression. *Psychometrika,* 1976, *41*, 9–34.

Werts, C. E., & Linn, R. L. Path analysis: Psychological examples. *Psychological Bulletin,* 1970, *74*, 193–212.

Wheaton, B., Muthén, B., Alwin, D. F., & Summers, G. F. Assessing reliability and stability in panel models. In D. R. Heise (Ed.), *Sociological methodology.* San Francisco: Jossey-Bass, 1977.

Wiley, D. E. The identification problem for structural equation models with unmeasured variables. In A. S. Goldberger & O. D. Duncan (Eds.), *Structural equation models in the social sciences.* New York: Academic, Seminar, 1973.

Woodward, J. A., & Overall, J. E. Factor analysis of rank-ordered data: An old approach revisited. *Psychological Bulletin,* 1976, *83*, 864–867.

Wright, S. Correlation and causation. *Journal of Agricultural Research,* 1921, *20*, 557–585.

Author Index

Subject Index